NEUROMODULATION

Neuromodulation

The Biochemical Control of Neuronal Excitability

LEONARD K. KACZMAREK
Yale University
and

IRWIN B. LEVITAN
Brandeis University

New York   Oxford
OXFORD UNIVERSITY PRESS
1987

Oxford University Press

Oxford   New York   Toronto
Delhi   Bombay   Calcutta   Madras   Karachi
Petaling Jaya   Singapore   Hong Kong   Tokyo
Nairobi   Dar es Salaam   Cape Town
Melbourne   Auckland

and associated companies in
Beirut   Berlin   Ibadan   Nicosia

Library of Congress Cataloging-in-Publication Data
Neuromodulation : the biochemical control of neuronal
excitability.
Bibliography: p.   Includes index.
1. Neurons.   2. Neural conduction.   3. Neural transmission—Regulation.
4. Neurophysiology.   5. Neurochemistry.   I. Kaczmarek, Leonard K.   II. Levitan, Irwin B.
QP363.N477   1987   591.1'88   86-5124
ISBN 0-19-504097-X

9 8 7 6 5 4 3 2 1

Printed in the United States of America

Preface

In the last several years it has become more and more apparent that the electrical properties of nerve cells may undergo marked changes, changes which are necessary for the cells to carry out their assigned functions in the nervous system. Such changes in neuronal excitability constitute **neuromodulation,** and this volume arose from the need to define some principles and boundaries of this rapidly emerging field. The term neuromodulation has been used in a number of different contexts, including changes in the properties of neuronal networks that regulate complex behaviors. The latter, however, is beyond the scope of this book; we will restrict ourselves here to modulation of the properties of individual neurons. Our goal is to introduce graduate students, and investigators who do not work in this area, to the way one thinks about and studies neuromodulatory phenomena at the cellular and molecular level. One of the characteristics of the field is that it is neither pure neurochemistry nor pure neurophysiology, but is at the interface between the two, and thus many of the practitioners do not talk the same language. Each of the editors has often found himself talking biochemistry to physiologists or physiology to biochemists, and we know it to be no easy task to make ourselves comprehensible. Accordingly, much of our effort in editing the contributed chapters, and in writing others, has gone into making complex concepts and approaches comprehensible to the novice in one or the other field.

The first five chapters are intended as an introduction to general principles of neuromodulation. In particular we have focused on the properties of ion channels, and on biochemical mechanisms of protein phosphorylation, since modulation of ion conductances by protein phosphorylation is the most thoroughly studied form of cellular neuromodulation. There follow several chapters describing specific examples of the above. Certainly other examples exist in the literature, and many are listed in Table 2.1; however, in this kind of volume it is impossible to discuss all of these in detail, and the examples in Chapters 6 through 11 serve to illustrate general approaches that also apply elsewhere. For instance, as emphasized in particular in Chapters 8, 10, and 11, neurons make a great deal of effort to regulate their intracellular calcium concentration by modulating the activity of specific ion channels, and the molecular details of this modulation are becoming rather well understood. In contrast, many of the functions of this intracellular calcium remain obscure. Chapter 12, for example, emphasizes the complexity of the role of intracellular calcium in the release of neurotransmitter, one of the most important but perhaps least well understood of the many calcium-dependent phenomena in neurons. Finally, Chapter 13 describes some fascinating neuromodulatory phenomena in the mammalian brain, phenomena that are begging for the kind of mechanistic investigations which have been possible in simpler systems. The development of concepts and techniques that will allow such investigations to be undertaken is a challenging task for the future.

We have made an effort to improve readability by editing the individual chapters seriously, to remove redundancy and excessive overlap between chapters and to emphasize general principles common to the different experimental systems. To allow the text to read smoothly we have limited the number of literature citations in the text and also have limited the number of specific experimental examples used to illustrate the general principles. We have done this quite ruthlessly and hope that authors who find their work described with only minimal attribution, or perhaps not described at all, will not be offended and will remember that any fault here lies with the editors and not with the individual contributors. To alleviate in part the dearth of references in the text, more extensive references are listed at the end of each chapter.

We are grateful to James Magno and Kathy Monaco for drawing or redrawing many of the figures, and to Maureen Delaney for typing and retyping many of the chapters. Finally, we thank our families for having endured a summer in Woods Hole, Massachusetts, so that we could prepare this volume.

July 1986   L. K. K.
                                                                     I. B. L.

Contents

Contributors

Dr. Paul R. Adams
Dept. of Neurobiology
State University of New York
Stony Brook, NY 11794

Dr. William B. Adams
The Biocenter, Klingelbergstrasse 70
Department of Pharmacology
University of Basel
CH-4056 Basel
Switzerland

Dr. Jack A. Benson
Agrochemical Research
CIBA GEIGY
Ch-4002 Basel
Switzerland

Dr. F. Edward Dudek
Tulane University Medical Center
Dept. of Physiology
School of Medicine
1430 Tulane Ave.
New Orleans, LA 70112

Dr. Douglas A. Ewald
Department of Pharmacology
University of Chicago
947 E. 58th Street
Chicago, IL 60637

Dr. Val Gribkoff
Tulane University Medical Center
Dept. of Physiology
School of Medicine
1430 Tulane Ave.
New Orleans, LA 70112

Dr. Richard L. Huganir
Laboratory of Molecular and Cellular
  Neuroscience
The Rockefeller University
1230 York Ave.
New York, NY 10021

Dr. Stephen W. Jones
Dept. of Neurobiology
State University of New York
Stony Brook, NY 11794

Dr. Leonard K. Kaczmarek
Depts. of Pharmacology and Physiology
Yale University School of Medicine
333 Cedar St.
New Haven, CT 06510

Dr. Irwin Levitan
Graduate Dept. of Biochemistry
Brandeis University
Waltham, MA 02254

Dr. Christopher Miller
Graduate Dept. of Biochemistry
Brandeis University
Waltham, MA 02254

Dr. Stephen A. Siegelbaum
Dept. of Pharmacology
Columbia University
College of Physicians and Surgeons
630 W. 168th St.
New York, NY 10031

Dr. Judith A. Strong
Dept. of Pharmacology
Yale University School of Medicine
333 Cedar St.
New Haven, CT 06510

Dr. Richard W. Tsien
Dept. of Physiology
Yale University School of Medicine
333 Cedar St.
New Haven, CT 06510

Dr. Robert S. Zucker
Dept. of Physiology and Anatomy
University of California
Berkeley, CA 94720

NEUROMODULATION

What Is Neuromodulation?

LEONARD K. KACZMAREK
IRWIN B. LEVITAN

An electrode advancing through a nervous system, be it the cerebral cortex of a human or the abdominal ganglion of an invertebrate, encounters neurons that display a variety of different types of electrical activity. Some neurons show no spontaneous activity, whereas others fire action potentials at fixed, regular intervals. Still others produce very irregular patterns of discharge. Some cells generate repetitive bursts of action potentials separated by profound hyperpolarizations of the membrane. The action potentials of different neurons in the same organism also display much heterogeneity in height, duration, and shape. Some neurons even fail to produce regenerative action potentials; transmission of information through such neurons is achieved by graded polarizations of the cell membrane.

Work with simple invertebrate systems has shown, in many instances, how the electrical characteristics of a given neuron are suited to its particular role in the control of a specific behavior or physiological function. For example, rapid transmission and electrical responses are required for the control of rapid motor acts such as those used in escape behavior. Feeding and reproductive behaviors, on the other hand, may use neurons with slower response characteristics. The characteristics of a neuron do not, however, remain fixed for all time.

NEUROMODULATION—A CHANGE IN THE ELECTRICAL PROPERTIES OF A NEURON

The term *neuromodulation* has been used loosely to describe a number of very different kinds of phenomena. In this book we define it, in a more restricted way, as the ability of neurons to alter their electrical properties in response to intracellular biochemical changes resulting from synaptic or hormonal stimulation. Defined this way, neuromodulation is one of the most important intrinsic properties of individual neurons. This property not only allows the nervous system to adapt its control of physiological functions to a continually changing environment, but it is also the basis for many long-lasting changes in animal behavior. Changes in behavior that can be

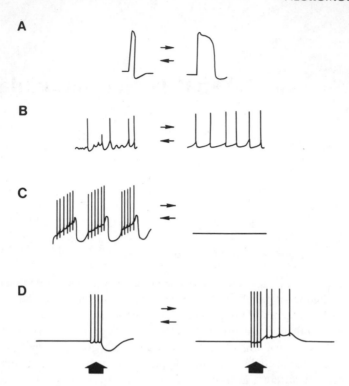

Fig. 1.1. Some of the changes that can be observed in the electrical properties of neurons. (A) Alterations in the shape of action potentials; (B) changes in frequency and pattern of firing; (C) inhibition and onset of bursting; (D) changes in response to stimulation *(arrow)*.

related directly to changes in the electrical responses of specific neurons include the triggering of long-lasting, but relatively fixed and innate, behaviors, such as feeding and reproductive behaviors, as well as alterations in behaviors that can be ascribed to learning. Because the modulation of neuronal electrical activity results in the choice of different patterns of behavior at different times, it is a fundamentally important aspect of neural activity.

CHANGES IN NEURONAL EXCITABILITY

Figure 1.1 shows some examples of various transitions in electrical excitability that can be observed in a single neuron. The width or height of its action potentials may increase and decrease. A neuron that is electrically silent may be induced to fire prolonged trains of action potentials or to burst repetitively. The first part of this chapter describes some of these changes that may be observed in the electrical properties of neurons, and indicates to some extent the physiological significance of these different types of transitions. The second part of the chapter summarizes some of the cellular and biochemical mechanisms that may be responsible for modulation of excitability. This sets the stage for the more detailed accounts of some of these topics in subsequent chapters.

Changes in the Shape of Action Potentials

A change in the width or height of the action potential results from synaptic or hormonal stimulation of many types of neurons in both vertebrates and invertebrates. One example of this can be observed in cells in the dorsal root ganglion, whose action potentials narrow in response to opioid peptides (see Chapter 11). Other examples are the action potential broadening seen in the bag cell neurons of *Aplysia* and certain sensory neurons from the same organism (Chapters 7 and 10).

At least two general consequences occur because of a change in action potential shape. First, since depolarization results in the opening of voltage-dependent calcium channels, a prolonged action potential duration will increase the amount of calcium that enters the cell during the action potential. Calcium entry triggers the release of neurotransmitters (Chapter 12). The prolonged action potential that occurs at a neurotransmitter release site will therefore directly increase the amount of neurotransmitter released. Conversely, in the case of the dorsal root ganglion cells, it is possible

Fig. 1.2. Effects of action potential width on propagation through a branched axonal network. On the left, a narrow action potential fails to propagate when it reaches branch points *(X)* at the terminal arborization of a hypothetical neuron. On the right, a broader action potential does propagate and reaches the terminals to release neurotransmitter.

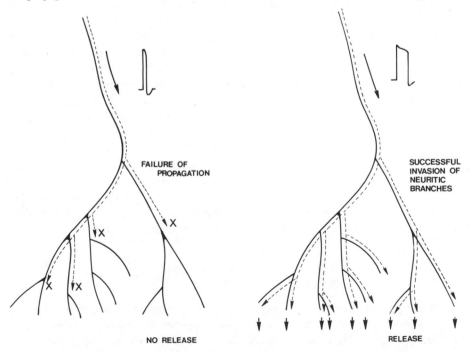

that the narrowing of the action potentials by opioid peptides inhibits transmitter release and attenuates the transmission of impulses corresponding to noxious stimuli.

The shape of an action potential will also influence the ability of an impulse to propagate through a highly branched axonal or dendritic network (Figure 1.2). It is known that an action potential traveling along a neuronal process may fail to propagate further when it reaches a branching point; this is particularly likely when an action potential traveling along a thin process attempts to invade a thicker process or network of processes. Such failure of propagation is, however, less likely to occur with a broad action potential than with a narrow one because the prolonged current flow during the broader action potential is more likely to depolarize the branch point to the threshold required for propagation (Westerfield et al., 1978).

A cell may use one of several different mechanisms for changing the shape of its action potential. These include directly altering the calcium current and modifying those potassium currents that act to repolarize the action potential. Such mechanisms will be addressed in more detail in Chapters 7, 10, and 11.

Control of Spontaneous Neuronal Discharge

The firing pattern of a neuron within the nervous system is determined both by mechanisms that are intrinsic to its own plasma membrane and by the synaptic inputs that it receives from other neurons. Changes in the pattern and the rate of firing of a neuron are the most basic mechanisms that the nervous system uses to encode and process sensory information and to generate motor output.

In some cases, it is possible to observe the electrical activity of a neuron in the absence of its synaptic inputs. This can be achieved by using pharmacological treatments to block synaptic inputs or by physically isolating a neuron, for example, by placing it in primary cell culture. From such studies it is apparent that some neurons display no spontaneous electrical activity whereas others can fire repetitively at fixed frequencies in the absence of synaptic input. As with the shape of the action potential, the nervous system can alter these intrinsic electrical properties of nerve cells so as to convert a silent neuron into a spontaneously active one and vice versa.

The biological significance of the onset of spontaneous discharge in a neuron depends on the nature of the cell in which it occurs. Neurons that control autonomic functions may undergo a change in the rate of their discharge to maintain homeostasis. On the other hand, "command" neurons, whose function it is to control the onset of specific animal behaviors (e.g., feeding), may be observed to undergo a transition from a silent to a discharging state in order to trigger such behaviors. One example of the cellular mechanisms that contribute to this form of transition is given in Chapter 7, which examines the bag cell neurons that control reproductive behavior in *Aplysia*.

Control of Neuronal Bursting

A special case of endogenously generated repetitive firing is the phenomenon of bursting. Bursting neurons generate trains of action potentials punctuated by periods of silence during which the cell membrane is usually hyperpolarized. Again, the

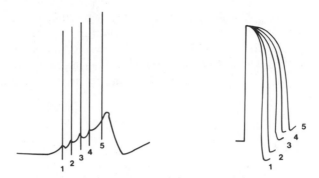

Fig. 1.3. Broadening of action potentials during a burst. On the left is shown a schematic representation of five successive action potentials in a burst. On the right, the action potentials are shown superimposed and on an expanded time scale.

nervous system uses biochemical mechanisms to turn on, turn off, and modulate the pattern of bursting. Chapters 6 and 8 deal with different aspects of the generation and biochemical modulation of endogenous neuronal bursting of single, identified molluscan neurons, in which such mechanisms have been studied in greatest detail.

Many of the neurons that display endogenous bursting are peptide-secreting cells. Periodic bursts of action potentials appear to be a more effective stimulus for the secretion of transmitters or hormones than a regular, pacing pattern of firing. This is true even when the mean frequency of action potentials (integrated over a long time) is the same in bursting and regularly firing cells (Dutton and Dyball, 1979). This enhanced release from bursting cells may result, at least in part, from the fact that in many neurons significant broadening of the later action potentials is observed during a burst of closely spaced action potentials (Figure 1.3). This broadening can result from progressive inactivation of the potassium currents that serve to repolarize the action potentials during the burst (see Chapter 2), which then leads to enhanced influx of calcium ions during the action potentials. In addition, it is possible that a bursting pattern may influence secretion by some other effect on cellular metabolism.

A second use that the nervous system has found for neuronal bursting is to control rhythmic motor output, as in many aspects of locomotion, respiration, and digestion. In general, such rhythmicity is the result of synaptic interactions among many different neurons. The understanding of such firing patterns therefore requires complete knowledge of the detailed synaptic interactions of neurons in a circuit, as well as of their intrinsic membrane properties and how they can be modulated. Although much excellent research has been done on the regulation of such networks of neurons, particularly in crustaceans and leeches (see Selverston, 1985), this work is outside the scope of this book.

Altered Responses to Synaptic Stimulation

Biochemical changes occurring in either the presynaptic or postsynaptic neuron at a synaptic junction may alter the response of the postsynaptic cell without changing the shape of the action potentials of either cell or their patterns of ongoing discharge. Such changes may be brought about either by altering the amount of transmitter released presynaptically or by modulating specific ionic conductances in the postsynaptic neuron. Chapters 9 and 13 provide examples of such changes in excitability for synaptic responses in the sympathetic ganglion and for transmission at other vertebrate synapses.

MECHANISMS OF MODULATION

Biochemical changes that lead to alterations in the electrical characteristics of a neuron may be triggered in one of three ways: (1) by the action of neurotransmitters at specific synaptic junctions, (2) by neurotransmitters that have been secreted at less specialized release sites at a distance from the target neuron, and (3) by the action of hormones (Figure 1.4). Several different mechanisms also exist for transducing these extracellular signals to a neuron into a change in its excitability. The simplest of these is the case of the ligand-gated ion channel in which the receptor and ion channel are contained in one protein complex (Figure 1.5, *top*). The prototype of this

Fig. 1.4. Stimuli that can modulate neuronal activity. These are (1) synaptic release of neurotransmitter, (2) local release of agents from neuronal processes that are not in direct contact with the target cell, and (3) actions of hormones released from tissues other than the nervous system.

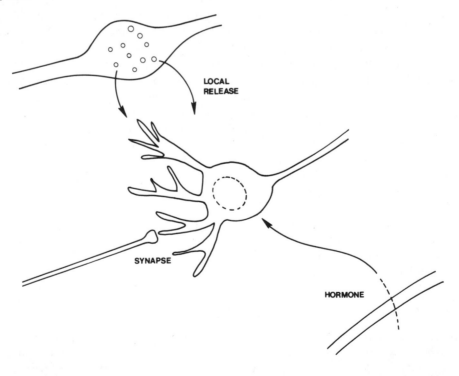

A

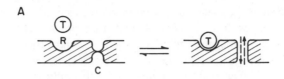

B

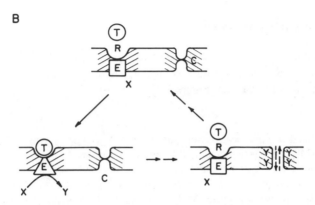

Fig. 1.5. Direct and indirect receptor-channel coupling. (A) A scheme depicting a *directly coupled* receptor/ion channel system. The receptor (R) and ion channel (C) are intimately associated, perhaps as parts of a single macromolecular complex, such that occupancy of the receptor by a transmitter *(T)* is linked directly to a change in ion flux through the channel. The change in ion flux is dependent on the continued occupation of the receptor by the transmitter and reverses when the receptor is no longer occupied. (B) A scheme depicting *indirect* receptor/ion channel coupling. Here the receptor and the ion channel are not part of the same molecular complex. Instead, the receptor is intimately associated with some enzyme *(E)*, which is activated when the receptor is occupied by transmitter. Active enzyme *E* converts a substrate *(X)* to a product *(Y)*, and *Y* acts as an intracellular second messenger to change ion flux through the ion channel. Such a change in ion channel properties can often outlast the initial stimulus, that is, the occupation of the receptor by the transmitter.

type of ion channel is the nicotinic acetylcholine receptor of the neuromuscular junction. Binding of a neurotransmitter to such a receptor results in an alteration in the flow of ions through the receptor–ion channel complex. Transmission at synapses that use this mechanism has traditionally been considered to be rather rapid and not to involve any long-term modification in the properties of the postsynaptic neuron. It is possible, however, that this type of electrical response can be modified by the actions of other agents that induce more generalized biochemical changes within a neuron (see Chapter 5).

The main focus of this book is on modulation of neuronal excitability occurring when transmitters act on receptors that trigger the formation of second messenger substances within the cell (Figure 1.5, *bottom*). These second messengers can engage a variety of biochemical pathways, most of which are linked to the activation of different classes of protein kinases. Such second messenger systems can therefore produce coordinated changes in the activity of more than one ion channel in the cell membrane and can, at the same time, influence other cellular processes not directly linked to ion fluxes. Although some of the second messenger pathways will be described in more detail in other chapters of this book, the following section gives a brief account of some of the different pathways believed to play important roles in the modulation of neuronal excitability.

SECOND MESSENGER SYSTEMS

The four second messenger systems, each of which may be linked to neurotransmitter or hormone receptors and which have been investigated for their roles in the control of neuronal excitability, are (see Figure 1.6) as follows:

Fig. 1.6. Simplified reaction schemes of four second messenger systems. (A) The adenylate cyclase/cyclic AMP-dependent protein kinase system; (B) guanylate cyclase and cyclic GMP-dependent protein kinase; (C) the inositol trisphosphate/diacylglycerol-protein kinase C system; (D) intracellular calcium ions as second messengers. Abbreviations: T, transmitter; R, Receptor; AC, adenylate cyclase; cA, cyclic AMP; PKA, cyclic AMP-dependent protein kinase; PP, phosphoprotein; GC, guanylate cyclase; cG, cyclic GMP; GK, cyclic-GMP-dependent protein kinase; PIP_2, phosphatidyl inositol 4,5-bisphosphate; PDE, phosphatidyl inositol, 4,5-biophosphate phosphodiesterase; DAG, diacylglycerol; PKC, protein kinase C; IP_3, inositol 1,4,5-trisphosphate; CC, calcium channels; CaK, calcium/calmodulin-dependent protein kinases; ISS, intracellular stores of calcium ions; CaM, calmodulin. For further details, see Chapter 4.

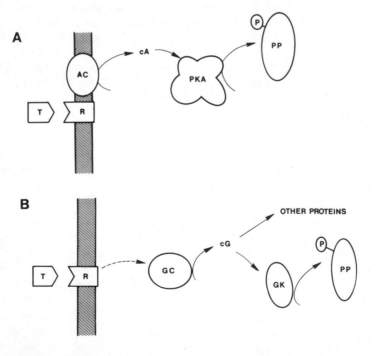

1. The adenylate cyclase/cyclic adenosine monophosphate (cyclic AMP)-dependent protein kinase system.
2. Guanylate cyclase and cyclic guanosine monophosphate (cyclic GMP)-dependent protein kinase.
3. The inositol trisphosphate/diacylglycerol-protein kinase C system.
4. Systems that are activated by calcium ions, including the calcium/calmodulin-dependent protein kinase systems.

The Adenylate Cyclase/Cyclic AMP-Dependent Protein Kinase System

Of the preceding four systems, the adenylate cyclase/cyclic AMP-dependent protein kinase system (Figure 1.6A) was the first to be described and has received the greatest attention from both biochemists and electrophysiologists. To a large extent, this is because the biochemistry of this pathway has been investigated very intensively and because highly specific reagents have been available to test the roles of cyclic

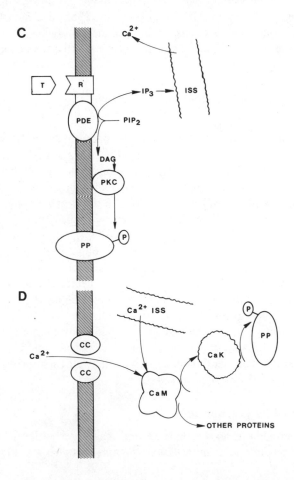

AMP and its kinase in the regulation of neuronal ion channels in a variety of independent ways. Figure 1.6A shows some of the major components of the cyclic AMP system. These include the neurotransmitter or hormonal receptors that are coupled to adenylate cyclase in the plasma membrane and the cyclic AMP-dependent protein kinase. The adenylate cyclase enzyme and the protein kinase that is activated following an elevation of cellular cyclic AMP levels are each composed of regulatory and catalytic subunits. Drugs and reagents that activate or inhibit each of these subunits, as well as some of the purified components themselves, are available and have allowed several independent tests for the involvement of this pathway in the control of a physiological response. Chapters 6, 7, 8, 10, and 11 each provide examples of electrophysiological responses mediated by cyclic AMP and its protein kinase.

Guanylate Cyclase and the Cyclic GMP-Dependent Protein Kinase

In contrast to that of the cyclic AMP system, the role of the second messenger cyclic GMP in the control of excitability is far from clear. (Figure 1.6B). Only in vertebrate photoreceptors does compelling evidence exist for the physiological regulation of a specific ion channel by cyclic GMP (Fesenko et al., 1985) and the role of the cyclic GMP-dependent protein kinase is unknown. Evidence in other systems indicates that cyclic GMP can exert some interesting physiological effects, but the ionic basis of these effects is not yet clear.

The Inositol Trisphosphate/Diacylglycerol-Protein Kinase C System

In recent years many neurotransmitters and hormones have been shown to stimulate the simultaneous formation of two substances within cells, diacylglycerol and inositol trisphosphate, each of which may act independently as a second messenger (Berridge, 1984; Nishizuka, 1984)(Figure 1.6C). Both substances are formed from a membrane phospholipid, phosphatidylinositol 4,5-bisphosphate, by the action of a receptor-linked phosphodiesterase. Diacylglycerol, which remains within the membrane, can activate a protein kinase (protein kinase C), while inositol trisphosphate, which is water soluble, can diffuse within the cytoplasm and release calcium ions from storage sites in intracellular membranes. Some emerging examples of the possible roles of protein kinase C in the regulation of neuronal ion channels are given in Chapters 7 and 11. Although no explicit examples of regulation by inositol trisphosphate are presented in this volume, good evidence exists for the activation of a sodium current in invertebrate photoreceptors by inositol trisphosphate (Fein et al., 1984; Brown et al., 1984). Because this is such a new and rapidly advancing area of research, it is certain that many more examples, as well as surprises, lie in store in the near future.

Systems Activated by Calcium Ions

It is clear that, in addition to the three second messenger systems just described, a change in the concentration of intracellular calcium ions also acts to transduce extracellular signals into cellular and electrical responses. The concentration of free calcium ions in a cell may change as a result of either the activation of calcium channels in the plasma membrane or the release of calcium ions from intracellular stores, for example, by the action of inositol trisphosphate. Calcium ions can act directly on specific ion channels in the membrane (Chapter 8) and can activate several different protein kinases (Chapter 4). Moreover, as is shown in Chapter 12, elevation of intracellular calcium at the nerve terminal is an essential step in the synaptic release of neurotransmitters.

Although the preceding are the second messenger systems best studied to date, other systems of intracellular biochemical reactions exist which may play roles in the modulation of neuronal activity, including those pathways involved in the formation of prostaglandins and related metabolites, the tyrosine kinase systems (See Chapter 4), and the methylation of proteins and lipids.

HOW MODULATION OF ELECTRICAL ACTIVITY IS ACHIEVED

A number of theoretical possibilities exist for the way in which the activation of a second messenger system can evoke a change in the electrical responses of a neuron. Because, as is described in the next chapter, the electrical activity of a neuron is directly regulated by the ion channels in its plasma membrane, the most direct way to influence excitability is to change the properties of one or more of its ion channels. This is the method of regulation this book addresses in most detail. It is also possible, however, to change the electrical responses of a neuron without a direct effect on any of its ion channels. This section contrasts the different classes of cellular mechanisms that can contribute to the modulation of neuronal activity.

Modulation of Ion Channels

In the simplest case, activation of a second messenger system can result directly in some covalent modification, for example phosphorylation, of an ion channel protein (Figure 1.7A). Both biochemical evidence and electrophysiological evidence indicate that this does occur (Chapters 5, 8, and 10). Unfortunately, the majority of ion channels, including all the different classes of potassium channels (see Chapter 2), have not yet been purified. This is, in part, because ion channels need be present in the plasma membrane only at low concentrations to produce major effects on electrical properties and are, therefore, relatively minor constituents of the cell. Thus, the chemical identity of nearly all those channels for which good evidence exists for physiological modulation by activation of protein kinases, is unknown and the possibility that they act as substrates for the kinases cannot be tested directly. An exception to this is one class of calcium channel, which may be modulated by cyclic AMP-dependent protein kinase and which has been purified (Curtis & Catterall, 1985). Unfortunately, for the two ion channels that have been best characterized biochemically, the acetylcholine receptor and the sodium channel, the physiological signifi-

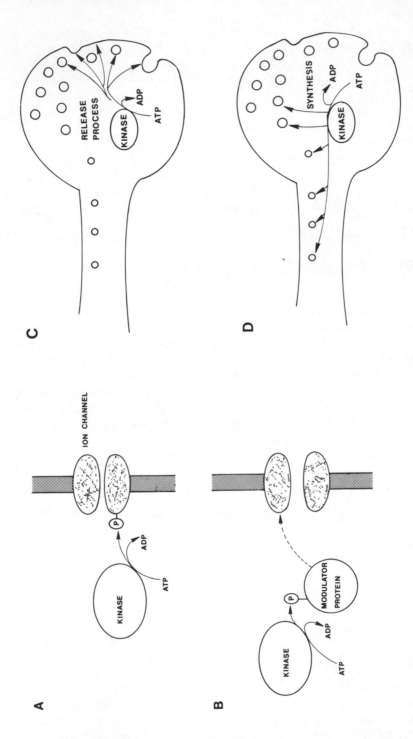

Fig. 1.7. Four mechanisms for the modulation of neuronal excitability by protein phosphorylation. (A) Direct phosphorylation of ion channels; (B) phosphorylation of other cellular constituents, which indirectly leads to the modulation of ion channel activity; (C) phosphorylation of intracellular components that control the release of neurotransmitter; (D) phosphorylation of intracellular components that control the synthesis and transport of neurotransmitter.

cance of their phosphorylation by protein kinases is not yet known (but see Chapter 5).

A second possibility, illustrated in Figure 1.7B, is that the ion channel itself is not directly modified by the second messenger system but its activity is modulated by some other membranous or cytoplasmic component that, in turn, is modified by activation of the second messenger pathway. It seems likely that a complete physiological response within a cell involves a combination of the mechanisms of Figure 1.7A and B. For example, it is known that phosphoprotein phosphatases, enzymes that catalyse the removal of phosphate groups from protein, are themselves substrates for different protein kinases and that their efficacy is altered by phosphorylation (Ingebritsen & Cohen, 1983). The characteristics of a physiological response that involves modulation of an ion channel may therefore also depend on the coordinate modulation of the activity of phosphatases or other cytoplasmic components (see Chapter 10).

Other Mechanisms for Modulation of Electrical Activity

Altering the properties of ion channels in a neuron is not the only way to change the electrical behavior of the cell. Other possible mechanisms that could influence excitability include changes in the morphology of the dendritic and axonal branches of a neuron, which could influence current flow through the cell without any modulation of its ion channels per se. A change in excitability also occurs when newly synthesized channels are inserted in the membrane, even if no modification of preexisting channels is made. Such transformations of electrical properties clearly occur and are of functional significance during development of the nervous system (Blair, 1983; O'Dowd, 1983).

One particularly important way in which the excitability of neurons may be influenced is by changes in the amount or type of neurotransmitter released at presynaptic sites (Figure 1.7C). Although the biochemical details are not fully understood, the release process is likely to be a prime target for modulation by neurotransmitters and by second messenger systems. Chapter 12 describes the role of calcium ions in the control of the secretory process and discusses some of the ways that the amount of release can be modified by prior activity in the presynaptic terminal. It has been reported that one form of calcium/calmodulin-dependent protein kinase may modulate release without any effect on ion channels of the presynaptic membrane (Llinas et al., 1985), perhaps through alterations in the properties of synaptic vesicles. The control of neurotransmitter release may be responsible for certain intriguing examples of neuromodulation that are not yet understood, for example, those in which long-lasting potentiation of synaptic efficacy occurs (Chapter 13).

In addition to the release process, the synthesis, transport, and processing of neurotransmitters and neuropeptides are candidates for modulation (Figure 1.7D). The alteration of these processes during the physiological activity of a neuron might directly affect the electrical response of its postsynaptic target and, in the case of a neuron that bears autoreceptors for its own transmitter, its own electrical properties.

CONCLUSIONS

The electrical properties of neurons are highly plastic. The form of their action potentials, their patterns of discharge, and how they respond to synaptic inputs may be modulated to allow the nervous system to respond appropriately to sensory stimuli, to generate motor output, and to control and change an animal's specific behavior. A variety of possible mechanisms exists to bring about such changes in excitability. Although future research into many of these possibilities promises to be highly fertile, most of them will not be discussed in this volume because their relevance to specific changes in neuronal excitability has yet to be investigated in detail. The best understood mechanisms are those in which the properties of specific ion channels are modified by the activation of different second messenger systems, which are linked to the activity of protein kinases. The next chapter introduces the different classes of ion channels within neurons, with emphasis on those whose properties can be modulated.

REFERENCES

Berridge, M.J. (1984) Inositol trisphosphate and diacylglycerol as second messengers. *Biochem. J. 220,* 345–360.

Blair, L.A. (1983) The timing of protein synthesis required for the development of the sodium action potential in embryonic spinal neurons. *J. Neurosci. 3,* 1430–1436.

Brown, J.E., Rubin, L.J., Ghalayini, A.J., Tarver, A.P., Irvine, R.F., Berridge, M.J., and Anderson, R.E. (1984) *Myo*-inositol polyphosphate may be a messenger for visual excitation in *Limulus* photoreceptors. *Nature 311,* 160–163.

Curtis, B.M. and Catterall, W.A. (1985) Phosphorylation of the calcium antagonist receptor of the voltage sensitive calcium channel by cAMP-dependent protein kinase. *Proc. Nat. Acad. Sci. USA 82,* 2528–2532.

Dutton, A. and Dyball, R.E.J. (1979) Phasic firing enhances vasopressin release from rat neurohypophysis. *J. Physiol. 290,* 433–440.

Fein, A., Payne, R., Corson, D.W., Berridge, M.J., and Irvine, R.F. (1984) Photoreceptor excitation and adaptation by inositol 1,4,5-trisphosphate. *Nature 311,* 159–160.

Fesenko, E.E., Kolesnikov, S.S., and Lyubarski, A.L. (1985) Induction by cyclic GMP of cationic conductance in plasma membrane of retinal rod outer segment. *Nature 313,* 310–313.

Gillette, R., Gillette, M.V., and Davis, W.J. (1980) Action potential broadening and endogenously sustained bursting are substrates of command ability in a feeding neuron of *Pleurobranchaea. J. Neurophysiol. 43,* 669–685.

Ingebritsen, T.S. and Cohen, P. (1983) Protein phosphatases: Properties and role in cellular regulation. *Science 221,* 331–338.

Kandel, E.R. (1976) *Cellular Basis of Behavior.* W.H. Freeman and Co., San Francisco.

Kravitz, E.A., Beltz, B.S., Glusman, S., Goy, M.F., Harris-Warrick, R.M., Johnson, M.F., Livingstone, M.F., Schwarz, T.L., and Siwicki, K.K. (1983) Neurohormones and lobsters: Biochemistry to behavior. *Trends in Neurosci. 6,* 346–349.

Kupfermann, I., Cohen, J.L., Mandelbaum, D.E., Schonberg, M., Susswein, A.J., and Weiss, K.R. (1979) Functional role of serotonergic neuromodulation in *Aplysia. Fed. Proc. 38,* 2095–2102.

Llinas, R., McGuinness, T.L., Leonard, C.S., Sugimori, M., and Greengard, P. (1985) *Proc. Nat. Acad. Sci. USA 82* 3035–3039.

Nishizuka, Y. (1984)The role of protein kinase C in cell surface signal transduction and tumour promotion. *Nature 308,* 693–697.

O'Dowd, D.K. (1983) RNA synthesis dependence of action potential development in spinal cord neurons. *Nature 303,* 619–621.

Selverston, A.I. (1985) *Model Neural Networks and Behavior.* Plenum Publishing Corp., New York.

Westerfield, M., Joyner, R.Y., and Moore, J.W. (1978) Temperature-sensitive conduction failure at axon branch points. *J. Neurophysiol. 41,* 1–8.

2

Ion Currents and Ion Channels: Substrates for Neuromodulation

IRWIN B. LEVITAN
LEONARD K. KACZMAREK

The electrical activity of nerve cells, and indeed of all cells, is determined by the net flow of current across the plasma membrane. Although some membrane current arises from the active transport of ions by electrogenic pumps, the major source of membrane current is the passive flow of ions down their concentration gradients through ion channels in the membrane. It is now known that the membranes of nerve cells contain a number of different populations of ion channels, each with its distinct ion selectivity, and also a number of different electrogenic ion pumps. As a result, the activities of many different pathways contribute to the net current flow across the membrane, and hence to the control of the cell's overall electrical activity.

Most examples of modulation of neuronal electrical activity that have been investigated occur by means of long-term changes in one or more of the membrane ion currents. Table 2.1 lists those ion currents that have been shown to be modulated by a particular biochemical mechanism, protein phosphorylation (see Chapter 4); many of these will be discussed in detail later in this volume. To date no firm evidence is available on the modulation of the activity of ion pumps in neurons, so the book will deal exclusively with the regulation of ion fluxes through ion channels. As is evident from Table 2.1 the modulation of calcium currents and several different kinds of potassium currents has been demonstrated in a variety of neuronal and nonneuronal systems. Although only limited evidence has been obtained for sodium and chloride, the two other ions that contribute substantially to the total membrane current, it is certainly conceivable that their flux is regulated in similar ways.

Specific components of ion current across a membrane, each representing the activity of a different kind of ion channel, can be differentiated from each other by their ion selectivities, voltage dependences, and sensitivity to various pharmacological agents. It was thought for many years that ion currents could be divided into two distinct classes, those activated by voltage and those activated by the binding of ligands (e.g., neurotransmitters), and that there was no overlap between these two classes. As will be seen below and in subsequent chapters, this distinction is no

Table 2.1. Ion currents whose activity has been shown to be modulated by protein phosphorylation.*

Cell type	Current modulated	Type of phosphorylation (see Chapter 4)
Aplysia bag cell neurons	Transient K^+ current $I_{K(A)}$	cAMP-dependent
	Delayed rectifying K^+ current $I_{K(V)}$ (slow)	cAMP-dependent
	Delayed rectifying K^+ current $I_{K(V)}$ (fast)	cAMP-dependent
	Ca^{++} current I_{Ca}	Protein kinase C
Aplysia sensory neurons	Serotonin-sensitive K^+ current $I_{K(S)}$†	cAMP-dependent
Aplysia neuron R15	Anomalously rectifying K^+ current $I_{K(r)}$	cAMP-dependent
Hermissenda photoreceptors	Transient K^+ current $I_{K(A)}$	cAMP-dependent
	Delayed rectifying K^+ current $I_{K(V)}$	Phosphorylase kinase
Helix neurons	Ca^{++} current I_{Ca}	cAMP-dependent
	Ca^{++}-dependent K^+ current $I_{K(Ca)}$†	cAMP-dependent
Squid giant axon	Delayed rectifying K^+ current $I_{K(V)}$	cAMP-dependent
Cardiac cells	Ca^{++} current I_{Ca}†	cAMP-dependent
Cultured cells	Gap junctional current	cAMP-dependent
		Tyrosine kinase

*For details of nomenclature of ion currents see text.
†Single channel measurements suggest the phosphorylation target is closely associated with the ion channel itself.

longer tenable. Many of the currents that can be modulated by ligands or by intracellular metabolic changes are indeed voltage dependent, and many of the classic voltage-dependent ion currents—for example, those that participate in the action potential—can be modulated. It is not inconceivable that, as technical and conceptual advances allow us to ask more detailed and sophisticated experimental questions, we will find that all ion currents are subject to some form of neuromodulatory influence.

This chapter will describe how ion currents can be measured in neuronal membranes and the properties of those individual ion currents that may be substrates for neuromodulation. In addition, it will describe a series of exquisitely sensitive and powerful new techniques to measure the activity of single ion channels that have permitted the testing of the hypothesis that ion channel proteins themselves might be molecular targets for neuromodulatory influences.

HOW TO MEASURE MEMBRANE ION CURRENTS

The ion current flowing across a membrane at a particular voltage can be measured by a technique known as voltage clamping. A voltage clamp system is built from three components (Figure 2.1). First, a microelectrode is inserted into the cell and connected to a voltage-measuring preamplifier. This allows measurement of the volt-

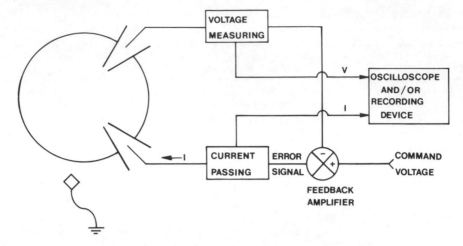

Fig. 2.1. Schematic representation of the components of a voltage clamp. A two-electrode voltage clamp of a neuronal membrane requires a voltage measuring preamplifier, a current-passing system, and a feedback amplifier that measures the difference between the measured voltage and the command voltage set by the experimenter. For a detailed description, see the text. This figure and much of the accompanying text description were kindly provided by J.A. Benson and W.B. Adams.

age across the cell membrane or, more precisely, of the voltage inside the cell compared to a reference electrode placed in the bathing medium. Under physiological conditions the electrical resistance of the cytoplasm is much smaller than the resistance of the cell membrane, so that the inside of the cell is essentially isopotential. (This is not true when the cell is not spherical but possesses a complex geometry; this complication is of practical importance in the voltage clamping of real cells, but it need not concern us for this theoretical discussion.) Next, a second microelectrode is placed in the cell and connected to a current-passing system (Figure 2.1). Finally, a feedback loop is created by adding a difference amplifier, which compares a voltage set by the experimenter ($V_{command}$) with the measured membrane voltage (V_{mem}). The difference between these two voltages is known as the error signal, and the purpose of the feedback system is to inject current through the current-passing electrode in order to maintain the error signal as close as possible to zero. This can be accomplished by making the gain in the current-passing amplifier sufficiently high so that V_{mem} is forced to be equal to $V_{command}$. By this means the membrane voltage is controlled by the experimenter, and the signal that is measured is the amount of membrane current required to maintain that voltage. This measured current may change with time after clamping to a particular voltage, as the individual ion channels that contribute to the total current activate and inactivate.

A graphical representation of the relationship between membrane current (measured) and membrane voltage (controlled) after the cell has been clamped at a particular voltage for a given length of time is known as a current-voltage or I-V curve. Chapter 6 describes the way in which the complicated I-V relationship of a real neuron can be thought of in terms of relatively simple combinations of individual conductance pathways. Readers not accustomed to thinking about ion currents and membrane I-V relationships might profit by reading about steady-state current voltage measurements in Chapter 6 before continuing here.

ION CURRENTS IN MOLLUSCAN NEURONS AND OTHER CELLS

The total membrane current is the sum of the currents carried by the various types of ion channels active at a given voltage. In order to examine in isolation the current carried by a particular ion channel, it is often necessary to use pharmacological agents that block certain ion channels selectively or to manipulate the ionic composition of the bathing medium, or both. This section will describe the ways in which these tricks can be used to measure the properties of sodium, calcium, and potassium currents in neuronal cell bodies. Chloride current also contributes to the total membrane current, but its properties and possible role in neuromodulation have been studied less thoroughly, and thus it will not be discussed here.

The central ganglia of many gastropod molluscs contain giant neurons, the spherical cell bodies of which can be 500 μm or more in diameter. Because these cell bodies are readily accessible on the ganglionic surface, and can be voltage clamped relatively easily, they have been the system of choice for investigating the properties of neuronal membrane ion currents (for a review see Adams et al. 1980). More recently, technical advances have permitted similar questions to be addressed in neurons in the brain and ganglia of several vertebrate species (Chapters 9, 11, and 13).

Sodium Current (I_{Na})

The sodium current is an inward current resulting from the flow of sodium into the cell down its concentration gradient (by convention inward currents are defined as negative, outward currents as positive). The classic description of the properties of the sodium current comes from the studies of Hodgkin and Huxley on the squid giant axon more than 30 years ago. More recent experiments on such systems as node of Ranvier and molluscan neuronal cell bodies have confirmed this general picture and have provided details of differences between cell types in the properties of sodium currents. Although there appear to be slowly activating sodium currents that may contribute to slow oscillatory activity in some cells, the best understood is the rapidly activating and inactivating sodium current, which contributes to the depolarizing phase of the action potential. At potentials more positive than a certain value, usually about -20 mV in molluscan neurons, the sodium current activates rapidly and then inactivates. Thus, during a depolarizing voltage pulse the current rises to a peak and then declines as inactivation occurs (Figure 2.2). Its activation shows a steep dependence on voltage (Figure 2.3), and both the extent and the rate of activation are voltage dependent. Inactivation is also voltage dependent (Figure 2.3), and as a result the sodium current is almost completely inactivated at the peak of the action potential. The I-V relationship for the sodium current at early times during a pulse, that is, at a time when inactivation does not yet play a major role, demonstrates that the current

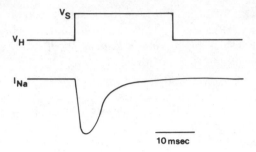

Fig. 2.2. Time course of sodium current during a depolarizing voltage pulse. When the membrane voltage is stepped from a hyperpolarized holding voltage V_H, to some voltage, V_S, sufficiently depolarized to activate sodium current, an inward current is seen that rises to a peak and then declines during the pulse. Calcium and potassium currents have been blocked by appropriate pharmacological agents for this and the next two figures. Figures 2.2 to 2.9 are schematic figures based on information and data in Adams and Benson (1985), Adams and Gage (1979 a, b), and Adams, Smith, and Thompson (1980).

rises to a peak and then declines as the voltage is increased (Figure 2.4). The rising limb of the curve reflects the voltage-dependent activation of the current, whereas the falling limb reflects the decreased driving force on sodium ions as the voltage approaches the sodium equilibrium potential (about $+50$ mV in most cells).

A number of creatures have evolved toxins that interfere with sodium channel function. For example, saxitoxin and tetrodotoxin (TTX), both of which bind tightly to the sodium channel and block the flow of sodium current, have been particularly useful pharmacological tools. As will be seen in subsequent chapters, these agents can be used to block sodium current in experiments designed to study individual ion

Fig. 2.3. Voltage dependence of activation and inactivation of the sodium current. The degree of steady-state activation (————) and inactivation (– – – – –) of sodium current as a function of membrane voltage. Note that inactivation is almost complete at all voltages at which activation occurs, indicating that the steady-state sodium current will always be very close to zero.

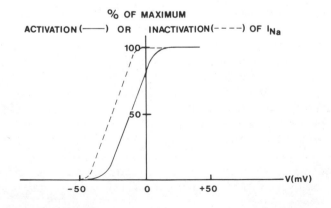

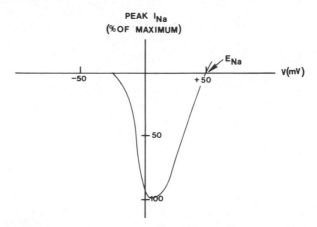

Fig. 2.4. I-V relationship for the sodium current. The peak inward current, at a time when inactivation is not yet significant, is plotted against the membrane voltage. Note the decline in current as the voltage approaches E_{Na}.

currents in isolation. In addition, the binding of radioactive saxitoxin has been used as a convenient assay for sodium channels during purification (reviewed by Catterall, 1984). The purified sodium channel protein is an excellent substrate for phosphorylation by cyclic AMP-dependent protein kinase (see Chapter 5), but to date no evidence for neuromodulation by phosphorylation of sodium channels has been reported.

Calcium Current (I_{Ca})

The other major inward current elicited by depolarization is the voltage-dependent calcium current. Although calcium does not make any substantial contribution to the squid axon action potential, it is the major and in some cases the only inward current underlying action potentials in cardiac cells (see Chapter 11) and in the cell bodies of many molluscan neurons. Furthermore, calcium does not act simply as a charge carrier; rather, the calcium that enters the cell can regulate the function of other ion channels (see below and Chapter 8) and can play an important role in many other intracellular events.

The calcium current can be measured when sodium current has been blocked by tetrodotoxin, and outward potassium currents have been blocked by appropriate pharmacological tools (see below). Like the sodium current, calcium current (Figure 2.5A) is activated by voltages more positive than about − 20 mV, and activation is maximal above about + 30 mV. The I-V relationship also exhibits a decline in current as the calcium equilibrium potential is approached at very positive voltages (Figure 2.5B). In some cells calcium current shows little or no inactivation, even during a prolonged depolarizing pulse. In other cells, including many molluscan neurons, the calcium current does inactivate (e.g., Figure 2.5A), but the inactivation is not directly dependent on voltage. An elegant series of experiments (reviewed by Eckert & Chad,

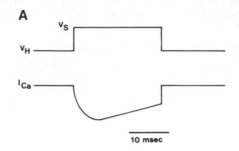

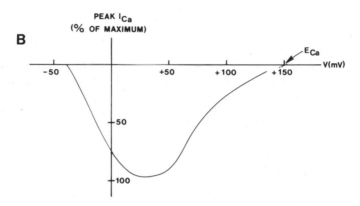

Fig. 2.5. Time course and voltage dependence of the calcium current. (A) When the sodium and potassium currents are blocked, stepping the membrane voltage from a holding potential V_H to a pulse potential V_S elicits an inward calcium current that exhibits some steady-state inactivation. (B) A plot of peak inward calcium current versus membrane voltage. Note the decline in current as the voltage approaches E_{Ca}.

1984) has demonstrated that the calcium that enters the cell during a depolarizing voltage pulse can feed back and inhibit the voltage-dependent calcium channels. This calcium-dependent inactivation of calcium current, which is an excellent example of modulation of a membrane ion current, will be discussed in more detail in Chapter 8.

A number of pharmacological probes that perturb calcium channel function are also available. Inorganic cations such as cadmium, cobalt, and lanthanum are excellent blockers of calcium current. Although they may have some effects on other ion currents as well, they have been used widely in attempts to examine other currents in isolation from calcium current. Barium, on the other hand, carries current through calcium channels somewhat better than calcium itself, and thus "barium current" has often been measured in situations in which the calcium current is small and difficult to quantitate. Particularly important is the dihydropyridine group of compounds, some of which inhibit calcium current (antagonists) and others of which enhance it (calcium channel agonists). As will be described in Chapter 11, these agents have been enormously helpful in extending our understanding of how the opening and closing of calcium channels (channel "gating"—see Chapter 3) is regulated. In addition, the availability of a binding assay using radioactive dihydropyridines has allowed the recent purification of a functional calcium channel (Curtis & Catterall, 1985). A great deal of evidence exists that calcium channel function is subject to neuromodulatory influences (see Chapters 8 and 11), and the availability of one type of purified calcium channel protein should allow the molecular mechanisms of this modulation to be investigated in detail.

Calcium-Dependent Cation Current ($I_{cation(Ca)}$)

A third inward current, first described in cardiac cells (Kass et al., 1978), is carried by an ion channel that allows the flow of both sodium and potassium ions. As a result, its reversal potential is about -10 to -20 mV, approximately halfway between the sodium and potassium equilibrium potentials. Accordingly, it is an inward current in the resting range of membrane potential but is outward at depolarized potentials, for example, during an action potential. Activation of this cation current depends only weakly on voltage, but it does require intracellular calcium (see Chapter 8). The current may help to provide a depolarizing drive toward action potential threshold in cardiac cells and also appears to be important in generating rhythmic bursting activity in some molluscan neurons (Kramer & Zucker, 1985a,b; see Chapter 8).

Potassium Current (I_K)

At least six—and probably more—distinct voltage-dependent outward potassium currents exist in molluscan neurons and many other cell types. They can be observed best when the inward sodium and calcium currents are blocked by tetrodotoxin and cadmium or cobalt, respectively (but at least one of the potassium currents is calcium dependent and thus is not evoked by depolarizing voltage pulses when calcium entry is blocked; see below and Chapter 8). The various potassium currents can be distinguished by their voltage dependences, kinetics of activation and inactivation, and sensitivity to various pharmacological agents. However, there is sufficient overlap in their properties so that it is often difficult to study one particular current without some degree of contamination by one or more of the others. Most of these potassium currents will be discussed in detail in subsequent chapters, and thus only a brief introduction will be provided here.

One important question is why neuronal membranes contain so many distinct conductance pathways for a single ion. Although this is far from being understood, one attractive hypothesis from the perspective of this volume is that by having a series of potassium currents with different properties, the electrical activity of a neuron can be modulated in many different ways and over a wide range of voltages. Subsequent chapters will demonstrate that all the potassium currents described below are substrates of neuromodulation, and this may reflect the wide diversity of changes in excitability that neurons must undergo.

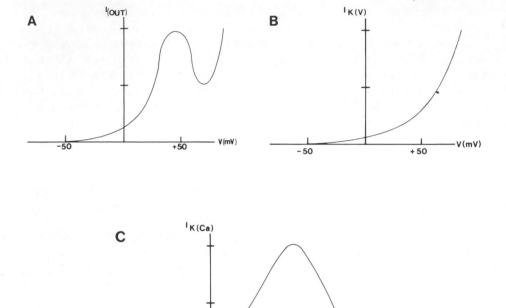

Fig. 2.6. I-V relationships for outward potassium currents. (A) Plot of the total steady-state outward current, elicited by depolarizing voltage steps, as a function of membrane voltage. This total current is the sum of at least two distinct current components. When the cell is injected with a high concentration of EGTA, or calcium entry is prevented with a blocker such as cobalt or cadmium, only the delayed rectifier component (B) is elicited by depolarization. The difference between A and B is the calcium-dependent potassium current (C). Note that its voltage dependence is similar to that of the calcium current (Figure 2.5B).

Delayed Rectifying Potassium Current ($I_{K(V)}$)

Again Hodgkin and Huxley provided a detailed description of the delayed rectifying potassium channel in squid axon, where it is the major outward current responsible for the repolarizing phase of the action potential. The delayed rectifier is also observed in molluscan neuronal cell bodies as one of the two delayed outward currents elicited by depolarizing pulses. The I-V curve for total outward current in these neurons has a characteristic ''N'' shape in the positive voltage range (Figure 2.6A), because it is the sum of at least two components. The delayed rectifier component itself often has the voltage dependence shown in Figure 2.6B, and the remaining current is the calcium-dependent potassium current (Figure 2.6C; see below). During prolonged depolarizations, the delayed rectifier current activates rapidly and then inactivates slowly. The inactivation is not complete as it is, for example, with sodium current, but rather the current declines to come nonzero value over a period of several seconds and remains there. Recovery from this steady-state inactivation is very slow, requiring as much as one minute in some cells. As a result, repetitive firing of action potentials can lead to cumulative inactivation of the delayed rectifier. Because this current is a major component of spike repolarization, such cumulative inactivation will result in spike broadening (Aldrich et al., 1979 a, b,). This, in turn, will alter calcium entry during a spike and the efficacy of release of neurosecretory products from the synaptic terminals of the cell (see Chapters 1, 10, and 12).

No selective and high-affinity pharmacological agents are known for the delayed rectifying potassium current. Tetraethylammonium ion (TEA) does block this current, but concentrations in the range of 5 mM or higher are required, and TEA also has effects on other potassium currents at these concentrations (see below). This lack of effective pharmacological tools has precluded any effort to purify delayed rectifier channels, and has contributed to the difficulties of examining individual potassium currents in isolation.

The delayed rectifier in some cells may be composed of more than one kinetically distinct current component, and, as will be discussed in detail in Chapter 7, two components of the delayed rectifier are among the several potassium currents subject to modulation in the neurosecretory bag cell neurons in *Aplysia*. Furthermore, although for many years the squid axon delayed rectifier was considered rather boring from the point of view of neuromodulation, recent experiments have provided evidence that protein phosphorylation can modulate the voltage dependence of both the activation and inactivation of this current (Bezanilla et al., 1985). Because these experiments are ongoing and preliminary, they will not be discussed elsewhere in this volume, but it is worth pointing out that the wealth of information available about squid axon potassium currents makes this system especially favorable for investigating the details of modulation of ion channel gating and conduction mechanisms.

Calcium-Dependent Potassium Current ($I_{K(Ca)}$)

The other outward current component that contributes to the N-shaped I-V curve at positive voltages is the calcium-dependent potassium current (Meech, 1978). This current is activated by the calcium that enters the cell through the voltage-dependent calcium channels during a depolarizing voltage pulse (Figure 2.7A). When this calcium is bound before it can activate the calcium-dependent potassium current—for example, by the intracellular injection of the calcium chelator ethylene glycol-bis (β-amino ethylether) N, N, N', N'-tetraacetic acid (EGTA) (Figure 2.7B)—the only outward current is that contributed by the delayed rectifier (Figure 2.6B). Subtracting the delayed rectifier component from the total outward current provides a measurement of the calcium-dependent potassium current (Figure 2.6C).

It will be noted that the voltage dependence of the calcium-dependent potassium current (Figure 2.6C) is very similar to that of the calcium current (Figure 2.5B), exhibiting a steep increase with depolarization and a decline at very positive potentials. This situation arises from the requirement for calcium entry to activate this current; at potentials approaching the calcium equilibrium potential, calcium current decreases and hence less intracellular calcium is available to activate the calcium-dependent potassium current. For the same reason, pharmacological agents that block

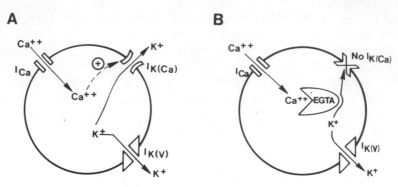

Fig. 2.7. Schematic representation of activation of potassium currents by depolarization. (A) Depolarization causes delayed rectifier channels to open and allows potassium current ($I_{K(v)}$) to flow. In addition, the depolarization opens voltage-dependent calcium channels; the resulting calcium current (I_{Ca}) provides intracellular calcium to activate the calcium-dependent potassium channels, producing another potassium current ($I_{K(Ca)}$). The sum of these two outward currents gives rise to the N-shaped I-V curve in Figure 2.6A. (B) When calcium is prevented from activating the calcium-dependent potassium current—for example, by intracellular injection of the calcium chelator EGTA—only the delayed rectifying potassium current is evoked by depolarization.

calcium current also block activation of the calcium-dependent potassium current by depolarization. However, the latter current can still be elicited by intracellular injection of calcium, even when the calcium current is blocked. This approach makes it possible to study the properties of the calcium-dependent potassium current without the complications associated with first having to elicit the calcium current.

As in the case of the delayed rectifier, the number of pharmacological probes for the calcium-dependent potassium current is rather limited. In some cells TEA blocks this current at concentrations below 1 mM, whereas in other cells TEA levels of 10 mM or higher are required. It is now becoming evident from single channel measurements (see below) that this occurs because at least two distinct types of calcium-dependent potassium channel that can give rise to calcium-dependent potassium current exist, and one of these channels is more sensitive than the other to TEA. The recent discovery and purification of charybdotoxin, a scorpion venom component that binds with high affinity to and blocks one of the types of calcium-dependent potassium channel (Miller et al., 1985), has opened up new possibilities for pharmacologically manipulating calcium-dependent potassium current and perhaps for purifying this potassium channel.

The calcium-dependent potassium current is almost by definition a modulated current, since its activity is regulated by calcium, one of the major intracellular messengers (Chapter 1). In addition, as will be described in Chapter 8, this current can be modulated by cyclic AMP-dependent protein phosphorylation. Thus, the calcium-dependent potassium current is one cellular locus at which the calcium and cyclic AMP second messenger systems can interact to produce an integrated change in the cell's activity. Because the calcium-dependent potassium current contributes to spike

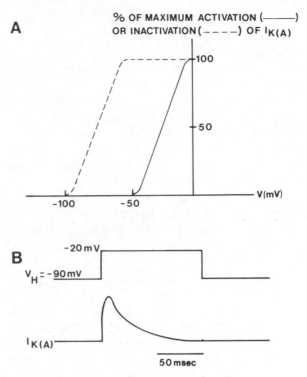

Fig. 2.8. Time course and voltage dependence of activation and inactivation of A-current. (A) The degree of steady-state activation (———) and inactivation (– – – – –) of A-current as a function of voltage. Note that, as in the case of the sodium current, at steady state the A-current will always be close to zero. (B) Time course of A-current, elicited by a step from a very hyperpolarized holding potential ($V_H = -90$ mV) to -20 mV. Note the complete inactivation of the current during the pulse.

repolarization, and is also responsible for the spike afterhyperpolarization that helps to control the frequency of repetitive firing (see Chapter 8), modulation of its activity can significantly alter neuronal activity.

Transient Potassium Current ($I_{K(A)}$)

A third outward potassium current that can be elicited by depolarizations is the rapidly activating and rapidly inactivating current often called A-current. A major difference between A-current and the delayed rectifying potassium current is in their voltage dependences. Although the exact voltage dependence varies from cell to cell, A-current is often largely inactivated at voltages more positive than about -40 mV (Figure 2.8A), close to the resting potential of many neurons. To elicit this current by depolarization, the membrane potential must first be set to a negative holding potential (typically more negative than -90 mV) for several hundred milliseconds to remove the steady-state voltage-dependent inactivation. Upon depolarization from these negative voltages to potentials more positive than about -45 mV, the A-current first undergoes rapid activation and then inactivates (Figure 2.8B). Activation can occur at fairly negative potentials (Figure 2.8A), often in a potential region subthreshold for action potential generation.

Because the A-current is active in this subthreshold region of membrane potentials, it is thought to play a role in determining the frequency of repetitive firing in neurons that are spontaneously active or that fire repetitively in response to tonic depolarization. Although in such cells the A-current may be largely inactivated at the potential threshold for action potential generation, the hyperpolarization that follows the action potential may remove some of the inactivation. During the subsequent depolarization preceding the next action potential, the A-current thus may be transiently activated before again undergoing inactivation. This transient activation of an outward current will slow the return of the membrane potential toward the action potential threshold and will serve to prolong the interspike interval. This possibility is discussed in more detail in Chapter 7, which also describes the modulation of the activity of the A-current by cyclic AMP.

Anomalously Rectifying Potassium Current ($I_{K(r)}$)

The term *anomalous* or *inward* rectification refers to a *decrease* in the slope of a cell's I-V relationship upon depolarization (Figure 2.9A). This may be compared with normal rectification, such as that exhibited by the delayed rectifying potassium current, which involves an *increase* in slope with depolarization (Figure 2.6B). In the hyperpolarized range of membrane potentials, the total membrane I-V curve of many cells displays anomalous rectification. As discussed in detail in Chapter 6, this might arise in several ways. In some cells anomalous rectification is due to the presence of an anomalously rectifying potassium current with an I-V curve such as that shown in Figure 2.9B. The voltage dependence of the anomalously rectifying potassium current differs from that of the other currents we have discussed earlier in that it is active at hyperpolarized voltages and becomes less active on depolarization. Furthermore, its voltage dependence is not absolute but is influenced by extracellular potassium, and thus it can be thought of as a potassium-dependent potassium current. When the potassium equilibrium potential, E_K, is altered by changing the extracellular potassium concentration, the current always begins to inactivate at E_K whatever this voltage happens to be, and thus the position of the I-V curve can shift to the left or right along the voltage axis depending on the value of E_K.

The anomalously rectifying potassium current is not a perfect rectifier, and thus it can pass some outward current in the voltage range up to about 30 mV positive of E_K (Figure 2.9B). Although the amount of current is not large, very few other ion currents are active in this range of membrane potentials; thus, the anomalous rectifier can contribute significantly to the membrane potential in the resting range. As will be discussed in Chapter 6, modulation of the anomalous rectifier by protein phosphorylation can result in a profound modulation of neuronal activity.

M-Current ($I_{K(M)}$)

Another potassium current that is active in the hyperpolarizing range of membrane potentials is M-current, which has been described in vertebrate brain and sympathetic ganglion (see Chapter 9). This current begins to activate at voltages more positive

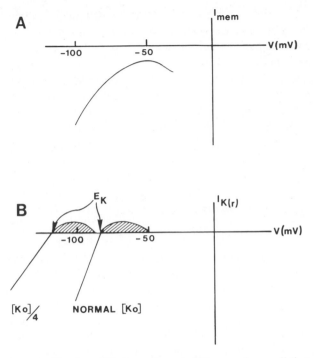

Fig. 2.9. Anomalous rectification. (A) A steady-state I-V curve for a cell that displays inward rectification in the hyperpolarized range of membrane potentials. Note the decrease in slope of the I-V curve upon depolarization. (B) I-V relationship for an anomalously rectifying potassium current, which contributes to the inward rectification of the total membrane I-V curve shown in A. The rectification is dependent on extracellular potassium and occurs at voltages positive to E_K; when E_K is changed by changing the extracellular potassium concentration (K_O), the I-V curve for the anomalous rectifier shifts along the voltage axis.

than about -50 mV, and activation is usually complete by about -20 mV. It does not inactivate, and thus even though it is a small current that activates relatively slowly following a depolarizing pulse, it can influence significantly the activity of the cell in the resting range.

A rich pharmacology is associated with the M-current, and it is an excellent example of a voltage-dependent ion current that can be modulated by neurotransmitters. It is turned off by a number of agents, including *m*uscarinic acetylcholine receptor agonists (hence the name *M*-current), and a variety of putative peptide neurotransmitters. As will be shown in Chapter 9, this modulation of M-current activity is probably responsible for several slow excitatory responses in vertebrate neurons.

S-Current ($I_{K(S)}$)

Another membrane ion current that can be inhibited by a neurotransmitter is the S-current in *Aplysia* sensory neurons, so named because it is decreased by serotonin (Klein et al., 1982). S-current exhibits some voltage dependence, but this is not very steep; it begins to activate at about -50 mV, and activation is complete by about 0 mV. No significant inactivation occurs, even during prolonged depolarizations; as a result, S-current remains active during action potentials and contributes to spike re- polarization. That this contribution is significant is shown by the finding that, when S-current is inhibited by serotonin, the duration of action potentials in the sensory neurons is enhanced. As will be described in Chapter 10, this modulation by seroto- nin results in an increase in neurotransmitter release at the synaptic terminals of sensory neurons, with a consequent modulation of behavioral responses in which the sensory neurons participate. Chapter 10 will also discuss details of the molecular mechanism of this neuromodulatory action of serotonin.

MEASUREMENT OF THE ACTIVITY OF SINGLE ION CHANNELS

As described previously, most of the membrane ion current arises from the trans- membrane movement of ions through a class of membrane spanning proteins known as ion channels. Although some of the properties of ion channels can be inferred from the measurement of membrane ion current (so-called macroscopic current mea- surements), the information that can be obtained about the channels themselves is limited and indirect. Much of what we know today about ion channels (see the fol- lowing chapter) has come from the measurement of individual ion channel activity, using powerful techniques developed during the last ten years. It should be noted that these techniques are probably the most sensitive in biological science, because it is the activity of a single molecule (or macromolecular complex) that is being monitored. These ''microscopic'' measurements of the current passing through an individual ion channel provide a different kind of information than the macroscopic currents, which represent the average behavior of a large population of channels. The ways in which single channel measurement can be used to elucidate information about the molecular details of ion channel gating and conduction will be described in Chapters 3 and 11.

Membrane Patch Recording

When a fire-polished glass electrode is brought up against the extracellular surface of a neuron or other cell, a very tight seal will sometimes form between the glass and the membrane. The membrane surfaces of some cells, particularly those in tissue culture, are often ''clean'' enough to allow seal formation, but in many cases it is necessary to mistreat the cell surface with a protease or other hydrolytic enzyme to allow the electrode sufficiently close access to the membrane surface. Under ideal conditions the electrode and membrane are so closely apposed that the so-called seal resistance, the resistance for ion flow between the glass and the membrane, can be as high as 10^{10} to 10^{11} ohms (10 to 100 gigohms). This means that most of the ions flowing through the ''patch'' of membrane under the electrode will not leak away through the seal, but will be detected by appropriate recording apparatus connected to the inside of the electrode (Figure 2.10A). Present limits of detection are such

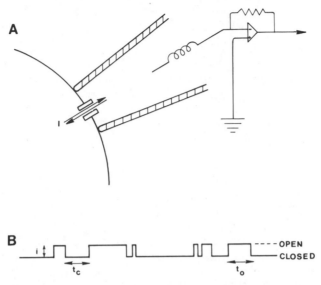

Fig. 2.10. Single channel recording in membrane patches. (A) Schematic representation of a "patch" of cell membrane, containing a single ion channel, under a fire-polished glass electrode. If the seal between the glass and the membrane is sufficiently high, the current passing through the ion channel can be detected by a sensitive current-to-voltage converter connected to the electrode. (B) An idealized single channel recording. When the channel goes from a closed to an open state, a step change in the current corresponds to the single channel current (i). In addition to the value of i, information about the mean channel open (t_0) and closed (t_c) times can be obtained from such records. Analysis of the t_0 and t_c values from many opening and closing transitions can provide information about channel gating mechanisms.

that, if there is a single ion channel in the patch of membrane, the current passing through this channel when it is open can be measured. As a result, one sees step changes in the current with time as the channel opens and closes (Figure 2.10B). From such records one can measure the amplitude of the single channel current, how long the channel stays open, and how long it is closed between channel openings (Figure 2.10B). Appropriate analysis of this information obtained under a variety of experimental conditions can provide fundamental information about the properties of ion channels.

This patch recording technique, which was introduced by Neher and Sakmann and their colleagues (Hamill et al., 1981), has revolutionized neurophysiology and has profoundly influenced other branches of biology. Elaborations of this technique have also proven to be particularly useful for studies of neuromodulation. The seal between the glass electrode and the membrane is not only electrically tight but also mechanically tight, so that the patch of membrane often can be pulled off the cell with the cytoplasmic membrane surface exposed to the bathing medium (Figure 2.11A). This "inside-out patch" configuration (Hamill et al., 1981) allows experimental control of the ion concentrations on both sides of the membrane, and in addition permits application of putative modulatory agents (e.g., calcium, and protein kinases or other

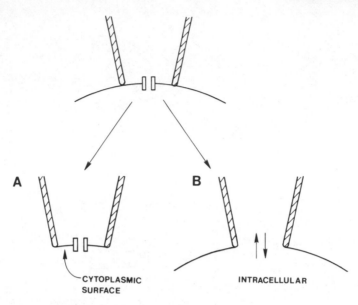

Fig. 2.11. Variations on the patch recording technique. (A) The inside-out detached patch has the cytoplasmic membrane surface exposed to the bathing medium. This configuration is useful for examining the effects of intracellular messengers on ion channel activity. (B) The whole cell configuration provides a low resistance pathway for voltage clamping and allows replacement of the cell's cytoplasmic contents.

enzymes) directly on the patch of membrane containing the ion channel of interest (see Chapters 8, 10, and 11). Another variation involves breaking the patch of membrane occluding the electrode to give the "whole cell clamp" configuration (Figure 2.11B). This does not permit the measurement of single ion channel activity but rather provides highly favorable conditions for voltage clamping and measuring the whole cell macroscopic current while allowing replacement of the cell's intracellular milieu with the contents of the electrode. This configuration has also been extremely useful for studies of neuromodulation (Chapters 7 and 11).

Reconstitution in Artificial Phospholipid Bilayers

Another technique that permits the measurement of single ion channel activity is the insertion of a channel into a synthetic membrane bilayer consisting of phospholipid. There are many possible variations on this approach (for a review see Miller, 1983), but the most popular has been to use a bilayer that occludes a small hole in a partition separating two aqueous solutions (Figure 2.12). A number of methods can be used either to insert a purified ion channel into such a bilayer or to allow the fusion of membrane vesicles containing ion channels with the bilayer (the latter method is illustrated in Figure 2.12). Because the bilayer membrane itself provides a very high resistance barrier to ion flow, considerations similar to those described for membrane patch recording apply, and the currents passing through individual ion channels in

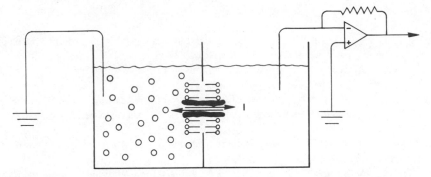

Fig. 2.12. Single channel recording in a planar bilayer. A phospholipid bilayer formed across a hole in a partition separating two aqueous solutions provides a high resistance barrier to ion flow. Membrane vesicles added to one side of the partition may fuse with the bilayer; if the vesicle that fuses happens to contain an ion channel, single channel currents across the bilayer may be recorded. One useful variation of this approach is to form the bilayer on the tip of a patch recording electrode.

the bilayer can be measured using relatively simple electronics (Figure 2.12). This technique allows the analysis of ion channels that are components of intracellular membrane systems and are not accessible to patch recording electrodes. Furthermore, it provides a simplified experimental system and, consequently, excellent experimental control, but it lacks the comfort of physiological reality provided by the native biological membrane; thus, it is probably most powerful when used in conjunction with the membrane patch approach (see, e.g., Chapter 8).

CONCLUSIONS

The membranes of neurons and many other cells contain multiple conductance pathways for ions such as sodium, calcium, chloride, and potassium. The ion currents that arise from the movement of these ions down their concentration gradients, through specific ion channels in the membrane, are responsible for the cell's electrical activity. The raison d'etre for this volume is that the ion channels are not simply inert pores in the membrane but are, in fact, *regulatable* pores. Rapid transitions of ion channels between different functional states can be regulated by the transmembrane voltage or by the binding of a ligand such as calcium or a neurotransmitter. Furthermore, these rapid transitions are themselves subject to long-term modulation, which may persist for minutes or hours and can result in profound changes in the activity of the cell. This chapter has described the properties, and especially the diversity, of the ion conductance pathways in nerve cell membranes. Subsequent chapters will present the details of the modulation of particular ion currents and ion channels to provide an appreciation of how this diversity allows the exquisitely sensitive "fine tuning" of neuronal activity.

REFERENCES

Adams, D.J. and Gage, P.W. (1976) Gating currents associated with sodium and calcium current in an *Aplysia* neurone. *Science 192*, 783–784.

Adams, D.J. and Gage, P.W. (1979a) Ionic currents in response to membrane depolarization in an *Aplysia* neurone. *J. Physiol. London 289*, 115–142.

Adams, D.J. and Gage, P.W. (1979b) Characteristics of sodium and calcium conductance changes produced by membrane depolarization in *Aplysia* neurone. *J. Physiol. London 289*, 143–162.

Adams, D.J and Gage, P.W. (1979c) Sodium and calcium gating currents in an *Aplysia* neurone. *J. Physiol. London 291*, 467–482.

Adams, D.J., Smith, S.J., and Thompson, S.H. (1980) Ionic currents in molluscan soma. *Ann. Rev. Neurosci. 3*, 141–167.

Adams, W.B. (1985) Slow depolarizing and hyperpolarizing currents which mediate bursting in *Aplysia* neurone R15. *J. Physiol. 360*, 51–68.

Adams, W.B. and Benson, J.A. (1985) The generation and modulation of endogenous rhythmicity in the *Aplysia* bursting pacemaker neurone R15. *Prog. Biophys. Molec. Biol. 46*, 1–49.

Adams, W.B. and Levitan, I.B. (1985) Voltage and ion dependences of the slow currents which mediate bursting in *Aplysia* neurone R15. *J. Physiol. 360*, 69–93.

Ahmed, Z. and Connor, J.A. (1979) Measurement of calcium influx under voltage clamp in molluscan neurones using the metallochromic dye arsenazo III. *J. Physiol. London 286*, 61–82.

Akaike, N., Lee, K.S., and Brown, A.M. (1978) The calcium current of *Helix* neuron. *J. Gen. Physiol. 71*, 509–531.

Aldrich, R.W., Jr., Getting, P.A., and Thompson, S.H. (1979a) Inactivation of delayed outward current in molluscan neurone somata. *J. Physiol. London 291*, 507–530.

Aldrich, R.W., Jr., Getting, P.A., and Thompson, S.H. (1979b) Mechanism of frequency-dependent broadening of molluscan neurone soma spikes. *J. Physiol. London 291*, 531–544.

Alkon, D.L. (1984) Calcium-mediated reduction of ionic currents: A biophysical memory trace. *Science 226*, 1037–1045.

Benson, J.A. and Levitan, I.B. (1983) Serotonin increases an anomalously rectifying K^+ current in the *Aplysia* neuron R15. *Proc. Natl. Acad. Sci. USA 80*, 3522–3525.

Bezanilla, F., DiPolo, R., Caputo, C., Rojas, H., and Torres, M.E. (1985) K^+ current in squid axon is modulated by ATP. *Biophys. J. 47*, 222a.

Catterall, W.A. (1984) The molecular basis of neuronal excitability. *Science 223*, 653–661.

Connor, J.A. (1978) Slow repetitive activity from fast conductance changes in neurons. *Fed. Proc. 37*, 2139–2145.

Connor, J.A. and Stevens, C.F. (1971a) Inward and delayed outward membrane currents in isolated neural somata under voltage clamp. *J. Physiol. London 213*, 1–20.

Connor, J.A. and Stevens, C.F. (1971b) Voltage clamp studies of a transient outward current in gastropod neural somata. *J. Physiol. London 213*, 21–30.

Connor, J.A. and Stevens, C.F. (1971c) Prediction of repetitive firing behaviour from voltage clamp data on an isolated neurone soma. *J. Physiol. London 213*, 31–53.

Curtis, B.M. and Catterall, W.A. (1985) Phosphorylation of the calcium antagonist receptor of the voltage-sensitive calcium channel by cAMP-dependent protein kinase.*Proc. Natl. Acad. Sci. USA, 82*, 2528–2532.

Eckert, R. and Chad J.E. (1984) Inactivation of calcium channels. *Prog. Biophys. Molec. Biol. 44*, 215–267.

Eckert, R. and Lux, H.D. (1975) A non-inactivating inward current recorded during small depolarizing voltage steps in snail pacemaker neurons. *Brain Res. 83*, 486–489.

Eckert, R. and Lux, H.D. (1976) A voltage-sensitive persistent calcium conductance in neuronal somata of *Helix. J. Physiol. London 254*, 129–151.

Eckert, R. and Lux, H.D. (1977) Calcium-dependent depression of a late outward current in snail neurons. *Science 197*, 472–475.

Eckert, R. and Tillotson, D. (1978) Potassium activation associated with intraneuronal free calcium. *Science 200*, 437–439.

Fenwick, E.M., Marty, A., and Neher, E. (1982) Sodium and calcium channels in bovine chromaffin cells. *J. Physiol. 331*, 599–635.

Gola, M., Ducreux, C., and Chagneux, H. (1977) Ionic mechanism of slow potential wave production in barium-treated *Aplysia* neurons. *J. Physiol. Paris 73*, 407–440.

Gorman, A.L. and Thomas, M.V. (1978) Changes in the intracellular concentration of free calcium ions in a pacemaker neurone, measured with metallochromic indicator dye arsenazo III. *J. Physiol. London 275*, 357–376.

Hagiwara, S., Kusano, K., and Saito, N. (1961) Membrane changes of *Onchidium* nerve cell in potassium-rich media. *J. Physiol. London 155*, 470–489.

Hamill, O.P., Marty, A., Neher, E., Sakmann, B., and Sigworth, F.J. (1981) Improved patch-clamp techniques for high-resolution current recording from cells and cell-free membrane patches. *Pflugers Arch. 391*, 85–100.

Hermann, A. and Gorman, A.L.F. (1979) External and internal effects of tetraethylammonium on voltage-dependent and Ca-dependent K^+ current components in molluscan pacemaker neurons. *Neurosci. Lett. 12*, 87–92.

Heyer, C.B. and Lux, H.D. (1976) Control of the delayed outward potassium currents in bursting pacemaker neurones of snail *Helix pomatia. J. Physiol. London 262*, 349–382.

Hodgkin, A.L. and Huxley, A.F. (1952) A quantitative description of membrane current and its application to conduction and excitation in nerve. *J. Physiol. London 117*, 500–544.

Hodgkin, A.L., Huxley, A.F., and Katz, B. (1952) Measurement of current-voltage relations in the membrane of the giant axon of *Loligo. J. Physiol. London 116*, 424–448.

Kandel, E.R. (1976) *Cellular Basis of Behavior*. Freeman Press, San Francisco.

Kass, R.S., Tsien, R.S., and Weingart, R. (1978) Ionic basis of transient inward current induced by strophanthidin in cardiac purkinje fibres. *J. Physiol. London 281*, 209–226.

Klein, M., Camardo, J., and Kandel, E.R. (1982) Serotonin modulates a specific potassium current in the sensory neurons that show presynaptic facilitation in *Aplysia. Proc. Natl. Acad. Sci. USA 79*, 5713–5717.

Kostyuk, P.G. and Krishtal, O.A. (1977) Effects of calcium and calcium-chelating agents on the inward and outward current in the membrane of the mollusc neurones. *J. Physiol. London 270*, 569–580.

Kostyuk, P.G., Krishtal, O.A., and Doroshenko, P.A. (1974) Calcium currents in snail neurones. I. Identification of calcium current. *Pflugers Arch. 348*, 83–93.

Kostyuk, P.G., Krishtal, O.A., and Shakhovalov, Y.A. (1977) Separation of sodium and calcium currents in the somatic membrane of mollusk neurones. *J. Physiol. London 270*, 545–568.

Kramer, R.H. and Zucker, R.S. (1985a) Calcium-dependent inward current in *Aplysia* bursting pace-maker neurones. *J. Physiol. London 362*, 107–130.

Kramer, R.H. and Zucker, R.S. (1985b) Calcium-induced inactivation of calcium current causes the inter-burst hyperpolarization of *Aplysia* bursting neurones. *J. Physiol. London 362*, 131–160.

Lee, K.S., Akaike, N., and Brown, A.M. (1978) Properties of internally perfused, voltage-clamped, isolated nerve cell bodies. *J. Gen. Physiol. 71*, 489–507.

Lux, H.D. and Heyer, C.B. (1977) An aequorin study of a facilitating calcium current in bursting pacemaker neurons of *Helix. Neuroscience 2*, 585–592.

Meech, R.W. (1978) Calcium-dependent potassium activation in nervous tissues. *Ann. Rev. Biophys. Bioeng. 7*, 1–18.

Meech, R.W. and Standen, N.B. (1975) Potassium activation in *Helix aspersa* neurones under voltage clamp; a component mediated by calcium influx. *J. Physiol. London 249*, 211–239.

Miller, C. (1983) Integral membrane channels: Studies in model membranes. *Physiol. Revs. 63*, 1209–1242.

Miller, C., Moczydlowski, E., Latorre, R., and Phillips, M. (1985) Charybdotoxin, a protein inhibitor of single Ca^{2+}-activated K^+ channels from mammalian skeletal muscle. *Nature 313*, 316–318.

Neher, E. (1971) Two fast transient current components during voltage clamp on snail neurons. *J. Gen. Physiol. 58*, 36–53.

Neher, E. and Lux, H.D. (1969) Voltage clamp on *Helix pomatia* neuronal membrane: Current measurement over limited area of the soma surface. *Pflugers Arch. 311*, 272–277.

Neher, E. and Lux, H.D. (1972) Differential action of TEA^+ on two K^+ current components of a molluscan neurone. *Pflugers Arch. 336*, 87–100.

Partridge, L.D. and Stevens, C.F. (1976) A mechanism for spike frequency adaptation. *J. Physiol. London 256*, 315–332.

Partridge, L.D., Thompson, S.H., Smith, S.J., and Connor, J.A. (1979) Current-voltage relationships of repetitively firing neurons. *Brain Res. 164*, 69–79.

Reuter, H. (1983) Calcium channel modulation by neurotransmitters, enzymes and drugs. *Nature 301*, 569–574.

Standen, N.B. (1974) Properties of a calcium channel in snail neurones. *Nature 250*, 340–342.

Standen, N.B. (1975) Voltage-clamp studies of the calcium inward current in an identified snail neurone: Comparison with the sodium inward current. *J. Physiol. London 249*, 253–268.

Thomas, M.V. and Gorman, A.L.F. (1977) Internal calcium changes in a bursting pacemaker neuron measured with arsenazo III. *Science 196*, 531–533.

Thompson, S.H. (1977) Three pharmacologically distinct potassium channels in molluscan neurones. *J. Physiol. London 265*, 465–488.

Thompson, S.H. and Smith, S.J. (1976) Depolarizing afterpotentials and burst production in molluscan pacemaker neurons. *J. Neurophysiol. 39*, 153–161.

Tillotson, D. (1979) Inactivation of Ca conductance dependent on entry of Ca ions in molluscan neurons. *Proc. Natl. Acad. Sci. USA 76*, 1497–1500.

Tsien, R.W. (1983) Calcium channels in excitable cell membranes. *Ann. Rev. Physiol. 45*, 341–358.

Wilson, W.A. and Wachtel, H. (1974) Negative resistance characteristic essential for the maintenance of slow oscillations in bursting neurons. *Science 186*, 932–934.

Wilson, W.A. and Wachtel, H. (1978) Prolonged inhibition in burst firing neurons: Synaptic inactivation of the slow regenerative inward current. *Science 202*, 722–775.

3

How Ion Channel Proteins Work

CHRISTOPHER MILLER

Membrane proteins of a single class—the ion channels— underlie all electrical excitation phenomena. The ion currents responsible for voltage changes in electrically active cells are mediated by these proteins and, as far as we know, by these proteins alone. Although ion channels were originally considered to be highly specialized transport systems for the highly specialized cells involved in electrical signaling, it is now clear that they are ubiquitous, being found in prokaryotes, plants, intracellular organelles, and nonexcitable tissues such as epithelia, erythrocytes, and exocrine glands.

The purpose of this chapter is to outline the fundamental mechanisms of operation of ion channel proteins, the most basic functional elements of the integrated nervous sytem. Inasmuch as the brain—or even a ganglion—is a computer, the ion channels are the transistors. However, unlike transistors with their fixed, hard-wired properties, ion channels are cellular macromolecules and as such are subject to regulation. On a priori grounds alone, therefore, we may safely expect that in many cases channels will be found to have their basic properties modulated by biochemical events occurring in the cell in response to external signals. Indeed, the contributions to this volume illustrate numerous examples of modulation of channel proteins involved in electrical excitation phenomena. The present summary of basic channel mechanisms will therefore be slanted toward a discussion of how biochemical modulation of channel proteins may lead to changes in channel behavior.

HOW WE KNOW CHANNELS ARE CHANNELS

The defining characteristic of an ion channel is the formation of a *hydrophilic pore* right through the heart of the protein, and hence across the membrane the protein spans. This definition is by now so commonplace that one easily forgets how amazing it is that we can make the definition at all. Remember that in no case has the structure of an integral membrane channel protein been determined; indeed, of the scores of ion channel proteins known to exist, only three—the nicotinic acetylcholine receptor, the excitable membrane sodium channel, and a variety of porins from bacterial or mitochondrial outer membranes—have been subjected to intense biochemical investigation. How, then, is it possible for us to define this class of proteins in terms of their structures?

The answer to this question is that there are certain unique properties that channels display in their observed behavior, properties which can be rationalized only in terms of an underlying pore structure. What are these properties? How does one know that channels are channels? The idea that ionic currents in nerve membranes are in fact mediated by porelike structures was initially suggested by Hodgkin and Keynes (1955) and was generally accepted by the time of Armstrong's (1975) review of this issue. In the following sections the four independent lines of evidence that, taken together, account for the acceptance of this picture of channel protein structure in the absence of any direct demonstration are discussed..

High Unitary Transport Rates

Of the many results arising from techniques for detecting the properties of single ion channels in neurons (Katz & Miledi, 1970; Anderson & Stevens, 1973; Hamill et al., 1981), one of the most important is the realization that channel-mediated ion transport rates are very high. The unitary current through an open channel, now so familiar in the torrent of single channel studies during the past decade, is really a measure of the turnover number of the transport mechanism, the number of ions processed per second by the channel. Single channel currents are typically in the range of 1 to 20 pA, equivalent to unitary transport rates of 0.6 to 12×10^7 ions per second. These rates are enormous compared with the typical turnover rates for other types of membrane transport proteins or for enzymes and with rates theoretically expected for a simple "carrier" mechanism.

Let us consider, first, a hypothetical ferryboat mechanism, in which a low-molecular-weight molecule binds the ion, diffuses across the membrane, and releases it to the other side, as with classic ionophores such as valinomycin. How rapidly might we expect such a transporter to operate? We can get a rough idea of the expected turnover rate by considering how long it would take for this complex to diffuse across a membrane. For simple diffusion, the average (actually, the root mean square) distance, $<x>$, traveled by a molecule diffusing for a given time, t, is

$$<x> = [2Dt]^{1/2}, \tag{1}$$

where D is the diffusion coefficient. Thus, we can calculate the time it would take this carrier complex to diffuse across the 5-nm width of a typical membrane, since the diffusion coefficient, in the transverse direction, cannot be larger than the lateral diffusion coefficient of a typical phospholipid (which must get out of the way of the carrier), 10^{-8} cm^2 sec. Plugging in these numbers, we find that, on the average, it takes the carrier complex at least 12 μsec to diffuse across the membrane. Therefore, a single such carrier cannot possibly shuttle more than 10^5 ions per second; the maximum conceivable "single-carrier" turnover number is 100 to 1000 times lower than the values observed for single channels.

If a ferryboat mechanism seems a straw man set up only to be discredited, let us consider a more realistic alternative mode of ion transport by an integral membrane protein. No theoretical consideration is appropriate here, but there is an ample body of precedent to convince us that channel-mediated transport rates are unusually high. The range of turnover rates for enzymes and for membrane transporters distinct from channels is wide, but no such system displays anything as high as channel-mediated transport rates. Carbonic anhydrase and acetylcholine esterase are among the fastest enzymes known (and were designed by evolution specifically to be very fast), with maximum turnover rates of 10^5 turnovers per second. Typical rates for ion pumps such as the sodium/potassium adenosintriphosphatase (ATPase) and calcium ATPase are in the order of 100 ions moved per second, and the fastest non-channel transporter known, the band-3 Cl^- shuttle of erythrocytes, moves about 10^4 Cl^- ions per second at 25° (Knauf, 1979). Thus, we see that an empirical upper limit of about 10^5 per second appears to constrain the turnover rates of known membrane transporters other than channels.

What is different about enzymes, pump or shuttle-type transporters, and molecular ferryboats that lead to turnover rates so much lower than those of channels? It is simply that all of these alternative mechanisms require grosser motions involving the movements of much more massive groups for each turnover than do ion channels. With the ferryboat mechanism, large lipid molecules must get out of the way for the carrier to hop into a vacancy on its way across the membrane; with enzymes and transporters, concerted movements of whole protein domains must occur stoichiometrically with the processing of each substrate or the movement of each ion. Such large motions will have to surmount much larger energy barriers than will the diffusion of ions through a water-filled pore of fixed structure.

The very high channel turnover rate is the very property that allows us to detect single channels at all. Present recording techniques are inadequate to permit the direct observation of a "single carrier" current, which would be at most 0.001 pA. The uniquely high turnover rates for ion channels, therefore, provide the single most important piece of evidence that these proteins do form porelike structures; if the unitary current can be observed directly, in a patch recording, for example, then it must be mediated by a pore structure of some kind.

Low Temperature Coefficients

In the very earliest days of modern electrophysiology, Hodgkin, Huxley, and Katz (1952) noted that the ionic currents involved in the squid axon action potential are unusually insensitive to temperature. The "Q_{10}" temperature coefficient for both sodium and potassium currents was found to be only 1.2 to 1.4, exactly the same value as for unrestricted diffusion in aqueous solution, and equivalent to an enthalpic barrier for movement of only about 5 kcal/mol. This is a general property of ion currents flowing through conducting channels (Parsegian, 1969; Hille, 1984). This simple observation argues that the ion movements mediated by such proteins cannot involve any large changes of protein conformation, the energy barriers for which would be expected to be much higher than 5 kcal/mol; on the other hand, a mechanism akin to aqueouslike diffusion is much more naturally suggested, in which the protein structure is essentially fixed, while the ion moves by breaking and making weak electrostatic interactions with water and protein liganding groups.

Ion-Ion Flux Coupling

In some of the first attempts to measure radioactive fluxes through ion channels, Hodgkin and Keynes (1955) argued that potassium fluxes through delayed rectifier potassium channels of squid axon involve diffusion through a pore. They observed several types of "long-pore" effects which suggested that potassium ions move in a single file through the transporter. The key observation was based on the measurement of how the "flux ratio"—the ratio of the unidirectional inward and outward fluxes—varies with applied voltage. Ussing (1949) had shown that such a measurement provides information about the valence of the transported species for passive ion transporters, independent of the specific mechanism of transport. In the squid axon potassium channel, it was found (Hodgkin & Keynes, 1955; Begenisich & DeWeer, 1980) that the flux ratio varies with voltage as if potassium were a species of valence $+2$ to $+3$! The interpretation was given that two or three potassium ions occupy a pore and cannot pass one another; for a potassium ion to transverse the membrane, it must "push" one or two other potassium ions ahead of it. The inward rectifier of muscle is now known to display this flux coupling as well. Such ion-ion flux coupling could conceivably be explained by a carrier mechanism, in which two or three potassium ions must simultaneously bind to a carrier before transport can take place. When taken in combination with the known high unitary transport rates, however, this long-pore effect strengthens the accepted view of channel structure. Not all channels will display this behavior, only those in which multiple ions can reside simultaneously in a region of restricted diffusion.

Ion-Water Flux Coupling

The open pores of ion channels contain water in addition to ions. For sufficiently narrow pores (<0.5 nm in diameter), the water molecules and ions do not have room to pass one another and are forced to position themselves in single file. For any channel with such single-filing regions, a remarkable phenomenon will be observed—ion-water flux coupling. When a potassium-selective channel is observed, for instance, in a membrane separating two identical solutions of a potassium salt, normally no current flows through the channel at zero voltage: there is no thermodymanic driving force on the potassium ion. However, if the water activity on one side of the membrane is lowered—for instance, by adding a nonelectrolyte such as urea—then potassium will flow through the channel at zero voltage, *even though there is no thermodynamic gradient for* potassium. An example of such an effect is shown in Figure 3.1, with a potassium channel from sarcoplasmic reticulum. The reason for this "uphill" potassium current is that *water* flows through the channel down its thermodynamic gradient, and since water and potassium lie in single file within the channel, potassium is dragged through as well. A voltage may be applied to reduce the potassium current to zero, and from the value of this voltage (the "streaming potential"), the number of water molecules constrained to line up in single file with a potassium ion may be determined (Rosenberg & Finkelstein, 1978).

One integral membrane channel—the potassium channel of sarcoplasmic reticulum (SR)—has been subjected to his sort of analysis (Miller, 1982) in which it was

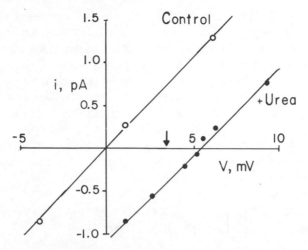

Fig. 3.1. Ion-water flux coupling in a potassium channel. The single channel current voltage curve is shown for the SR potassium channel inserted into planar bilayer membranes. The control curve refers to symmetrical solutions of 250 mM potassium. The curve labeled " +Urea" represents the same aqueous conditions, except that 1.9-molal urea was added to one side of the membrane to lower the activity of water. (From Miller, 1982.)

found that at most only two water molecules and a potassium ion share a single-filing region. That the method actually works (as it must, since it is based on a purely thermodynamic effect) was shown earlier with a model peptide channel of known structure, gramicidin A (Rosenberg & Finkelstein, 1978); here, the finding of about nine water molecules in single file agrees very well with the known length of the channel, 2.6 nm. In the absence of structural information, the observation of ion-water flux coupling is good evidence for the existence of a pore. Carrier mechanism, too, could predict such coupling (e.g., if the ion were shuttled in a hydrated form), but in combination with the high unitary flux rates, it further confirms the pore model. Virtually all channels with high ionic selectivity are expected to display this effect, which is easily detected with modern single channel methods.

These four lines of argument have been reviewed to show that ion channels constitute a unique class of transport proteins and that there is very good reason to view the ion conduction process as occurring through a water-filled pore of essentially fixed structure. The movement of each ion does not require the individual attention of the protein through a cycle of conformational changes, as with enzymes, pumps, and other types of transporters. The abundance of examples of "artificial" channels further confirms this picture. The existence of gramicidin A is particularly pertinent; this peptide antibiotic of known pore structure has been studied in great depth (Finkelstein & Andersen, 1981) and shows exactly the same sorts of behavior as integral membrane channels of excitable cells—high unitary transport rates, low temperature coefficients, and flux coupling with water and other ions.

Ion channel proteins in the nervous system perform two fundamental tasks. First, they must be able to switch rapidly between conducting and nonconducting states in response to external signals such as changes in voltage or binding of ligands. Second, when in its conducting state, an ion channel must be able to discriminate among the plethora of small inorganic ions with which it is presented, allowing the rapid passage of only one or a few species and excluding all others. These two tasks—rapid gating and ionic selectivity—are essential to the proper functioning of the nerve cell. All neuronal electrical behaviors, from the dedicated axonal propagation of the motor neuron to the modulatable patterns of bursting pacemakers, are ultimately traceable to the ion conduction and gating characteristics of each cell's ensemble of channels. In the following sections, current views of the ion conduction and gating processes of ion channels will be discussed, so that we are in a position to speculate on how biochemical signals may affect these fundamental processes.

BASIC MECHANISM OF ION CONDUCTION

It is a truth universally acknowledged that studies of kinetic processes tell us very little about structure and mechanism of transport proteins. For example, the enormous amount of literature on the kinetics of ion transport and ATPase reactions in ion pumps has given us no idea of what these proteins actually "look like" on the molecular level. The failure to achieve a molecular picture of these types of transport proteins is a result of a single characteristic of the reactions they catalyze: complexity. Ion pumping, substrate cotransport, and solute "carrier" processes are very complicated, each requiring the intimate participation of the transport protein in a *stoichiometric cycle* of substrate binding, transport, and release; every transporter of this kind must carry its own specific set of gears, springs, dashpots, and ratchets uniquely designed and assembled for the task at hand.

But this is not true of ion channels. These proteins catalyze what is by far the simplest type of solute transport: ion *diffusion* through a hydrophilic pore of basically fixed structure. The protein need not give its undivided attention to each ion moving through. It is because of this simplicity of the underlying ion transport mechanism that kinetic analysis of ion conduction through channels has led to structural pictures of the channel proteins. The intention of this section is to outline our understanding of ion conduction through channels, with an emphasis on the question of how channel proteins interact with and select small inorganic ions.

The Free Energy Profile

It is easy to picture a channel as an aqueous hole through the membrane, but this picture can be a little misleading, because our mental images tend to carry with them our own experience of the macroscopic world. It is important to avoid thinking of the conduction pathway of a neuronal channel as merely a plug of aqueous electrolyte solution; such an analogy contains two major errors, at least from the point of view of an ion. First, an ion in dilute aqueous solution experiences only the average, smeared-out forces due to solvation by water and the average "ion cloud" around it; an individual ion from its own vantage point is the only thing in the universe, being surrounded by a wholly isotropic aqueous medium, extending infinitely in all directions. This is not the case of an ion inside a channel protein. Here, the ion and its surrounding water molecules are confined in a small space; even for the quite unselective acetylcholine receptor channel, the pore is about 0.7 nm in diameter along much of its length (Horn & Stevens, 1980). Thus, a potassium ion (0.27 nm in diameter) in the middle of this pore can move only slightly more than 0.2 nm of space to either side (about the size of a single water molecule) before encountering the proteinaceous channel wall. Thus, the "solvent" seen by this ion is quite unlike water in aqueous solution. Not only is the ion's environment very nonisotropic, but a large part of its "solvent" is not water at all but rather protein residues. Even when not directly in contact with the channel wall, the ion is often only a single water molecule's distance from it. Such water in the first layer of hydration of an ion has a dielectric constant lower than the value of 80 in bulk water. Because of this, the forces of the protein groups are much less strongly shielded from an ion in the channel than we might expect if we imagined the pore as a plug of normal electrolyte solution. In other words, an ion inside the confines of a channel's conduction pathway will experience strong forces from its immediate surroundings; because these surroundings change along the conduction pathway, according to the local protein structure, *an ion moving through a channel experiences a wildly varying set of forces.* In this sense, the ion does not have a solvent at all but rather a solvation structure that varies with its position within the channel. This is very different from the situation in a region of simple aqueous electrolyte.

The second error resulting from picturing the channel as simply a plug of solution resides in our intuitive notions of electroneutrality. In our macroscopic image, a plug of electrolyte solution is electrically neutral, with equal numbers of anions and cations. But because the distances involved in channel structures are small—on the order of nanometers—electroneutrality does not hold here. A cation, for instance, can enter a channel protein and traverse it without requiring the movement of a counterion. But this means that ions inside channels will set up and experience large electric fields in their vicinity, that they will exert forces on other ions inside of, or about to enter, the pore structure. In other words, inside channels, *ions do not move independently of one another*.

What does all this mean? First, it means that we must not consider a channel as a plug of normal water. More specifically, it means that we must picture the conduction pathway of a channel something like the active site of an enzyme. To see this, let us refer to Figure 3.2, which presents a cartoon of a hypothetical pore structure, with various protein groups. This pore is broken into several regions for reference, so that we can consider the forces on a cation in each region. We set the energy level of the ion in the external aqueous solution equal to zero. In region 1, the ion enters the pore and in this more restricted space must lose some of its normal water of hydration while keeping its primary hydration shell. In general, the ion will have to overcome a repulsive force here since, in exchanging its old solvent (water) for the new (water and protein), it is entering a region of somewhat lower dielectric constant. The energy (actually molar Gibbs free energy) of the ion increases. Once inside the channel, however, having taken on this new "solvent," the ion may feel specific interactions as a result of the protein structure. In region 2, for example, two negatively charged groups lie in proximity on one side of the channel wall; the cation

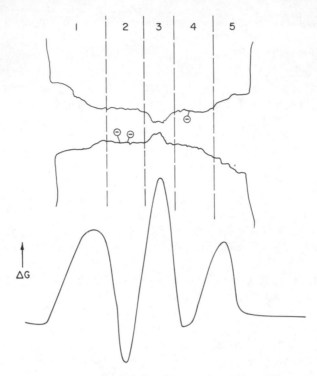

Fig. 3.2. An energetic journey through a pore. A hypothetical pore structure is drawn and broken into five regions, as described in the text. The free energy experienced by a cation moving through this structure is illustrated below the cartoon.

can approach this "chelating" group while remaining hydrated with water on its back side. This is a favorable interaction, with the ion in a place where it likes to be inside the pore. It is an energy well.

Further along, in region 3, the channel narrows drastically; it is here that the ion must lose nearly all its water to squeeze through. If this narrow region were not built out of very polar groups, the ion would simply never enter it: dehydrating the ion in its immediate vicinity would cost too much energy without paying back energy by resolvation with polar groups. Therefore, this narrow "selectivity filter" is drawn as containing carbonyl groups as well as a carboxylate, so that the ion will be able to get through this inherently unfavorable place. The energy here is still somewhat unfavorable in balance although not impossibly so. As the ion leaves the selectivity constriction and enters region 4, it can again become hydrated and also interact with a polar group, as shown, residing at a favorable place in the channel. Finally, the ion leaves the channel, overcoming an electrostatic barrier on the way out (region 5) similar to the one it felt on the way in, and regains its fully hydrated state in aqueous solution.

The ion has negotiated a series of energy peaks (unfavorable transition states) and wells (favorable binding sites) in its journey along the diffusion pathway. The rate of "hopping" from one energy well to the next is controlled by the height of the barrier over which the ion must jump: as the barrier height increases, the rate decreases. A quantitative theory that accounts for these rates in terms of the "free energy profile" of the pore structure is Eyring rate theory (Hille, 1975).

Ion Occupancy and the Single Ion Channel

In the preceding example, we considered a channel with two "binding sites" within the same pore. Can both of these sites be occupied simultaneously? To answer this, we need to consider what the free energy profile looks like to a second ion about to enter the pore already occupied by one ion. Because of the lack of requirement for electroneutrality, it is clear that the *second* ion sees a much different free energy profile than the first, simply because of the repulsive electrostatic forces exerted by the occupant ion on the ion aspiring to enter. The second ion will see a more unfavorable (higher energy) profile than did the first. Indeed, if the diffusion pathway is short, so that the aspirant ion is physically near the occupant ion, the repulsive forces will be so strong that the second ion cannot enter as long as the channel is occupied. In this case, ion-ion interactions inside the pore have established a "single ion rule"— the pore can be unoccupied or occupied by one ion but never by more than one even though it contains two binding sites.

This is an important case to consider because it leads to simple and intuitively understandable behavior for the conduction of ions. It is also important because a number of well-studied channels are observed to behave in this way. The single ion channel has been treated in detail in several places (Lauger, 1973; Hille, 1975; Coronado et al., 1980), and this exposition is meant only to illustrate qualitatively the properties of this system. The most important characteristic of the single ion channel is that it behaves as a Michaelis-Menten enzyme with respect to the ion concentration. Let us assume that we can measure the current through the channel with identical salt solutions on both sides of the membrane and that only one type of ion, say potassium, is permeant. It can then be shown that the channel conductance, γ (extrapolated to zero voltage), saturates with ion concentration according to a simple rectangular hyperbola:

$$\frac{\gamma}{\gamma^{\max}} = \frac{c/K_m}{[1 + c/K_m]}, \tag{2}$$

where c and K_m are the ion concentration and the apparent dissociation constant, and $\gamma^{\max}$ is the maximum conductance at very high ion concentration. As shown in Figure 3.3, several channels for which the experiment has been done actually do follow such a prediction. It is important to realize that a plug of aqueous solution would never behave in this way!

How can we interpret behavior like this? Clearly, some kind of change in rate-determining step, or saturation, is occurring; in fact, this is a direct consequence of the single ion rule for the channel. At low ion concentration, the channel is usually unoccupied, and so the current through it is low and proportional to the fraction of time an ion actually resides within the channel. As concentration increases in this

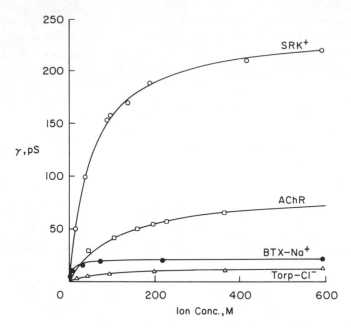

Fig. 3.3. Saturation of single ion channels. Saturation curves of several ion channels are presented, each being fit with a rectangular hyperbola. The data are taken from Coronado et al. (1980) for the SR potassium channel (potassium as the permeant ion), from Horn and Patlak (1980) for the acetylcholine receptor (sodium), from White and Miller (1981) for the Torpedo chloride channel (chloride), and from Moczydlowski et al. (1984) for the batracho-toxin-activated sodium channel (sodium).

low range, the occupancy, and hence the conductance, increases linearly. But eventually the concentration gets so high that the channel is occupied by an ion almost all the time. Under these conditions, the rate of ions getting through the channel is limited by the rate at which the ion can leave the channel, thus making room for the next ion to enter. The maximum conductance is thus a measure of the exit rate from the channel, whereas the initial slope of the curve of Figure 3.3, γ^{max}/K_m, measures the second-order rate constant of ion entry into the channel. When these measurements are extrapolated to zero voltage (and most of the time real measurements made at 30 mV or lower are good approximations), the "Michaelis constant," K_m, is a measure of the true dissociation constant of the ion from the channel's binding sites (Hille, 1975).

How are measurable conduction parameters related to the free energy profile? For a single ion channel, the correspondence is made easily. The maximum conductance is related to the highest barrier within the channel, that is, the energy difference between the highest peak and deepest well. The initial slope of Figure 3.3, the "entry rate," refers to the extreme condition in which the ion concentration is so low that the slowest, or rate-limiting, step is a jump from the aqueous solution over the highest energy peak; thus, γ^{max}/K_m is related only to the energy of the highest peak (referred to the external solution). The half-saturation constant K_m is related only to the depths of the wells. Thus, by analyzing the conductance-concentration relation, we can get a rough idea of a channel's free energy profile, whether it has relatively deep wells or high peaks.

Biochemists encountering saturation curves for channels as in Figure 3.3 are often struck by the seemingly low affinities of the conducting ions for the channels. Values of K_m are typically in the range of 10 to 100 mM, whereas enzymes often attain maximum rates in the micromolar range of substrate concentrations. A biochemist might ask why channels display such very low affinities for their ion substrates. There is a very simple reason for this: channels bind their substrates 1000-fold less tightly than enzymes do because channels operate at turnover rates 1000-fold higher than those of enzymes, as we have seen. For a channel to be half saturated at $1\mu M$, for instance, the conducting ion would get stuck in a deep energy well of about 7 kcal/mol; the maximum conductance of the channel in such a case would be 1000-fold smaller than a "typical" channel conductance. In other words, because tight binding implies low maximal rates, channels must bind their conducting ions loosely.

The point of this qualitative discussion is to establish that a channel's free energy profile derived from conduction studies is not a mere plaything of biophysicists but carries real meaning in terms of the underlying structure of the channel. Although conduction studies do not allow us to deduce details of the pore structure, they can give us a gross picture of it. This is much easier to do for single ion channels, but even with multiple ion channels such free energy profiles can be derived (Hille & Schwarz, 1978; Hess & Tsien, 1984).

Selectivity Regions in Ion Channels

In the hypothetical channel of Figure 3.2, we imagined that at a critical point, the pore narrows and thus creates a region of high energy for a permeating ion. It is reasonable to assume that the narrowest point in the channel will be the most unfavorable place for the ion, since ionic dehydration will be most severe here. Therefore, in such a view, this "selectivity filter" is where the channel most effectively discriminates among similar ions. Hille (1971, 1973, 1975) pioneered the study of ionic conduction processes and showed that channel selectivity filters can actually be sized. By measuring the permeabilities of a large number of poorly permeant small organic cations, Hille (1971) showed that the narrowest place in the axonal sodium channel is a hole of 0.3 × 0.5 nm, just large enough for a sodium ion and a water molecule to fit simultaneously but too small to accommodate a potassium ion and water molecule. Thus, potassium, which does permeate the channel at a low rate, can fit through sterically, but to do so it must shed more of its water than sodium, as shown in Figure 3.4. Thus, in this case, the ionic selectivity is determined by the energetics of dehydration of these small cations.

Sodium ions are smaller than potassium ions in naked size. How can we explain the selectivity *against* sodium by potassium channels of nerve? Again, Hille (1973), by sizing the selectivity of the delayed rectifier potassium channel of nerve, provided a satisfying solution to this puzzle. He found that the potassium channel, which is

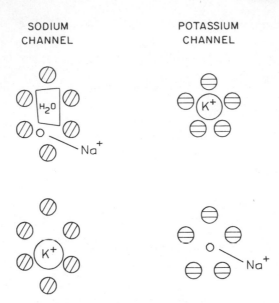

Fig. 3.4. Selectivity filters of sodium and potasssium channels. These cartoons illustrate Hille's (1975) picture of the exclusion of sodium from potassium channels and the exclusion of potassium from sodium channels. The sizes of the selectivity filters are based on Hille (1975), and the sodium and potassium ions are placed in the most favorable interaction configuration for each.

very selective for potassium, with sodium having no measurable permeability at all, has a smaller constriction, 0.3×0.3 nm, than does the sodium channel (see Figure 3.4). This is only slightly larger than the unhydrated diameter of the potassium ion, and it is clear that to go through this hole potassium must shed all the water around its periphery in exchange for "solvation" by liganding groups on the proteins. Why does sodium not do the same thing? It certainly could fit through the potassium channel selectivity filter on steric grounds, and yet it does not permeate measurably. The reason for the failure of sodium to pass this selectivity region is very simple: the energy it has to pay in shedding its water is not sufficiently paid back by liganding to the selectivity filter, because the naked sodium ion is too small, 0.08 nm smaller in diameter than potassium. Thus, if sodium were positioned in the center of the selectivity target, there would be about 0.04 nm of empty space on all sides, space which could easily add 10 kcal/mol of unfavorable electrostatic energy to the interaction of the sodium ion with this site (Armstrong, 1975a). In other words, for a highly dehydrated ion to pass a selectivity constriction, it must make a very tight fit with the liganding groups there. It also follows from this argument that the selectivity filter of the potassium channel is rigid; if it had much conformational freedom or floppiness, it would be able to contract around the sodium ion, "solvate" it well, and allow permeation.

Figure 3.5 illustrates the dimensions of the selectivity filters of those channels that have been sized to date. The results make sense: the smallest hole (in the delayed

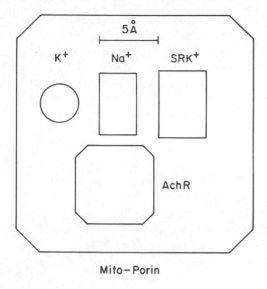

Fig. 3.5. A compendium of known channel cross sections. Scale drawings of the narrowest cross sections of five ion channels for which the determination has been made: sodium and potassium channels of frog node of Ranvier, the nicotinic acetylcholine receptor, the potassium channel of sarcoplasmic reticulum, and mitochondrial portin.

rectifier potassium channel) is the most selective, and the largest hole (in mitochondrial porin) is the least.

GATING PROCESSES

Until now, we have been discussing the process of ions diffusing through open channels. The process of opening and closing the channel, often called "gating," is an equally important aspect of ion channel function. For the same reasons that we can use ionic conduction studies to reveal molecular structure, it is nearly impossible to make structural conclusions from channel gating studies. The gating process is a direct expression of conformational changes within the channel protein, and therefore is complicated, with no underlying simplicity to guide us in our interpretation of experimental results. The phenomena here ultimately rely on the architechture of the particular protein under study. Thus, the very few generalizations we can make about gating are quite unhelpful in yielding molecular detail. Nevertheless, it is worthwhile to summarize briefly those aspects of gating processes that we can easily imagine to be modulatable.

In its essence, the gating of an ion channel can be best viewed in terms of a simple conformational equilibrium process in which two distinguishable states of the protein exist:

$$\text{Closed} \rightleftharpoons \text{Open} \tag{3}$$

(Of course, most if not all channels operate in more complicated ways, with multiple open and closed states, but a discussion of schemes more complicated than scheme 3 will add no enlightenment here). Underlying such a scheme is molecular chaos, and the advent of single channel recording techniques has allowed us to observe this chaos directly. When we say that some external variable "causes" a channel to open, we really mean, and really observe at the single channel level, that application of this variable *biases* the statistics of opening—that is, it makes the free energy of the open state relatively more favorable with respect to the closed state. This can be done by either stabilizing the open state or destabilizing the closed state; only the energy difference matters.

Voltage-Dependent Channels

Proteins residing in membranes are unique in that they live out their lives in the presence of intense electric fields. A typical excitable membrane at rest maintains an electric field in the order of 10 million V/m. This is an enormous value, close to the dielectric breakdown point, where electrostatic forces literally rip molecules apart; the sparks from a van de Graaff generator to a grounded lead (e.g., one's finger held a meter away) attest to the dielectric breakdown and resulting ionization of gas molecules in air. While *all* membrane proteins have had to evolve to survive this intense external force, many ion channels of excitable membranes have evolved to exploit it. Voltage-dependent channels are simply proteins built so that, when the conformational change leading to channel opening occurs, fixed charged groups on the protein move transversely to the membrane surface so as to move net charge in the membrane field. Electric charge moving in a voltage gradient gives rise to a change in energy. Therefore, if charge moves when the protein changes shape upon opening, an electrostatic energy is added to all the chemical energies involved in protein structure changes in reaction 3. The equilibrium can be thus biased toward opening or closing just by changing the electric field within the membrane, that is, changing the applied voltage. In this way, membrane depolarization "causes" potassium channels, for instance, to open. This conclusion is general: an applied electric field will bias any reaction in which charge moves when the reaction proceeds.

Ligand-Gated Channels

Again, not much can be said about ligand-gated channels in general. Many channels are opened by the binding of a ligand, such as a neurotransmitter. One question that may be worth discussing concerns how such a thing can happen: how can the binding of a ligand stabilize the open state, say, of a channel protein?

A principle that is repeatedly confirmed in biochemistry is that protein conformational changes may be driven directly by the change in energy that occurs upon binding of a ligand. Part of the binding energy of a ligand with an inherently high affinity for a site may be used to "pay" for an inherently unfavorable conformational change. As a result, the observed affinity of the ligand is much lower than its inherent affinity for the site (Jencks, 1975). In other words, if the binding of the ligand could be uncoupled from the protein's change in structure, it would bind much more strongly than under normal conditions. This effect may operate in the opening and desensitization of the acetylcholine receptor. The observed affinity of acetylcholine in opening the channel is low: dissociation constants for the activated state in the order of 0.1 to 1 mM are found (Neubig et al., 1979; Aoshima et al., 1981). Upon prolonged exposure to agonist, however, the channel desensitizes, that is, it closes again and becomes locked into an agonist-binding state from which it can return only slowly. The dissociation constant of acetylcholine for this state is in the nanomolar range. It is as though the full, inherent affinity of the agonist for its site is expressed, since the twisting and turning of the protein necessary to open the channel does not have to be paid for.

MODULATION OF BASIC CHANNEL MECHANISMS

After a discussion of basic mechanisms of channel behavior, it would be a pleasant exercise to consider examples of know channel modulation, identifying the basic mechanism that is modified in each case. Unfortunately, this is impossible to do. Although much is known phenomenologically about the modulation of ionic currents, in no case has a mechanistic picture of a modulatory change in a channel's behavior been achieved. Successes of this kind, however, may be forthcoming in the near future, as the patch-recording method is brought increasingly to bear on modulated channels.

Calcium-Activated Potassium Channel

One case that may be considered an example of channel modulation in which some mechanistic information is available is the high-conductance calcium-activated potassium channel from rat skeletal muscle (Moczydlowski & Latorre, 1983). First observed in adrenal chromaffin cells (Marty, 1981), this channel is now known to be very widespread, being found in nonexcitable as well as excitable tissues (Latorre & Miller, 1983). Latorre and colleagues (1982) succeeded in reconstituting the calcium-activated potassium channel from rat muscle in planar lipid bilayers, where its properties are similar to those observed in its native membrane (Barrett et al., 1982). This

Fig. 3.6. Control of calcium-dependent potassium channel opening by voltage and calcium. Tracings of single calcium-dependent potassium channel fluctuations illustrating the activation by both calcium and depolarization. The data are taken from Moczydlowski and Latorre (1983) for rat muscle channels inserted in planar bilayer membranes.

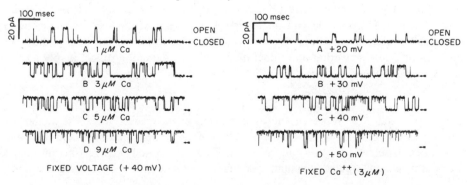

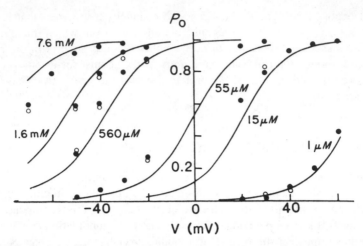

Fig. 3.7. Calcium-dependent potassium channel opening probability: effects of voltage and calcium. Data from Moczydlowski and Latorre (1983) showing the activation of the calcium-dependent potassium channel in planar bilayer membranes as influenced by both voltage and calcium concentration. The abscissa (P_o) shows the probability of the channel being open as a function of voltage (V), at the indicated calcium concentrations between 1 μM and 7.6 mM. The solid curves are drawn according to scheme 4 in the text.

channel, as Figure 3.6 shows, is activated by both voltage and cytoplasmic calcium. It thus appears to be both voltage gated and ligand gated. In Figure 3.7, the combined effects of voltage and calcium on the equilibrium probability of opening are shown; the channel opens with depolarization (e-fold per 12 mV at all calcium concentrations), and calcium simply shifts these curves to the left along the voltage axis. The most straightforward reading of these results would be to say that the channel has an inherently voltage-dependent gating mechanism involving charge movement on the protein and that calcium acts by enhancing the chemical stability of the open state with respect to the closed state. We might further say, based on inspection of these curves, that since calcium does not affect the slopes of these curves, this ion does not appear to be involved in voltage dependence per se. This is apparently a clear case of simple modulation by a classic second-messenger, calcium ion.

Moczydlowski and Latorre (1983) showed that this interpretation is too facile, that something more subtle and interesting is occurring in the relationship between voltage and calcium activation. By performing a detailed kinetic analysis of the channel's gating, they arrived at a minimal model of this channel, a model involving four states of the protein:

$$C \rightleftharpoons C:[Ca] \rightleftharpoons O:[Ca] \rightleftharpoons O:[Ca]_2 \qquad (4)$$

Here, "C" and "O" represent closed and open states, respectively. The model proposes that a single calcium ion must bind before the channel can open and that, once it is open, a second calcium ion can bind. Thus, at a fixed voltage, this appears to be a simple ligand-gated channel; calcium causes activation by driving the above

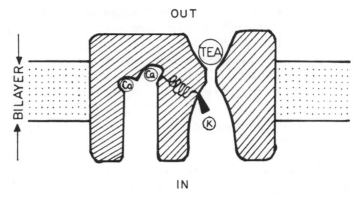

Fig. 3.8. A voltage-dependent calcium-binding reaction. The cartoon illustrates how the binding of calcium to a site on a membrane protein could be voltage dependent. The site is assumed to be located in a hydrophilic cavity of the protein, which extends deeply across the membrane. In this way, the binding site will sense the electric field applied across the membrane.

reactions to the right, into the two open states (which have identical conductances). The questions were then posed: What is the effect of voltage? Which of the above steps are voltage dependent?

Our earlier simple idea of a voltage-dependent conformational change being modulated by calcium tells us that the second reaction, the conformational change from the closed to the open channel, should be the voltage-dependent step. This is not the case. Instead, it was found that this step is completely independent of voltage while the *other* two steps contain all the voltage dependence. This means that this is not a voltage-dependent channel! Instead, it is the *binding* of calcium to the channel protein that senses the applied voltage. The channel itself is voltage independent but is subject to voltage-dependent modulation by a second messenger.

How can a calcium-binding step sense the voltage across the membrane? As discussed by Moczydlowski and Latorre (1983), one way would be for the calcium binding site to be located in a cavity buried deeply within the protein (Figure 3.8), but still accessible from the cytoplasmic side. If this site were thus located within the transmembrane electric field, the binding constant for calcium would vary with applied voltage, becoming increasingly favorable with depolarization. Quantitative treatment of the data indicates that the site would have to be located about 80% of the way across the membrane (Figure 3.8) to account for the steepness of channel opening with voltage. This is not the only possible explanation for voltage-dependent calcium binding, but it is the most economical one.

Channel Phosphorylation: Some Hypothetical Mechanisms of Modulation

There now exist several examples that are documented at the single-channel level, in which a phosphorylation reaction changes the properties of an ion channel (see Chapters 8, 10, and 11). In this section, we will consider some possible hypothetical mechanisms by which phosphorylation might affect channel behavior and what experimental tests might be applied to try to choose among competing mechanisms. This section is totally speculative and is meant only to illustrate some of the ways we might think about the modulation of fundamental mechanisms by phosphorylation and to suggest how we might try to test such ideas.

Effects of Phosphorylation on Gating

Any covalent modification of a channel occurring near regions of the protein that move during the conformational change leading to opening will contribute to energy differences between the open and closed states. In other words, such a modification will generally stabilize one state in relation to the other. If such energies are greater than 0.5 kcal/mol (a small value), then a change in opening probability should be easily observable. Thus, if phosphorylation of a two-state channel (scheme 3), normally open 10% of the time, stabilizes the open state by 1 kcal/mol, the channel's opening probability would increase to 37%. A stabilization of 5 kcal/mol would cause the channel to be open more than 99% of the time—that is, it would apparently be "locked" into its open state. Likewise, if a channel normally open 90% of the time were phosphorylated such that its closed state were stabilized by 5 kcal/mol, it would then open only 0.2% of the time; in such a case, we might say that the channel had been "knocked out" by phosphorylation.

Thus, very large and dramatic effects we observe on the level of ionic currents and single channels can be due to relatively small energy contributions at the molecular level. Suppose that the opening of a channel moves an aspartate residue to within 0.3 nm of a serine hydroxyl (Figure 3.9); such an interaction might help to stabilize a channel's open state, by virtue of an H-bond shared by these groups in the open state (but not in the closed state, where the groups would be too far away from each other). Now, suppose further that this serine became phosphorylated. Not only would this wreak havoc on the favorable H-bonding interaction, but it would place a negatively charged phosphoserine near a carboxylate group. This could easily destabilize the open state by 5 kcal/mol (Kirkwood & Westheimer, 1938), and therefore "cause" the channel to close.

There is no general way to test whether such a picture is correct, short of knowing the detailed structure of the channel protein in its open and closed states, phosphorylated and unphosphorylated. Some simple cases, however, lend themselves to experimental approaches aimed at measuring the degree of putative conformational stabilization due to phosphorylation. If, in the last example, the channel opening reaction were voltage dependent (activation upon depolarization, say), then it should be possible to reopen the channel closed by phosphorylation by stronger depolarization; that is, the energy resulting from the phosphoryl group destabilizing the open state could be overcome by a compensatory energy from applied voltage. In this case, phosphorylation would have the effect of simply shifting the voltage activation curve to the right along the voltage axis. Unfortunately, the quantitative analysis of such an experiment will depend completely on the specific model chosen for channel gating. For this reason, it is necessary to begin with a deeply studied channel, for

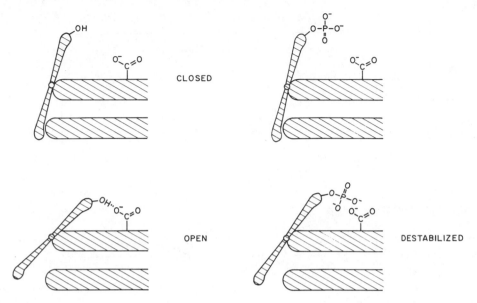

Fig 3.9. Conformational destabilization by phosphorylation. A conceivable way in which phosphorylation of a serine residue could lead to destabilization of the open state of a channel protein.

which a detailed gating model has been derived, before one can ask which specific step in the model is affected by phosphorylation.

Electrostatic Effects of Phosphorylation

Phosphorylation adds fixed negative charge to proteins. One possible effect of converting an uncharged to a charged group is to create new electrostatic interactions that can lead to observable effects on a channel's gating and conduction properties. The electrostatic effect to be discussed here is the tendency of cations to accummulate near a region of local negative charge density. Near a uniformly charged surface, for instance a membrane containing acidic phospholipids, the concentration of cations will be much higher (and that of anions much lower) than the concentration added to bulk solution (McLaughlin, 1977). This "electrical double-layer" may be studied quantitatively in ideal systems such as charged membranes (infinite planar sheets of uniform charge density), but even in a system as nonideal (and unknown) as a protein surface, the same phenomena will apply qualitatively.

Let us consider a calcium-activated potassium channel that is phosphorylated near the calcium-activation site. In this case, the concentration of calcium seen at the site will be increased by the phosphorylation event, just by this electrostatic mechanism, and the channel will be activated. Further study would show that the activation is due to an enhanced apparent increase in the affinity of calcium for the channel, as has in fact been proposed by DePeyer et al. (1982) for calcium-activated potassium currents in perfused *Helix* neurons.

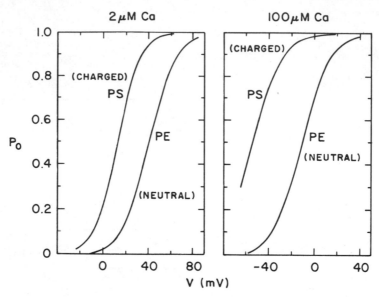

Fig. 3.10. Electrostatic ennhancement of calcium activation in calcium-dependent potassium channels. Activation curves (P_0 versus V as in Figure 3.7) for the calcium-dependent potassium channel from rat muscle plasma membranes were determined after reconstitution into neutral (pure PE) and negatively charged (pure PS) bilayers. (From Moczydlowski & Latorre, 1985).

How might we try to test whether an enhancement in calcium affinity of this kind is due to the electrostatic effect described? This is a very difficult problem to settle with certainty, but one type of experiment can shed some light on it. The efficacy of an electrostatic mechanism in raising the local calcium concentration depends strongly on the ionic strength of the aqueous medium. Local electrostatic potentials are weakened as ionic strength is raised and strengthened as it is lowered. (More precisely, the *distance* over which local electrostatic forces operate decreases with increasing ionic strength.) In testing an idea of this kind, therefore, the channel should be examined in a system in which ionic strength can be systematically varied. If such a test could be performed, we would expect to observe larger effects of phosphorylation on the calcium affinity at low salt than at high salt.

Moczydlowski and Latorre (1985) have observed an electrostatic effect on the calcium-dependent potassium channel reconstituted in planar bilayer membranes. In their case, they examined the effect of the local electrostatic potential not by inducing a change in phosphorylation but by comparing the voltage dependence of channel open probability in uncharged and negatively charged phospholipid membranes. They found a change in voltage dependence as shown in Figure 3.10, equivalent to an approximately tenfold increase in calcium affinity, in negatively charged membranes.

A second consequence of a local electrostatic potential due to phosphoryation could be on the conductance of the channel itself. Near a negatively charged phosphoryl group, the local potassium concentration will be elevated. If this site is close

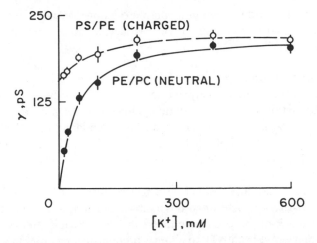

Fig. 3.11. Electrostatic enhancement of potassium channel conductance. The data show the single channel conductance of the SR potassium channel, reconstituted into planar bilayer membranes, as a function of potassium concentration. Closed circles: neutral membranes (PE/PC). Open circles: negatively charged membranes containing 70% PS. The curves represent a rectangular hyperbola (for the neutral membranes) and the same rectangular hyperbola modified by an electrostatic effect due to the negatively charged lipids. (From Bell & Miller, 1984).

to the mouth of the channel, the increased potassium concentration seen by the channel would lead to an increased conductance. This sort of effect would be particularly applicable to potassium channels, which carry outward current; phosphorylation on the cytoplasmic side would specifically enhance the conductance in the outward direction. This effect is complicated, however, by the fact that channel conductance saturates with ion concentration (as in Figure 3.2). Therefore, this effect will be significant only for channels that bind the conducting cation *weakly,* that is, those that do not normally operate near channel saturation. This point is illustrated in Figure 3.11, which shows the effect of negatively charged phospholipid membranes on the single channel conductance of a potassium channel from sarcoplasmic reticulum (Bell & Miller, 1984). In electrically neutral membranes, the conductance-concentration relation follows a rectangular hyperbola, as is shown in Figure 3.1. In negatively charged membranes, the conductance is enhanced at each potassium concentration, but this effect is much more pronounced at low potassium; virtually no difference in conductance is seen above 300 mM potassium, where the channel is saturated.

Both of these examples have referred to the phosphoryl group as being "near" a site. How close does a charged group have to be to a Ca^{++} activation site, say, in order to exert a direct electrostatic effect on it? In an ideal system, such as an infinite planar charged surface, we can answer this question precisely: electrostatic forces fall off with distance according to the "Debye length," a characteristic distance that depends on the ionic strength. In physiological salt solution (150 mM ionic strength), the Debye length is about 1 nm, whereas it is 0.3 nm at 1 M salt and 3 nm at 10 mM salt. Qualitatively, a similar situation will hold near charged groups on a protein:

a calcium binding site within 1 nm of a phosphorylation site will feel the full electro-static effect of the phosphoryl group at 10 mM salt, a partial effect at 150 mM, and very little at 1 M.

Direct Occlusion of the Pore

One mechanism that is quite unlikely but not impossible for the inhibition of a chan-nel by phosphorylation is the direct steric occlusion of the pore by the phosphoryl group. This group, with a diameter of 0.6 nm, is much larger than the hydroxyl (0.1 nm) it replaces. It is thus possible that a channel with a rather small opening to the external solution could be physically blocked by a suitably placed phosphorylation site.

Although this possibility has not been tested, it is worth discussing because it would be expected to give rise to an observable, and somewhat unusual, phenome-non: reversible block of the open channel by the *kinase itself*. Before a phosphoryl group can be transferred from ATP to a target protein substrate (S), the charged (i.e., phosphorylated) kinase (K~P) must bind to its target, as shown in scheme 5:

$$K{\sim}P + S \underset{k_{-1}}{\overset{k_1}{\rightleftharpoons}} K{\sim}P{:}S \underset{k_{-2}}{\overset{k_2}{\rightleftharpoons}} K{:}S{\sim}P \underset{k_{-3}}{\overset{k_3}{\rightleftharpoons}} K + S{\sim}P \qquad (5)$$

On average, the kinase-target complex has a certain lifetime before the complex dissociates or the phosphoryl transfer takes place, a lifetime related to the rate con-stants above. Not very many mechanistic enzymological studies have been carried out on protein kinase reactions, but those that have indicate the pertinent rate con-stants, k_{-1} and k_2, are rather slow, in the order of 10 sec^{-1}. Therefore, if the phos-phorylation site is near the channel mouth, we might expect the kinase itself to in-duce blocked states of the channel that are relatively long-lived ($\sim$100 msec). Such blocking events would be immediately apparent on the single channel level for a channel that, under unmodified conditions, is open most of the time, without "flick-ers" on the 100-msec time scale.

Modification of Gating Charge of
Voltage-Dependent Channels

One obvious means by which phosphorylation might affect a voltage-dependent ion channel's behavior would be by changing its "gating charge." If phosphorylation occurs at a region of the protein that moves in the membrane field upon opening, then the voltage dependence of the activation process would be changed. How rea-sonable is such a mechanism? Intuitively it seems likely that the structural changes involved in the gating of integral membrane channel proteins will turn out to be quite small—that critical groups will be found to move only small distances from the opened to the closed state. A channel with a voltage dependence of opening of e-fold per 12 mV, say, could be pictured as moving two charges across the entire membrane field, or 20 charges 10% of the way through the field. The latter picture seems much more plausible—that a voltage-gated channel will have a highly asymmetric distribution of fixed charge (a large dipole moment) that moves only a small distance upon gating. Thus, a phosphorylation reaction that adds one more charge to this highly charged region on the protein will not change the measured gating charge very much. Only if multiple phosphorylations were utilized, as is the case with vertebrate rhodopsin, is it likely that significant change in gating charge could be achieved.

CONCLUSIONS

This chapter has presented in a qualitative way some of the essential aspects of the fundamental processes governing the behavior of ion channel proteins. It has also attempted to anticipate some possible ways in which these processes might be changed by biochemical events targeted at channel proteins. Most of the experimental tests suggested here are not now feasible; only recently have modulation events been observed at the single channel level, and in none of these cases is the channel's behavior understood mechanistically. But it seems reasonable to believe that in the near future, with diligent application of patch-recording methods and reconstitution techniques that allow a great simplification of the experimental system, experiments to test some of these hypothetical mechanisms will enter the realm of possibility.

REFERENCES

Anderson, C.R. and Stevens, C.F. (1973) Voltage-clamp analysis of acetylcholine produced end-plate current fluctuations at frog neuromuscular junction. *J. Physiol. London 235,* 655–691.

Aoshima, H., Cash, D., and Hess, G.P. (1981) Mechanism of inactivation of acetylcholine receptor. Investigations by fast reaction techniques with membrane vesicles. *Biochemistry 20,* 3467–3474.

Armstrong, C.M. (1975a) Ionic pores, gates, and gating currents. *Q. Rev. Biophys. 7,* 179–210.

Armstrong, C.M. (1975b) Potassium pores of nerve and muscle membranes. In *Membranes, a Series of Advances* (ed. G. Eisenman), Vol. 3, pp. 325–358. Dekker, New York.

Barrett, J.N., Magelby, K.L., and Pallotta, B.S. (1982) Properties of single calcium-activated potassium channels in cultured rat muscle. *J. Physiol. London 331,* 211–230.

Begenisich, T.B. and De Weer, P. (1980) Potassium flux ratio in voltage-clamped squid axons. *J. Gen. Physiol. 76,* 83–98.

Bell, J.E. and Miller, C. (1984) Effects of phospholipid surface charge on ion conduction in the sarcoplasmic reticulum potassium channel. *Biophys. J. 45,* 279–288.

Coronado, R. and Miller, C. (1982) Conduction and block by organic cations in a potassium-selective channel from sarcoplasmic reticulum incorporated into planar bilayer membranes. *J. Gen. Physiol. 79,* 529–547.

Coronado, R., Rosenberg, R.L., and Miller, C. (1980) Ionic selectivity, saturation, and block in a potassium-selective channel from sarcoplasmic reticulum. *J. Gen. Physiol. 76,* 425–453.

DePeyer, J.E., Cachelin, A.B., Levitan, I.B., and Reuter, H. (1982) Ca^{2+}-activated potassium conductance in internally perfused snail neurons is enhanced by protein phosphorylation. *Proc. Natl. Acad. Sci. USA 79,* 4207–4211.

Dwyer, T.M., Adams, D.J., and Hillie, B. (1980) The permeability of the endplate channel to organic cations in frog muscle. *J. Gen. Physiol. 75,* 469–492.

Ewald, D., Williams, A., and Levitan, I.B. (1985) Modulation of single Ca^{2+}-dependent K^+ channel activity by protein phosphorylation. *Nature 315*, 503–506.

Finkelstein, A. and Andersen, O.S. (1981) The gramicidin A channel: A review of its permeability characteristics with special reference to the single file aspect of transport. *J. Membr. Biol. 59*, 155–171.

Hamill, O.P., Marty, A., Neher, E., Sakmann, B., and Sigworth, F.J. (1981) Improved patch-clamp techniques for high-resolution current recording from cells and cell-free membrane patches. *Pfluegers Arch. 391*, 85–100.

Hess, P. and Tsien, R.W. (1984) Mechanism of ion permeation through calcium channels. *Nature 309*, 453–456.

Hille, B. (1971) The permeability of the sodium channel to organic cations in myelinated nerve. *J. Gen. Physiol. 58*, 599–619.

Hille, B. (1973) Potassium channels in myelinated nerve. Selective permeability to small cations. *J. Gen. Physiol. 61*, 669–686.

Hille, B. (1975) Ionic selectivity of Na and K channels of nerve membranes. In *Membranes, a Series of Advances* (ed. G. Eisenman), pp. 255–323. Dekker, New York.

Hille, B. (1984) *Ionic Channels of Excitable Membranes*. Sinauer Associates, Sunderland, MA.

Hille, B. and Schwarz, W. (1978) Potassium channels as multi-ion single-file pores. *J. Gen. Physiol. 72*, 409–442.

Hodgkin, A.L., Huxley, A.F., and Katz, B. (1952) Measurements of current-voltage relations in the membrane of the giant axon of Loligo. *J. Physiol. London 116*, 424–448.

Hodgkin, A.L. and Keynes, R.D. (1955) The potassium permeability of a giant nerve fibre. *J. Physiol. London 128*, 61–88.

Horn, R. and Patlak, J. (1980) Single channel currents from excised patches of muscle membrane. *Proc. Natl. Acad. Sci. USA 77*, 6930–6934.

Horn, R. and Stevens, C.F. (1980) Relations between structure and function of ion channels. *Comm. Molec. Cell. Biophys. 1*, 57–70.

Jencks, W.P. (1975) Binding energy, specificity, and enzymatic catalysis: The Circe effect. *Adv. Enzymol. 43*, 219–410.

Katz, B. and Miledi, R. (1970) Membrane noise produced by acetylcholine. *Nature 226*, 962–963.

Kirkwood, J. and Westheimer, F.H. (1938) The electrostatic influence of substituents on the dissociation constant of organic acids. I. *J. Chem. Phys. 6*, 506–512.

Knauf, P.A. (1979) Erythrocyte anion exchange and the band 3 protein: Transport kinetics and molecular structure. *Curr. Top. Membr. Transp. 12*, 250–363.

Latorre, R. and Miller, C. (1983) Conduction and selectivity in potassium channels. *J. Membr. Biol. 71*, 11–30.

Latorre, R., Vergara, C., and Hidalgo, C. (1982) Reconstitution in planar bilayers of a Ca^{2+}-dependent potassium channel from transverse tubule membranes isolated from rabbit skeletal muscle. *Proc. Natl. Acad. Sci. USA 79*, 805–809.

Lauger, P. (1973) Ion transport through pores: a rate-theory analysis. *Biochim. Biophys. Acta. 311*, 423–441.

Marty, A. (1981) Calcium-dependent channels with large unitary conductance in chromaffin cell membranes. *Nature 291*, 497–500.

McLaughlin, S. (1977) Electrostatic potentials at membrane-solution interfaces. *Curr. Top. Membr. Transp. 9*, 71–144.

Miller, C. (1982) Coupling of water and ion fluxes in a potassium-selective channel of sarcoplasmic reticulum. *Biophys. J. 38*, 227–230.

Moczydlowski, E. and Latorre, R. (1983) Gating kinetics of Ca^{2+}-activated potassium channels from rat muscle incorporated into planar lipid bilayers: evidence for two voltage-dependent Ca^{2+} binding reactions. *J. Gen. Physiol. 82*, 511–542.

Moczydlowski, E., Alvarez, O., Vergara, C., and Latorre, R. (1985) Effect of phospholipid surface charge on the conductance and gating of a Ca^{2+}-activated potassium channel in planar lipid bilayers. *J. Membr. Biol. 83*, 273–284.

Moczydlowski, E., Garber, S.S., and Miller, C. (1984) Batrachotoxin-activated Na^+ channels in planar lipid bilayers. Competition of tetrodotoxin block by Na^+. *J. Gen. Physiol. 84*, 665–686.

Neubig, R.R., Krodel, E.K., Boyd, N.D., and Cohen, J.B. (1979) Acetylcholine and local anaesthetic binding to *Torpedo* nicotinic postsynaptic membranes after removal of non-receptor peptides. *Proc. Natl. Acad. Sci. USA 76*, 690–694.

Parsegian, A. (1969) Energy of an ion crossing a low dielectric membrane: solutions to four relevant electrostatic problems. *Nature 221*, 844–846.

Rosenberg, P.A. and Finkelstein, A. (1978) Interaction of ions and water in gramicidin A channels. Streaming potentials across lipid bilayer membranes. *J. Gen. Physiol. 72*, 327–340.

Shuster, M., Camardo, J.S., Siegelbaum, S.A., and Kandel, E.R. (1985) Serotonin-sensitive potassium channel of *Aplysia* neurons: Modulation by cAMP-dependent protein kinase in cell-free membrane patches. *Nature 313*, 392–395.

Ussing, H.H. (1949) The distinction by means of tracers between active transport and diffusion. The transfer of iodide across the isolated frog skin. *Acta Physiol. Scand. 19*, 43–56.

White, M.M. and Miller, C. (1981) Probes of the conduction process of a voltage-gated Cl^- channel from *Torpedo* electroplax. *J. Gen. Physiol. 78*, 1–18.

4

Biochemical Mechanisms That Regulate the Properties of Ion Channels

RICHARD L. HUGANIR

Extracellular signals such as those of neurotransmitters and hormones regulate physiological properties in specific target cells. Many of these extracellular signals produce their effects by regulating the levels of intracellular second messengers. The concept of second messengers was first introduced by Sutherland and his colleagues in the late 1950s. They demonstrated that the stimulation of glycogenolysis in the liver by the hormone epinephrine is mediated by an increase in the synthesis of an intracellular messenger, cyclic AMP. Krebs and his colleagues subsequently demonstrated that cyclic AMP activates a protein kinase in skeletal muscle and that the stimulation of glycogenolysis by epinephrine is mediated by this cyclic AMP-dependent protein kinase. More recent studies have shown that many hormones and neurotransmitters regulate the levels of cyclic AMP in their target cells and thereby regulate the activity of cyclic AMP-dependent protein kinase. In addition, many neurotransmitters and hormones have been demonstrated to regulate the levels of other intracellular second messengers such as cyclic GMP, calcium and diacylglycerol. It has become increasingly clear that all the actions of cyclic AMP, and many of the actions of cyclic GMP, calcium, and diacylglycerol are mediated by the activation of specific classes of protein kinases. Protein kinases that are dependent on cyclic AMP, cyclic GMP, calcium and diacylglycerol have been identified and shown to be activated by physiological concentrations of these second messengers.

Protein kinases are enzymes that catalyze the transfer of the terminal phosphate of ATP to serine, threonine, or tyrosine amino acid residues in specific substrate proteins in the target cells. The addition of the highly charged phosphate molecule alters the structure of the phosphorylated protein and thereby regulates its function. The phosphorylated protein then directly or indirectly modulates the physiological properties of the cell, including the activities of its ion channels. This process can be reversed by protein phosphatases that remove the phosphate from the substrate protein and return the substrate protein and the cell to their basal states.

The physiological response of neurons to many neurotransmitters and hormones therefore depends on which second messenger system or systems are activated by the

Table 4.1. Phosphoproteins of the nervous system

Enzymes involved in neurotransmitter biosynthesis	
Tyrosine hydroxylase	Joh et al., 1978; Edelman et al., 1981
Tryptophan hydroxylase	Yamauchi and Fujisawa, 1981; Kuhn and Lovenberg, 1982
Synaptic vesicle-associated proteins	
Synapsin I	Johnson et al., 1971; Ueda and Greengard, 1977
Protein III	Huang et al., 1982; Browning and Greengard, 1984
Cytoskeletal proteins	
MAP-2	See Nestler and Greengard, 1984
Tau	See Nestler and Greengard, 1984
Neurofilaments	See Nestler and Greengard, 1984
Myosin light chain	Hathaway et al., 1981
Actin	Demaille and Pechere, 1983
Tubulin	Goldenring et al., 1982
Neurotransmitter receptors	
Nicotinic acetylcholine receptor	Gordon et al., 1977a; Teichberg et al., 1977; Huganir et al., 1984
Muscarinic acetylcholine receptor	Burgoyne, 1983
β-Adrenergic receptor	Stadel et al., 1983
GABA receptor (GABA-modulin)	Wise et al., 1983
Ion channels	
Nicotinic acetylcholine receptor	Gordon et al., 1977a; Teichberg et al., 1977; Huganir et al., 1984
Voltage-dependent sodium channel	Costa et al., 1982; Costa and Catterall, 1984a,b
Voltage-dependent potassium channels	Kaczmarek et al., 1980; Castellucci et al., 1980, 1982; Adams and Levitan, 1982; dePeyer et al., 1982; Alkon et al., 1983
Voltage-dependent calcium channels	Osterrieder et al., 1982; DeRiemer et al., 1985; Curtis and Catterall, 1985

transmitter or hormone, which protein kinase system or systems are activated by the second messenger, and which substrate proteins are phosphorylated by the activated protein kinase(s) in the target cell. Phosphorylated proteins in the nervous system have been studied extensively and include many different nerve cell elements such as cytoskeletal proteins, synaptic vesicle-associated proteins, enzymes involved in neurotransmitter synthesis, membrane receptors, and ion channels (Table 4.1)

Within the past few years, many studies have demonstrated that protein phosphorylation is a major mechanism in the modulation of neuronal ion channels. Microinjection of various protein kinases or their inhibitors into excitable cells has provided direct evidence that protein phosphorylation regulates the function of voltage-dependent calcium and potassium channels. In addition, recent studies of identified ion channel proteins such as the nicotinic acetylcholine receptor and the voltage-dependent sodium channel have demonstrated that these identified ion channel proteins are multiply phosphorylated by different protein kinases (see Chapter 5).

This chapter deals with the biochemical mechanisms involved in the modulation of ion channel function by neurotransmitters and hormones. Specifically, the bio-chemical steps between the binding of neurotransmitter or hormone to its membrane receptor and the subsequent change in the functional state of the ion channel will be discussed in detail, with particular emphasis on the role of protein kinases.

CYCLIC AMP-DEPENDENT PROTEIN KINASE

Neurotransmitters and hormones regulate the intracellular levels of cyclic AMP through their interaction with specific receptors at the membrane surface. The binding of the neurotransmitter or hormone activates the receptor and eventually results in the stim-ulation or inhibition of cyclic AMP synthesis by adenylate cyclase within the cell. Receptors that stimulate adenylate cyclase include the β-adrenergic, dopamine (D1), and 5-HT receptors, whereas receptors that inhibit adenylate cylase include α-adrenergic, muscarinic cholinergic, and opiate receptors.

The signal produced by the binding of the neurotransmitter or hormone to the receptor at the membrane surface is transduced to the interior of the cell by a pair of guanine nucleotide-binding proteins, G_s and G_i (Rodbell, 1980; Gilman, 1984). Stim-ulatory receptors interact with the G_s protein and inhibitory receptors with the G_i protein. These activated G proteins regulate the activity of the catalytic subunit of adenylate cyclase, which catalyzes the synthesis of cyclic AMP from ATP. By stim-ulating (G_s) or inhibiting (G_i) adenylate cyclase, the G proteins regulate the intra-cellular levels of cyclic AMP.

Specific pharmacological agents, developed to interact with each component of the adenylate cyclase system, have been very useful in the study of the action of cyclic AMP *in vitro* and *in vivo*. The various receptors for neurotransmitters and hormones are the sites of action of numerous specific agonists and antagonists that activate or inhibit receptor activity. The G_s and G_i proteins are the sites of action for the bacterial toxins of cholera and pertussis, respectively (Gilman, 1984). These tox-ins cause the ADP-ribosylation of the G proteins and have characteristic effects on their function. Cholera toxin irreversibly activates the G_s subunit, bypassing the re-ceptor and stimulating cyclic AMP production (Gill & Meren, 1978; Cassel & Pfeuf-fer, 1978). Pertussis toxin irreversibly inactivates the G_i protein and prevents the inhibition of cyclic AMP synthesis by the inhibitory receptors (Katada & Ui, 1982). The catalytic subunit of adenylate cyclase is the site of action of the diterpene, for-skolin (Daly, 1984). As will be shown elsewhere in this volume, forskolin has proved to be an extremely useful pharmacological agent in intact cells because it is mem-brane permeant and directly activates the catalytic subunit of adenylate cyclase, by-passing the stimulatory receptors and G_s protein.

The action of cyclic AMP within the cell is most likely to be mediated exclu-sively by the activation of cyclic AMP-dependent protein kinase, because cyclic AMP-dependent protein kinase is the major intracellular receptor for cyclic AMP (Walter et al., 1977). After the initial discovery of cyclic AMP-dependent protein kinase in skeletal muscle by Krebs and his colleagues (Walsh et al., 1968), cyclic AMP-dependent protein kinase was found to be widespread throughout various tissues and phyla of the animal kingdom (Kuo & Greengard, 1969).

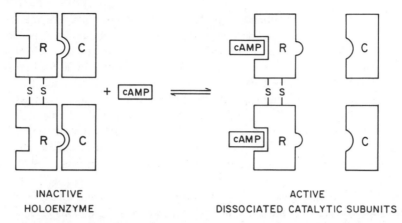

Fig. 4.1. Schematic diagram of cyclic AMP-dependent protein kinase and its dissociation and activation by cyclic AMP. R, regularly subunit; C, catalytic subunit; S–S, disulfide bonds. The cyclic AMP binding site is indicated by the rectangular indentation in the R subunits and the catalytic site is indicated by the semicircular indentation in the catalytic subunit.

Cyclic AMP-dependent protein kinase is a tetrameric complex of two types of subunits, a regulatory subunit (M—49,000 to 50,000), which binds cyclic AMP, and a catalytic subunit (M—40,000), which catalyzes the phosphorylation reaction (Figure 4.1) (Krebs &Beavo, 1979). The holoenzyme is inactive and contains two regulatory subunits linked covalently by disulfide bonds. These regulatory subunits interact noncovalently with two catalytic subunits (Beavo et al., 1975; Rosen et al., 1975). Binding of cyclic AMP to the regulatory subunits reduces the affinity between the regulatory and catalytic subunits and leads to the dissociation of the catalytic subunits (see Figure 4.1). These free catalytic subunits are then completely active. Many tissues contain small amounts of a heat-stable protein that specifically inhibits the catalytic subunit of cyclic AMP-dependent protein kinase (Walsh et al., 1971). Although the function of this inhibitor has not been determined, it may possibly serve to inhibit any free catalytic subunit present in the cell under resting conditions. Purified preparations of this protein kinase inhibitor (PKI) have been extremely useful in both the *in vivo* and *in vitro* studies of the action of cyclic AMP-dependent protein kinase.

Two types of cyclic AMP-dependent protein kinase have been reported, which have been termed type I and type II cyclic AMP-dependent protein kinase (Reimann et al., 1971). Both have identical catalytic subunits but contain different types of regulatory subunits, regulatory subunit type I (RI) (M—49,000) and regulatory subunit type II (RII) (M—52,000 to 55,000) (Hofmann et al., 1975; Nimmo & Cohen, 1977). The regulatory subunits RI and RII differ in many properties including their affinities for cyclic AMP and ATP, their tissue distribution, and their ability to be autophosphorylated (Krebs & Beavo, 1979). The RII regulatory subunit has been shown to be autophosphorylated by the catalytic subunit, and this autophosphorylation decreases the rate of the reassociation of RII with the catalytic subunit, thereby enhancing the response to cyclic AMP.

Although cyclic AMP-dependent protein kinase is a soluble enzyme in many tissues, it is distributed evenly between particulate and soluble fractions in brain (Maeno et al., 1971; Hofmann et al., 1977). The particulate and cytosolic forms of the type II enzyme seem to have identical biochemical and immunological properties, suggesting either that the kinase exists in equilibrium between the cytosolic and particulate forms or that some minor modification of the kinase is causing its association with the particulate fraction (Rubin et al., 1979; Lohmann et al., 1980). The association of the kinase with the particulate fraction has been shown to be dependent on the regulatory subunit because the addition of cyclic AMP releases the catalytic subunit but not the regulatory subunit from the membranes (Rubin et al., 1979; Corbin et al., 1977).

The highest specific activity of cyclic AMP-dependent protein kinase in the brain is in the cytosolic fraction and synaptic membrane-enriched fractions (Walter et al., 1978; Kelly et al., 1979). The enzyme is highly enriched in purified synaptic structures such as synaptic junctions, synaptic plasma membranes, and postsynaptic densities (Kelly et al., 1979; Ueda et al., 1979), suggesting an important role for this enzyme in the regulation of synaptic transmission. Other studies have demonstrated a specific interaction of the type II enzyme with microtubule-associated protein 2 (MAP-2) (Vallee et al., 1981; Theurkauf & Vallee, 1982). The association of cyclic AMP-dependent protein kinase with membranes and microtubule-associated proteins is most likely involved in compartmentalizing the effects of the enzyme. This would help to limit the specific response to cyclic AMP by maintaining a local concentration of cyclic AMP-dependent protein kinase in subcellular compartments of the cell near particular substrate proteins.

How a cell will respond to an increase in cyclic AMP is determined by the cell-specific substrate proteins that are phosphorylated by the cyclic AMP-dependent protein kinase. Cyclic AMP-dependent protein kinase has a broad substrate specificity and phosphorylates a wide variety of substrate proteins in many tissues. Many substrate proteins in neurons have been studied in detail. These include proteins involved in neurotransmitter release, neurotransmitter synthesis, and ion channel function. Ion channels known to be phosphorylated by the cyclic AMP-dependent protein kinase include the nicotinic acetylcholine receptor, the voltage-dependent sodium channel, and the voltage-dependent calcium channel (see Chapter 5). In addition, the catalytic subunit of cyclic AMP-dependent protein kinase has been shown to regulate the function of several different types of potassium channels (see Table 2.1 in Chapter 2).

Most of the identified substrates for cyclic AMP-dependent protein kinase are phosphorylated on serine residues although some are phosphorylated on threonine residues. The substrate specificity appears to be determined to a large extent by the primary sequence of the substrate protein (Krebs & Beavo, 1979). The amino acid sequences around the phosphorylation sites of several well-characterized substrate proteins are shown in Figure 4.2. These sequences all contain two to three basic amino acids (e.g., arginine or lysine) that precede the phosphorylated serine or threonine residue by one amino acid, suggesting that these residues are important in determining substrate specificity. Krebs and his colleagues have studied the primary sequence requirements of the cyclic AMP-dependent protein kinase by using synthetic peptides (Kemp et al., 1975). They have determined that the presence of two

AMINO ACID SEQUENCE

SUBSTRATE PROTEIN	AMINO ACID SEQUENCE
Phosphorylase kinase (α subunit)	PHE – ARG – ARG – LEU – SER(P) – ILE – SER – THR – GLU – SER – GLX
Regulatory subunit (R-II)	ASP – ARG – ARG – VAL – SER(P) – VAL
Synapsin I	TYR – LEU – ARG – ARG – ARG – LEU – SER(P) – ASP – SER – ASN – PHE
Pyruvate kinase (rat liver)	GLY – VAL – LEU – ARG – ARG – ALA – SER(P) – VAL – ALA – GLX – LEU
Phosphatase inhibitor-1	ILE – ARG – ARG – ARG – ARG – PRO – THR(P) – PRO – ALA – THR
DARPP-32	ARG – ARG – ARG – PRO – THR(P) – PRO – ALA – MET – LEU – PHE

Fig. 4.2. Amino acid sequences around the phosphorylation sites of physiological substrates for cyclic AMP-dependent protein kinase. SER(P) and THR(P) represent the amino acid residues that are phosphorylated (Nestler & Greengard, 1984; Czernik, Pang, & Greengard, in preparation).

to three basic residues preceding the phosphorylated serine or threonine residue by
one amino acid is critical to the recognition of the substrate protein by the kinase.
Basic amino acids preceding the phosphorylated serine or threonine residue are a
common feature of substrates for cyclic AMP, cyclic GMP, calcium/calmodulin, and
calcium/phospholipid-dependent protein kinases (see following sections). However,
it appears that the number and the relative position of the basic amino acid residues
may explain the very different substrate specificity of each of these kinases. In addition, the primary amino acid sequence surrounding the phosphorylated amino acid
is not the sole determinant of substrate specificity. Secondary and tertiary structure
are also likely to play a major role.

CYCLIC GMP-DEPENDENT PROTEIN KINASE

Neurotransmitters and hormones have been demonstrated to regulate the levels of the
intracellular second messenger cyclic GMP. These neurotransmitters and hormones
interact at the membrane surface with specific receptors, such as muscarinic cholinergic and α-adrenergic receptors, which then transduce the signal to the interior of
the cell. However, the actual transduction mechanism between the receptor and the
synthesis of cyclic GMP by guanylate cyclase in the cell is not well understood.
Most hormones and neurotransmitters appear to require the presence of extracellular
calcium to regulate the levels of cyclic GMP in cells, and it has been assumed that
an increase in cytoplasmic calcium is a primary and necessary step in coupling receptors to guanylate cyclase (Walter, 1981; Berridge, 1984). Many neurotransmitters
that stimulate phosphatidylinositol breakdown (see below) have been observed to
cause an increase in cyclic GMP levels (Berridge, 1984; Berridge & Irvine, 1984).
Studies demonstrating that guanylate cyclase can be activated by a variety of fatty
acids suggest that regulation of guanylate cyclase by metabolites of receptor-stimulated
phosphatidylinositol breakdown may be physiologically important (Berridge, 1984).
In contrast to the adenylate cyclase system, guanine nucleotide binding proteins have
not been demonstrated to be required in the coupling of activated receptors to the
regulation of intracellular levels of cyclic GMP. However, in the retina, light-acti-
vated rhodopsin has been shown to be coupled to a decrease in the level of cyclic
GMP by transducin, a guanine nucleotide-binding protein homologous to G_s and G_i
(Stryer et al., 1983).

   Many of the actions of cyclic GMP are presumably mediated by the activation
of cyclic GMP-dependent protein kinase (Kuo & Greengard, 1970) because cyclic
GMP-dependent protein kinase appears to be the major intracellular receptor for cyclic
GMP (Walter & Greengard, 1981). Recent evidence, however, has suggested that
cyclic GMP may directly activate ion channels in rod outer segments (Fesenko et al.,
1985), and it is possible that cyclic GMP may have other roles as well. Cyclic GMP-
dependent protein kinase was initially discovered in arthropods and has subsequently
been shown to be present in most mammalian tissues examined (Kuo, 1974; Lincoln
et al., 1976). In contrast to cyclic AMP-dependent protein kinase, cyclic GMP-
dependent protein kinase shows a very uneven tissue distribution. The brain contains
relatively low amounts of cyclic GMP-dependent protein kinase with large variations

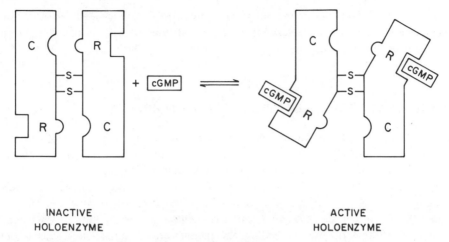

INACTIVE   ACTIVE
HOLOENZYME   HOLOENZYME

Fig. 4.3. Schematic diagram of cyclic GMP-dependent protein kinase and its activation by cyclic GMP. R, regulatory domain; C, catalytic domain; S–S disulfide bond. Cyclic GMP binding site is indicated by the rectangular indentation in the regulatory domain and the catalytic site is indicated by the seimcircular indentation in the catalytic domain.

in its levels in different areas of the brain (Schlichter et al., 1980). The highest levels occur in the cerebellum where cyclic GMP-dependent protein kinase is specifically localized in the Purkinje cells (Lohmann et al., 1981; De Camilli et al., 1984).

In most tissues that have been examined, cyclic GMP-dependent protein kinase appears to be primarily a soluble enzyme. It is a dimeric protein of identical subunits of $M_r \sim 74,000$ (Figure 4.3) (Lincoln & Corbin, 1983). Each subunit contains a cyclic GMP-binding domain similar in amino acid sequence to the regulatory subunit of the cyclic AMP-dependent protein kinase and a catalytic domain similar in amino acid sequence to the catalytic subunit of cyclic AMP-dependent protein kinase (Takio et al., 1984). In contrast with the latter enzyme, binding of cyclic GMP does not dissociate the subunits but induces a conformational change that exposes and activates the catalytic domain (see Figure 4.3) (Lincoln et al., 1978). Cyclic GMP-dependent protein kinase autophosphorylates in the presence of cyclic GMP, and this autophosphorylation appears to increase the V_{max} of the enzyme (de Jonge & Rosen, 1977; Hofmann & Flockerzi, 1983).

Much less is known about substrate proteins in cells for the cyclic GMP-dependent protein kinase, although it appears that it has narrower substrate specificity than the cyclic AMP-dependent enzyme (Lincoln & Corbin, 1983). All of the identified substrates for cyclic GMP-dependent protein kinase are phosphorylated on serine or threonine residues. By using purified exogenous substrates such as histones, Glass and Krebs (1979) have shown that cyclic GMP-dependent protein kinase has a substrate specificity that is similar to, although distinct from, the cyclic AMP-dependent kinase. In addition, these authors have studied the primary sequence requirements for substrates of cyclic GMP-dependent protein kinase with synthetic peptide substrates. As with the cyclic AMP-dependent protein kinase, it appears that basic amino acids such as arginine and lysine immediately preceding the phosphorylated serine or threonine residue are important determinants of the substrate specificity of cyclic GMP-dependent protein kinase.

CALCIUM/CALMODULIN-DEPENDENT PROTEIN KINASES

Many neurotransmitters and hormones, as well as the nerve impulse itself, produce changes in the intracellular levels of calcium. Intracellular calcium exerts its physiological effects in cells through a variety of molecular mechanisms. However, many of the effects of calcium are mediated by the calcium binding protein, calmodulin (Cheung, 1980; Klee et al., 1980). Calmodulin is a ubiquitous, small, heat-stable protein that, in the presence of micromolar concentrations of calcium, can activate a number of different enzymes including phosphodiesterases, adenylate cyclases, protein phosphatases, and protein kinases. Calcium binding to calmodulin induces a large conformational change in calmodulin, which exposes a hydrophobic domain that interacts with and activates the calcium/calmodulin-dependent enzymes.

Many of the effects of calcium/calmodulin in the nervous system appear to be mediated by the activation of a class of calcium/calmodulin-dependent protein kinases. In contrast with the cyclic nucleotide-dependent protein kinases, many types of calcium/calmodulin-dependent protein kinases exist. Four different types have been identified in brain: calcium/calmodulin-dependent protein kinase I, calcium-calmodulin-dependent protein kinase II, myosin light chain kinase, and phosphorylase kinase (Nairn et al., 1985). Myosin light chain kinase and phosphorylase kinase do not appear to have any neuron-specific role in the modulation of neuronal function and will not be discussed in detail here.

Calcium/Calmodulin-Dependent Protein Kinase II

Calcium/calmodulin-dependent protein kinase II is the major calcium/calmodulin-dependent protein kinase in brain and may comprise aproximately 0.4% of the brain protein (Bennett et al., 1983; McGuinness et al., 1985). In different brain regions the enzyme exists as specific isozymic forms, which are similar to the multifunctional calcium/calmodulin-dependent protein kinases present in many species and tissues (Palfrey et al., 1983; Gorelick et al., 1983; McGuinness et al., 1983).

Within the brain, calcium/calmodulin-dependent protein kinase II is found in particulate and soluble fractions. The soluble and particulate forms of the enzyme appear to have identical biochemical properties, suggesting that the kinase exists in equilibrium between the cytosolic and particulate forms or that some minor modification of the enzyme determines its distribution (Walaas et al., 1983a,b; Kennedy et al., 1983). Calcium/calmodulin-dependent protein kinase II is present in the presynaptic nerve terminal and in synaptic vesicle preparations, and it has recently been shown to be a major component of the postsynaptic density protein (Kennedy et al., 1983; Kelly et al., 1984; Goldenring et al., 1984). These results suggest that the enzyme may play a role in both presynaptic and postsynaptic regulation of synaptic function.

Calcium/calmodulin-dependent protein kinase II isolated from rat forebrain has a native molecular weight of 550,000 to 600,000 and contains major subunits of M_r $\sim$ 50,000 (α) and M_r $\sim$ 58,000 to 60,000 (β) in a net ratio of 3:1. Peptide maps of the subunits show that the α and β subunits, although similar in structure, are distinct polypeptides. The heterogeneity of the β subunit appears to be due to partial proteolysis of the M_r $\sim$ 60,000 protein. Each subunit autophosphorylates in a calcium/calmodulin-dependent manner and binds calmodulin, suggesting that each subunit in the complex contains a regulatory and a catalytic domain (Bennett et al., 1983; McGuinness et al., 1985).

Calcium/Calmodulin-Dependent Protein Kinase I

Calcium/calmodulin-dependent protein kinase I has a widespread species and tissue distribution (Nairn & Greengard, 1983) and is predominantly a cytosolic enzyme in all tissues examined. Although this enzyme phosphorylates the synaptic vesicle-associated protein synapsin I, its role in neuronal function remains to be investigated.

Substrates

Calcium/calmodulin-dependent protein kinase II, like cyclic AMP-dependent protein kinase, appears to be a multifunctional protein kinase that is able to phosphorylate a broad array of tissue-specific substrates. Many of these substrate proteins have been characterized in detail; they include proteins involved in neurotransmitter release, neurotransmitter synthesis, and the cytoskeleton. In contrast, calcium/calmodulin-dependent protein kinase I, like cyclic GMP-dependent protein kinase, appears to be a protein kinase with a limited substrate specificity.

Most of the calcium/calmodulin-dependent protein kinases phosphorylate substrate proteins or serine residues although some are phosphorylated on threonine residues. The amino acids surrounding the phosphorylation sites of some well-characterized substrate proteins for various calcium/calmodulin-dependent protein kinases are shown in Figure 4.4. Although these substrates are phosphorylated by different calcium/calmodulin-dependent protein kinases, a basic amino acid preceding the serine by two amino acids is a common feature in all of the substrates. Using synthetic peptides, Kemp et al. (1982) have looked at the substrate specificities of myosin light chain kinase and concluded that the basic residues preceding the phosporylated amino acids are important determinants of the specificity of the kinase for the substrates. In addition, as for the cyclic nucleotide-dependent protein kinases, the primary amino acid sequence surrounding the phosphorylated amino acid probably is not the sole determinant of substrate specificity; secondary and tertiary structure may also play a major role in the substrate specificity of the calcium/calmodulin-dependent protein kinases.

PROTEIN KINASE	SUBSTRATE PROTEIN	AMINO ACID SEQUENCE
Calcium/calmodulin-dependent protein kinase II	Synapsin I	GLY – PRO – THR – ARG – GLN – ALA – SER(P) – GLN – ALA – GLY – PRO
Phosphorylase kinase	Phosphorylase	GLU – LYS – ARG – LYS – GLN – ILE – SER(P) – VAL – ARG – GLY – LEU – ALA – GLY – VAL
Myosin light-chain kinase	Myosin light chain kinase	ARG – PRO – GLN – ARG – ALA – THR – SER(P) – ASN – VAL – PHE – SER
Glycogen synthase kinase	Glycogen synthase (site 2)	PRO – LEU – SER – ARG – THR – LEU – SER(P) – VAL – SER – SER – LEU – PRO – GLY – LEU

Fig. 4.4. Amino acid sequences around the phosphorylation sites of physiological substrates for calcium/calmodulin-dependent protein kinases. SER(P) represents the amino acid that is phosphorylated (Czernik, Pang, & Greengard, in preparation; Cohen, 1980; Kemp et al., 1982; Soderling & Payne, 1981).

CALCIUM/PHOSPHOLIPID-DEPENDENT PROTEIN KINASE
(PROTEIN KINASE C)

Many neurotransmitters and hormones have been shown to increase the breakdown of inositol-containing phospholipids through interactions with specific receptors in the target cell membranes (Berridge, 1984; Berridge & Irvine, 1984). Binding of the neurotransmitters and hormones to their specific receptors, such as muscarinic cholinergic and α_1-adrenergic receptors, causes the rapid breakdown of triphosphatidylinositol into diacylglycerol and inositol trisphosphate by a triphosphatidylinositol-specific phosphodiesterase. The mechanism of the coupling of receptor activation to activation of this specific phosphodiesterase is not clear, although recent evidence has suggested that a guanine nucleotide-binding protein similar to the G proteins is involved (Cockcroft & Gomperts, 1985). Both products of phosphatidylinositol hydrolysis appear to have second messenger roles. Inositol trisphosphate is a soluble intracellular messenger that causes release of intracellular stores of calcium from the endoplasmic reticulum, while diacylglycerol acts as a second messenger within the plane of the membrane to activate calcium/phospholipid-dependent protein kinase (protein kinase C) in the presence of normal intracellular concentrations of calcium (Nishizuka, 1984). The molecular mechanism of the release of intracellular calcium by inositol trisphosphate is unknown. The calcium released from intracellular stores by inositol trisphosphate may play a role in the activation of protein kinase C (see below) as well as activate calcium/calmodulin-dependent protein kinases in the cell.

Protein kinase C was purified initially as a cyclic nucleotide-independent protein kinase that could be activated irreversibly by proteolysis (Inoue et al., 1977). It appeared, at first, that second messengers had no role in the regulation of its activity. This enzyme was later shown to be activated, reversibly, by calcium and phospholipid in the absence of calmodulin, establishing it as a new type of calcium-dependent protein kinase that does not require calmodulin (Takai et al., 1979). Further work has demonstrated that this enzyme is activated by diacylglycerol in the presence of phospholipid and low levels of calcium (Nishizuka, 1984). As indicated previously, diacylglycerol is one of the earliest products of neurotransmitter and hormone-stimulated phosphatidylinositol breakdown, and it therefore has been proposed that diacylglycerol is an intracellular second messenger.

Phorbol esters have diverse effects on cellular function. Protein kinase C has recently been demonstrated to be the major phorbol ester receptor in cells and may mediate many of these diverse effects of phorbol esters (Castagna et al., 1982; Niedel et al., 1983, Leach et al. 1983). Phorbol esters appear to activate protein kinase C by mimicking diacylglycerol (Nishizuka, 1984), and because they are membrane premeant, they have been extremely useful in studying the activation of this enzyme *in vivo*.

Protein kinase C is widely distributed in various tissues and is highly enriched in brain (Kuo et al., 1980; Minakuchi et al., 1981; Walaas et al., 1983a,b). When tissues are homogenized in the presence of divalent cation chelators, protein kinase C is found primarily in the soluble fraction. However, in the presence of activators such as calcium, diacylglycerol, or phorbol esters, the kinase is largely associated with the membrane fractions. This suggests that on physiological activation the enzyme may translocate from cytosol to membranes (Kraft & Anderson, 1983; Kikkawa et al., 1982).

The purified enzyme from brain is a protein of M_r 80,000 to 87,000 (Kikkawa et al., 1982). Partial proteolysis yields a calcium/phospholipid-independent protein kinase with an $M_r \sim 51,000$. It has been suggested that the intact enzyme contains a hydrophobic regulatory domain that interacts with the membrane phospholipid and calcium and a hydrophilic catalytic domain. Protein kinase C autophosphorylates in a calcium/phospholipid-dependent manner.

Protein kinase C is activated by micromolar levels of calcium in the presence of phospholipid, with phosphatidylserine being the most efficient (Takai et al., 1979). However, addition of small amounts of diacylglycerol or phorbol esters decreases the Ka for calcium to the $10^{-7}M$ range (Nishizuka, 1984). Diacylglycerol therefore activates the kinase at resting cell calcium levels and acts as a second messenger for neurotransmitters that activate phosphatidylinositol breakdown. It is possible that increases in the level of intracellular calcium may activate protein kinase C even in the absence of increased levels of diacylglycerol.

Protein kinase C appears to be a multifunctional protein kinase and, like the cyclic AMP-dependent enzyme and calcium/calmodulin-dependent protein kinase II, it has a broad substrate specificity. As will be shown in the following chapter, the ion channels known to be phosphorylated by protein kinase C include the nicotinic acetylcholine receptor and the voltage-dependent sodium channel. Protein kinase C also regulates the voltage-dependent calcium channel in *Aplysia* bag cell neurons, presumably by direct phosphorylation of the channel (see Chapters 7 and 11).

Most of the substrates phosphorylated by protein kinase C have been reported to be phosphorylated on serine residues although some are phosphorylated on threonine residues (Nishizuka, 1984). The enzyme has a substrate specificity distinct from that of the cyclic AMP-, cyclic GMP-, or the calcium/calmodulin-dependent protein kinases. However, protein kinase C and cyclic AMP-dependent protein kinase phosphorylate the same sites on histones (Nishizuka, 1980) and tyrosine hydroxylase (Albert et al., 1984). In addition, as in substrates for the cyclic AMP-, cyclic GMP-, and calcium/calmodulin-dependent protein kinase, the amino acid sequences around the phosphorylated serine or threonine residues of characterized substrate proteins for protein kinase C are very rich in the basic amino acids arginine and lysine (Nishizuka, 1980; Hunter et al., 1984).

TYROSINE-SPECIFIC PROTEIN KINASES

Tyrosine-specific protein kinases are a unique class of protein kinases that phosphorylate tyrosine residues exclusively (Sefton & Hunter, 1984). Tyrosine-specific protein kinases have not been demonstrated to be regulated by neurotransmitters or any identified second messengers, but they have been shown to be regulated directly by certain growth factors and peptide hormones. The membrane receptors for epidermal growth factor, platelet-derived growth factor and insulin are tyrosine-specific protein kinases that are directly activated by their respective physiological ligands (Cohen et al., 1980; Heldin et al., 1983; Kasuga et al., 1983). The brain has been reported to contain insulin receptors and may contain epidermal growth factor receptors, which suggests that receptor-stimulated tyrosine phosphorylation may be involved in the regulation of neuronal function.

Other tyrosine kinases include the viral gene products that mediate cell transformation by a number of retroviruses (Sefton & Hunter, 1984). The most well characterized of these is the SRC gene product pp60^{vsrc} of Rous sarcoma virus. This tyrosine kinase is homologous to a normal cellular enzyme, pp60^{csrc}, which is present in low levels in a variety of normal vertebrate cells. The level of pp60^{csrc} in vertebrate brain is higher than in any other nontransformed tissue (Barnekow et al., 1982; Cotton & Brugge, 1983). The presence of tyrosine kinase activity in brain and in other nonproliferating tissue suggests that tyrosine-specific phosphorylation may be involved in processes other than cell proliferation.

Tyrosine-specific protein kinases appear to have a relatively limited substrate specificity. Many endogenous substrates for tyrosine-specific protein kinases have been well characterized and include cytoskeletal proteins and glycolytic enzymes (Sefton & Hunter, 1984) and the nicotinic acetylcholine receptor (see Chapter 5). The substrate specificity of tyrosine-specific kinases, like that of the serine- and threonine-specific protein kinases, depends on the primary sequence of the amino acids surrounding the phosphorylated residue. However, in contrast with phosphorylatable serine and threonine residues, the tyrosine residues on many well-characterized substrates of tyrosine-specific protein kinases are preceded by the acidic amino acids glutamic acid and aspartic acid (Sefton & Hunter, 1984; Patschinsky et al., 1982). Studies using synthetic peptides as substrates for the tyrosine kinases have shown that the acidic amino acid residues are important in the recognition of these peptides by the tyrosine kinases (Hunter, 1982; Pike et al., 1982).

CONCLUSIONS

The modulation of ion channel activity is one of the major mechanisms in the regulation of neuronal function. In this chapter, the biochemical mechanisms involved in the regulation of ion channel function by neurotransmitters and hormones have been reviewed. In most cases, the modulatory hormone or neurotransmitter binds to a specific membrane receptor that regulates the intracellular levels of second messenger substances such as cyclic AMP, cyclic GMP, calcium, or diacylglycerol. Many of the actions of the second messengers are mediated by specific protein kinases, which are activated by changes in the intracellular concentrations of these second messengers. The activated protein kinase then phosphorylates specific substrate proteins in the target cells. Ultimately, the physiological response evoked in target cells depends on what substrate proteins are phosphorylated in the cell. Presumably, when neurotransmitters, second messengers, or protein kinases modulate ion channel function, the ion channel itself or a closely associated protein is one of the specific substrates for these protein kinases.

REFERENCES

Adams, W.B. and Levitan, I.B. (1982) Intracellular injection of protein kinase inhibitor blocks the serotonin-induced increase of K conductance in *Aplysia* neuron R14. *Proc, Natl, Acad. Sci. USA 79,* 3877–3880.

Adelstein, R.S. (1982) Calmodulin and the regulation of the actin-myosin interaction in smooth muscle and non-muscle cells. *Cell 30,* 349–350.

Albert, K.A., Helmer-Matyjek, E., Nairn, A.C., Muller, T.H., Haycock, J.W., Greene, L.A., Goldstein, M., and Greengard, P. (1984) Calcium/phospholipid-dependent protein kinase (protein kinase C) phosphorylates and activates tyrosine hydroxylase. *Proc. Natl. Acad. Sci. USA 81,* 7713–7717.

Albert, K.A., Wu, W.C.S., Nairn, A.C., and Greengard, P. (1984b) Inhibition by calmodulin of calcium/phospholipid-dependent protein phosphorylation. *Proc. Natl. Acad. Sci. USA 81,* 3622–3625.

Alkon, D.L., Acosta-Urguidi, J., Olds, J., Kuzma G., and Neary, J.T. (1983) Protein kinase injection reduces voltage-dependent potassium currents. *Science 219,* 303–306.

Barnekow, A., Schartl, M., Anders, F., and Bauer, H. (1982) Identification of a fish protein associated with a kinase activity and related to the Rous sarcoma virus transforming protein. *Cancer Res. 42,* 2429–2433.

Beavo, J.A., Bechtel, P.J., and Krebs, E.G. (1975) Mechanisms of control for cyclic AMP-dependent protein kinase from skeletal muscle. *Adv. Cyclic Nucleotide Res. 5,* 2241–251.

Bennett, M.K., Erondu, N.E., and Kennedy, M.B. (1983) *J. Biol. Chem. 258,* 12735–12744.

Berridge, M.J. (1984) Inositol trisphosphate and diacylglycerol as second messengers. *Biochem. J. 220,* 345–360.

Berridge, M.J. and Irvine, R.F. (1984) Inositol trisphosphate, a novel second messenger in cellular signal transduction. *Nature 312,* 315–321.

Browning, M.D. and Greengard, P. (1984) A family of synaptic vesicle-associated phosphoproteins: Synapsin 1a, synapsin 1b, protein IIIa, and protein IIIb. *Soc. Neurosci. Abstr. 10,* 196.

Browning, M.D., Huganir, R., and Greengard, P. (1985) Protein phosphorylation and neuronal function. *J. Neurochem., 45,* 11–23.

Burgoyne, R.D. (1983) Regulation of the muscarinic acetylcholine receptor: Effects of phosphorylating conditions on agonist and antagonist binding. *J. Neurochem. 40,* 324–331.

Casnellie, J.E., and Greengard, P. (1974) Guanosine 3′:5′-cyclic monophosphate-dependent phosphorylation of endogenous substrate proteins in membranes of mammalian smooth muscle. *Proc. Natl. Acad. Sci. USA 71,* 1891–1895.

Cassel, D. and Pfeuffer, T. (1978) Mechanism of cholera toxin action: Covalent modification of the guanyl nucleotide-binding protein of adenylate cyclase. *Proc. Natl. Acad. Sci. USA 75,* 2669–2673.

Castagna, M., Takai, Y., Kaibuchi, K., Sano, K., Kikkawa, U., and Nishizuka, Y. (1982) Direct activation of calcium-activated, phospholipid-dependent protein kinase by tumor-promoting phorbol esters. *J. Biol. Chem. 257,* 7847–7851.

Castellucci, V.F., Kandel, E.R., Schwartz, J.H., Wilson, F.D., Nairn, A.C., and Greengard, P. (1980) Intracellular injection of the catalytic subunit of cyclic AMP-dependent protein kinase simulates facilitation of transmitter release underlying behavioral sensitization in *Aplysia*. *Proc. Natl. Acad. Sci. USA 77,* 7492–7496.

Castellucci, V.F., Nairn, A., Greengard, P., Schwartz, J.H., and Kandel, E.R. (1982) Inhibitor of adenosine 3′:5′-monophosphate-dependent protein kinase blocks presynaptic facilitation in *Aplysia*. *J. Neurosci. 2,* 1673–1681.

Cheung, W.Y. (1980) Calmodulin plays a pivotal role in cellular regulation. *Science 207*, 19–27.

Cockcroft, S., and Gomperts, B.D. (1985) Role of guanine nucleotide binding protein in the activation of polyphosphoinositide phosphodiesterase. *Nature 314*, 534–536.

Cohen, P. (1980) Well established systems of enzyme regulation by reversible phosphorylation. *Mol. Aspects Cell Reg. 1*, 1–10.

Cohen, S., Carpenter, G., and King, L., Jr. (1980) Epidermal growth factor-receptor-protein kinase interactions. *J. Biol. Chem. 235*, 4834–4842.

Corbin, J.D., Sugden, P.H., Lincoln, T.M., and Keely, S.L. (1977) Compartmentalization of adenosine 3':5'-monophosphate and adenosine 3':5'-monophosphate-dependent protein kinase in heart tissue. *J. Biol. Chem. 252*, 3854–3861.

Costa, M.R., Casnellie, J.E., and Catterall, W.A. (1982) Selective phosphorylation of the alpha subunit of the sodium channel by cAMP-dependent protein kinase. *J. Biol. Chem. 257*, 7918–7921.

Costa, M.R. and Catterall, W.A. (1984a) Cyclic AMP-dependent phosphorylation of the a-subunit of the sodium channel in synaptic nerve ending particles. *J. Biol. Chem. 259*, 8210–8218.

Costa, M.R., and Catterall, W.A. (1984b) Phosphorylation in the a subunit of the sodium channel by protein kinase C. *Cell. Mol. Neurobiol. 4*, 291–297.

Cotton, P.C. and Brugge, J.S. (1983) Neural tissues express high levels of the cellular src gene product pp60. *Mol. Cell Biol. 3*, 1157–1162.

Curtis, B.M., Catterall, W.A (1985) Phosphorylation of the calcium antagonist receptor of the voltage-sensitive calcium channel by cAMP-dependent protein kinase. *Proc. Natl. Acad. Sci. USA 82*, 2528– 2532.

Daly, J.W. (1984) Forskolin, adenylate cyclase and cell physiology: An overview. In *Advances in Cyclic Nucleotide and Protein Phosphorylation Reseach*. Vol. 17. (ed. P. Greengard), Raven Press, New York.

De Camilli, P., Miller, P.E., Levitt, P., Walter, U., and Greengard, P. (1984) Anatomy and projections of cerebellar Purkinje cells in the rat determined by a specific immunohistochemical marker. *Neuroscience 11*, 761–817.

de Jonge, H.R., and Rosen, O.M. (1977) Self-phosphorylation of cyclic guanosine 3':5'-monophosphate-dependent protein kinase from bovine lung. *J. Biol. Chem. 252*, 2780–2783.

Demaille, J.G. and Pechere, J.-F. (1983) The control of contractility by protein phosphorylation. *Adv. Cyclic Nucleotide Res. 15*, 337–371.

dePeyer, J.E., Cachelin, A.B., Levitan, I.B., and Reuter, H. (1982) Ca^{2+}-activated K^+ conductance in internally perfused snail neurons is enhanced by protein phosphorylation. *Proc. Natl. Acad. Sci. USA 79*, 4207–4211.

DeRiemer, S.A., Strong, J.A., Albert, K.A., Greengard, P., and Kaczmarek, L.K. (1985) Enhancement of calcium current in *Aplysia* neurons by phorbol ester and protein kinase C. *Nature 313*, 313–316.

Edelman, A.M., Raese, J.D., Lazar, M.A., and Barchas, J.D. (1981) Tyrosine hydroxylase: Studies on the phosphorylation of a purified preparation of the brain enzyme by the cyclic AMP-dependent protein kinase. *J. Pharmacol. Exp. Ther. 216*, 647–653.

Fesenko, E.F., Kolesnikov, S.S., and Lyubarsky, A.L. (1985) Induction by cyclic GMP of cationic conductance in plasma membrane of retinal rod outer segment. *Nature 313*, 310–313.

Gill, D.M. and Meren, R. (1978) ADP-ribosylation of membrane proteins catalyzed by cholea toxin: Basis of the activation of adenylate cyclase. *Proc. Natl. Acad. Sci. USA 75*, 3050–3054.

Gilman, A.G. (1984) G proteins and dual control of adenylate cyclase. *Cell 36*, 577–579.

Glass, D.B. and Krebs, E.G. (1979) Comparison of the substrate specificity of adenosine 3^+:5 monophosphate- and guanosine 3':5'-monophosphate-dependent protein kinases. *J. Biol. Chem. 254*, 9728–9738.

Goldenring, J.R., Gonzalez, B., and DeLorenzo, R.J. (1982) Isolation of brain Ca-calmodulin tubulin kinase containing calmodulin binding proteins. *Biochem. Biophys. Res. Commun. 108*, 421–428.

Goldenring, J.R., McGuire, J.S., and Delorenzo, R.J. (1984) Identification of the major postsynaptic density protein as homologous with the major calmodulin-binding subunit of a calmodulin-dependent protein kinase. *J. Neurochem. 42*, 1077–1084.

Gordon, A.S., Davis, C.G., Milfay, D., and Diamond, I. (1977a) Phosphorylation of acetylcholine receptor by endogenous membrane protein kinase in receptor-enriched membranes of *Torpeda californica*. *Nature 267*, 539–540.

Gorelick, F.S., Cohn, J.A., Freedman, S.D., Delahunt, N.G., Gershoni, J.M., and Jamieson, J.D. (1983) Calmodulin-stimulated protein kinase activity from rat pancreas. *J. Cell. Biol. 97*, 1294–1298.

Greengard, P. (1976) Possible role for cyclic nucleotides and phosphorylation of membrane proteins in the postsynaptic actions of neurotransmitters. *Nature London 260*, 101–108.

Greengard, P. (1978) Phosphorylated proteins as physiological effectors. *Science 199*, 146–152.

Greengard, P. (1981) Intracellular signals in the brain. *Harvey Lecture Series 75*, 277–331.

Hathaway, D.R., Adelstein, R.S., and Klee, C.B. (1981) Interaction of calmodulin with myosin light chain kinase and cAMP-dependent protein kinase in bovine brain. *J. Biol. Chem. 256*, 8183–8189.

Heldin, C.-H., Ek, B., and Ronnstrand, L. (1983) Characterization of the receptor for platelet-derived growth factor on human fibroblasts. *J. Biol. Chem. 16*, 10054–10061.

Hofmann, F., Beavo, J.A., Bechtel, P.J., and Krebs, E.G. (1975) Comparison of adenosine 3':5'-monophosphate-dependent protein kinases from rabbit skeletal and bovine heart muscles. *J. Biol. Chem. 250*, 7795–7801.

Hofmann, F., Bechtel, P.J., and Krebs, E.G. (1977) Concentrations of cyclic AMP-dependent protein kinase subunits in various tissues. *J. Biol. Chem. 252*, 1441–1447.

Hofmann, F. and Flockerzi, V. (1983) Characterization of phosphorylated and native cGMP-dependent protein kinase. *Eur. J. Biochem. 130*, 599–603.

Huang, C.-K., Browning, M.D., and Greengard, P. (1982) Purification and characterization of protein IIIb, a mammalian brain phosphoprotein. *J. Biol. Chem. 257*, 66524–66525.

Huganir, R.L., Miles, K., and Greengard, P. (1984) Phosphorylation of the nicotinic acetylcholine receptor by an endogenous tyrosine-specific protein kinase. *Proc. Natl. Acad. Sci. USA 81*, 6963–6972.

Hunter, T. (1982) Synthetic peptide substrates for a tyrosine protein kinase. *J. Biol. Chem. 257*, 4843–4848.

Hunter, T., Ling, N., and Cooper, J.A. (1984) Protein kinase C phosphorylation of the EGF receptor at a threonine residue close to the cytoplasmic face of the plasma membrane. *Nature 311*, 450–483.

Ingebritsen, T.S., and Cohen, P. (1983) Protein phosphatases: Properties and role in cellular regulation. *Science 221*, 331–338.

Inoue, M., Kishimoto, A., Takai, Y., and Nishizuka, Y. (1976) Guanosine 3':5'-monophosphate-dependent protein kinase from silkworm, properties of a catalytic fragment obtained by limited proteolysis. *J. Biol. Chem. 252*, 4476–4478.

Inoue, M., Kishimoto, A., Takai, Y., and Nishizuka, Y. (1977) Studies on a cyclic nucleotide-independent protein kinase and its proenzyme in mammalian tissues. II. Proenzyme and its activation by calcium-dependent protease from rat brain. *J. Biol. Chem. 251,* 7610–7616.

Joh, T.H., Park, D.H., and Reis, D.J. (1978) Direct phosphorylation of brain tyrosine hydroxylase by cyclic AMP-dependent protein kinase: Mechanism of enzyme activation. *Proc. Natl. Acad. Sci. USA 75,* 4744–4748.

Johnson, W.M., Maeno, H., and Greengard, P. (1971) Phosphorylation of endogenous protein of rat brain by cyclic adenosine 3':5'-monophosphate-dependent protein kinase. *J. Biol. Chem. 246,* 7731–7739.

Kaczmarek, L.K., Jennings, K.R., Strumwasser, F., Nairn, A.C., Walter, U., Wilson, F.D., and Greengard, P. (1980) Microinjection of catalytic subunit of cyclic AMP-dependent protein kinase enhances calcium action potentials of bag cell neurons in cell culture. *Proc. Natl. Acad. Sci USA 77,* 7487–7491.

Kasuga, M., Fujita-Yamaguchi, Y., Blithe, D.L., and Kahn, C.R. (1983) Tyrosine-specific protein kinase activity is associated with the purified insulin receptor. *Proc. Natl. Acad. Sci. USA 80,* 2137–2141.

Katada, T. and Ui, M. (1982) ADP ribosylation of the specific membrane protein of C6 cells by islet-activating protein associated with modification of adenylate cyclase activity. *J. Biol Chem. 257,* 7210–7216.

Kelly, P.T., Cotman, C.W., and Largen, M. (1979) Cyclic AMP-stimulated protein kinases at brain synaptic junctions. *J. Biol Chem. 254,* 1564–1575.

Kelly, P.T., McGuinness, T.L., and Greengard, P. (1984) Evidence that the major postsynaptic density protein is a component of a Ca/calmodulin-dependent protein kinase. *Proc. Natl. Acad. Sci. USA 81,* 945–949.

Kemp, B.E., Bylund, D.V., Huang, T.S., and Krebs, E.G. (1975) Substrate specificity of the cAMP-dependent protein kinase. *Proc. Natl. Acad. Sci. USA 72,* 3448–3452.

Kemp, B.E., Graves, D.J., Benjamin, E., and Krebs, E.G. (1977) Role of multiple basic residues in determining the substrate specificity of cyclic AMP-dependent protein kinase. *J. Biol Chem. 252,* 4888–4894.

Kemp, B.E., Pearson, R.B., and House, C. (1982) Phosphorylation of a synthetic heptadecapeptide by smooth muscle myosin light chain kinase. *J. Biol Chem. 257,* 13349–13353.

Kemp, B.E., Pearson, R.B., and House, C. (1983) Role of basic residues in the phosphorylation of synthetic peptides by myosin light chain kinase. *Biochemistry 80,* 7471–7475.

Kennedy, M.B., Bennett, M.K., and Erondu, N.E. (1983) Biochemical and immunochemical evidence that the "major postsynaptic density protein" is a subunit of a calmodulin-dependent protein kinase. *Proc. Natl. Acad. Sci. USA 80,* 7357–7361.

Kikkawa, U., Takai, Y., Minakuchi, R., Inohara, S., and Nishizuka, Y. (1982) Calcium-activated, phospholipid-dependent protein kinase from rat brain. Subcellular distribution, purification, and properties. *J. Biol Chem. 257,* 13341–13348.

Klee, C.B., Crouch, T.H., and Richman, P.G. (1980) Calmodulin, *Ann. Rev. Biochem. 49,* 489–515.

Kraft, A.S. and Anderson, W.B. (1983) Phorbol esters increase the amount of Ca, phospholipid-dependent protein kinase associated with plasma membrane. *Nature 301,* 621–623.

Krebs, E.G., and Beavo, J.A. (1979) Phosphorylation-dephosphorylation of enzymes. *Annu. Rev. Biochem. 48,* 923–959.

Kuhn, D.M., and Lovenberg, W. (1982) Role of calmodulin in the activation of tryptophan hydroxylase. *Fed. Proc. 41,* 2258–2264.

Kuo, J.F. (1974) Guanosine 3':5'-monophosphate-dependent protein kinase in mammalian tissues. *Proc. Natl. Acad. Sci. USA 71,* 4037–4041.

Kuo, J.F., Andersson, R.G.G., Wise, B.C., Mackerlova, L., Salomonsson, I., Brackett, N.L., Katoh, N., Shoji, M., and Wrenn, R.W., (1980) Calcium-dependent protein kinase: Widespread occurrence in various tissues and phyla of the animal kingdom and comparison of effects of phospholipid, calmodulin, trifluoperazine. *Proc. Natl. Acad. Sci. USA 77,* 7039–7043.

Kuo, J.F., and Greengard, P. (1969) Cyclic nucleotide-dependent protein kinases. IV. Widespread occurrence of adenosine 3':5'-monophosphate-dependent protein kinase in various tissues and phyla of the animal kingdom. *Proc. Natl. Acad. Sci. USA 64,* 1349–1355.

Kuo, J.F., and Greengard, P. (1970) Cyclic nucleotide-dependent protein kinases. VI. Isolation and partial purification of a protein kinase activated by guanosine 3',5'monophosphate. *J. Biol Chem. 245,* 2493–2498.

Leach, K.L., James, M.L., and Blumberg, P.M. (1983) Characterization of a specific phorbol ester aporeceptor in mouse brain cytosol. *Proc. Natl. Acad. Sci. USA 80,* 4208–4212.

Lincoln, T.M. and Corbin, J.D. (1983) Characterization and biological role of the cGMP-dependent protein kinase. *Adv. Cyclic Nucleotide Res. 15,* 139–192.

Lincoln, T.M., Flockhart, D.A., and Corbin, J.D. (1978) Studies on the structure and mechanism of activation of the guanosine 3':5'-monophosphate-dependent protein kinase. *J. Biol Chem. 253,* 6002–6009.

Lincoln, T.M., Hall, C.C., Park, C.R., and Corbin, J.D. (1976) Guanosine 3':5'-cyclic monophosphate binding proteins in rat tissues. *Proc. Natl. Acad. Sci. USA 73,* 2559–2563.

Lohmann, S.M., Walter, U., and Greengard, P. (1980) Identification of endogenous substrate proteins for cAMP-dependent protein kinase in bovine brain. *J. Biol Chem. 255,* 9985–9992.

Lohmann, S.M., Walter, U., Miller, P.E., Greengard, P., and De Camilli, P. (1981) Immunohistochemical localization of cyclic GMP-dependent protein kinase in mammalian brain. *Proc. Natl. Acad. Sci. USA 78,* 653–657.

Maeno, H., Johnson, E.M., and Greengard, P. (1971) Subcellular distribution of adenosine 3':5'-monophosphate-dependent protein kinase in rat brain. *J. Biol Chem. 246,* 134–142.

McGuinness, T.L., Lai, Y., Greengard, P., Woodget, J.R., and Cohen, P. (1983) A multifunctional calmodulin-dependent protein kinase: Similarities between skeletal muscle glycogen synthase and brain synapsin I kinase. *FEBS Lett. 163,* 329–334.

McGuinness, T.L., Lai, Y., Greengard, P. (1985) Ca/calmodulin-dependent protein kinase II. *J. Biol Chem. 260,* 1696–1704.

Minakuchi, R., Takai, Y., Yu, B., and Nishizuka, Y. (1981) Widespread occurrence of calcium activated, phospholipid-dependent protein kinase in mammalian tissues. *J. Biochem. 89,* 1651–1654.

Nairn, A.C. and Greengard, P. (1983) Purification and characterization of brain Ca^{2+}/calmodulin-dependent protein kinase I that phosphorylates synapsin I. *Soc. Neurosci. Abstr. 9,* 1029.

Nairn, A.C., Hemmings, H.C., Jr., and Greengard, P. (1985) Protein kinases in the brain. *Annu. Rev. Biochem. 54,* 931–976.

Nestler, E.J., and Greengard, P. (1983) Protein phosphorylation in the brain. *Nature 305,* 538–588.

Nestler, E.J. and Greengard, P. (1984) *Protein Phosphorylation in the Nervous System.* John Wiley & Sons, New York.

Nestler, E.J., Walaas, S.I., and Greengard, P. (1984) Neuronal phosphoproteins: Physiological and clinical implications. *Science 225,* 1357–1364.

Niedel, J.E., Kuhn, L.J., and Vandenbark, G.R. (1983) Phorbol diester receptor copurifies with protein kinase C. *Proc. Natl. Acad. Sci. USA 80*, 36–40.

Nimmo, H.G., and Cohen, P. (1977) Hormonal control of cAMP-dependent protein kinase. *Adv. Cyclic Nucleotide Res. 8*, 145–266.

Nishizuka, Y. (1984) The role of protein kinase C in cell surface signal transduction and tumour promotion. *Nature 308*, 693–698.

Nishizuka, Y. (1980) Three multifunctional protein kinase systems in transmembrane control. In *Molecular Biology Biochemistry and Biophysics, Vol. 32, Chemical Recognition in Biology*. (eds. F. Chapeville and A.-L. Hernani), Springer-Verlag, Berlin and Heidelberg.

Noda, M., Takahashi, H., Tanabe, T., Toyosato, M., Furutani, Y., Hirose, T., Asai, M., Inayama, S., Miyata, T., and Numa, S. (1982) Primary structure of α subunit precursor of *Torpedo californica* acetylcholine receptor deduced from cDNA sequence. *Nature 299*, 793–797.

Osterrieder, W., Brum, B., Hescheler, J., Trautwein, W., Flockerzi, V., and Hofman, F. (1982) Injection of subunits of cyclic AMP-dependent protein kinase into cardiac myocytes modulates Ca current. *Nature 298*, 576–578.

Palfrey, H.C., Rothlein, W.J.E., and Greengard, P. (1983) Calmodulin-dependent protein kinase and associated substrates in *Torpedo* electric organ. *J. Biol Chem. 258j*, 9496–9503.

Patschinsky, T., Hunter, T., Esch, F.S., Cooper, J.A., and Sefton, B.M. (1982) Analysis of the sequence of amino acids surrounding sites of tyrosine phosphorylation. *Proc. Natl. Acad. Sci. USA 79*, 973–977.

Pike, L.J., Gallis, B., Casnellie, J.E., Bornstein, P., and Krebs, E.G. (1982) Epidermal growth factor stimulates the phosphorylation of synthetic tyrosine-containing peptides by A431 cell membranes. *Proc. Natl. Acad. Sci. USA 79*, 1443–1447.

Rall, T.W., Sutherland, E.W., and Berthet, J. (1957) Relationship of epinephrine and glucogen on the reactivation of phosphorylase in liver homogenates. *J. Biol Chem. 224*, 463–475.

Reimann, E.M., Walsh, D.A., and Krebs, E.G. (1971) Purification and properties of rabbit skeletal muscle adenosine 3':5'-monophosphate-dependent protein kinase. *J. Biol Chem. 246*, 1986–1995.

Robison, G.A., Butcher, R.W., and Sutherland, E.W. (1971) *Cyclic AMP*. Academic Press, New York.

Rodbell, M. (1980) The role of hormone receptors and GTP-regulatory proteins in membrane transduction. *Nature 284*, 17–22.

Rosen, O.M., Erlichmann, J., and Rubin, C.S. (1975) Molecular structure and characterization of bovine heart protein kinase. *Adv. Cyclic Nucleotide Res. 5*, 253–263.

Ross, E.M., and Gilman, A. (1980) Biochemical properties of hormone-sensitive adenylate cyclase. *Annu. Rev. Biochem. 49*, 533–564.

Rubin, C.S., Rangel-Aldao, R., Sarkar, D., Erlichman, J., and Fleischer, N. (1979) Characterization and comparison of membrane-associated and cytosolic cAMP-dependent protein kinases. *J. Biol Chem. 254*, 3797–3805.

Schlichter, D.J., Detre, J.A., Aswad, D.W., Cherazi, B., and Greengard, P. (1980) Localization of cyclic GMP-dependent protein kinase and substrate in mammalian cerebellum. *Proc. Natl. Acad. Sci. USA 77*, 5537–5541.

Schulman, H. and Greengard, P. (1978a) Ca-dependent protein phosphorylation system in membranes from various tissues, and its activation by "calcium-dependent regulator." *Proc. Natl. Acad. Sci. USA 75*, 5432k–5436.

Schulman, H. and Greengard, P. (1978b) Stimulation of brain membrane protein phosphory-
    lation by calcium and an endogenous heat-stable protein. *Nature 271*, 478–479.
Sefton, B.M. and Hunter, T. (1984) Tyrosine protein kinases. In *Advances in Cyclic Nucleo-
    tide and Protein Phosphorylation Research*. (eds. P. Greengard and G.A. Robison),
    18, 195–226. Raven Press, New York.
Soderling, T.R., and Payne, M.E. (1981) Rabbit liver calmodulin-dependent glycogen syn-
    thase kinase. *Cold Spring Harbor Conf. Cell Prolif. 8*, 413–423.
Stadel, J.M., Nambi, P., Short, R.G.E., Sawyer, D.J., Caton, M.G., and Lefkowitz, R.J.
    (1983) Catecholamine-induced desensitization of turkey erythrocyte adenylate cyclase
    is associated with phosphorylation of the b-adrenergic receptor. *Proc. Natl. Acad. Sci.
    USA 80*, 3173–3177.
Stryer, L. (1983) Transducin and the cyclic GMP phosphodiesterase: Amplifier proteins in
    vision. *Cold Spring Harbor Symp. Quant. Biol. 48*, 841–852.
Sutherland, E.W. and Rall, T.W. (1958) Fractionation and characterization of a cyclic aden-
    osine ribonucleotide formed by tissue particles. *J. Biol Chem. 232*, 1077–2091.
Takai, Y., Kishimoto, A., Iwasa, Y., Kawahara, Y., Mori, T., and Nishizuka, Y. (1979)
    Calcium-dependent activation of a multifunctional protein kinase by membrane phos-
    pholipids. *J. Biol Chem. 254*, 3692–3695.
Takio, K., Wade, R.D., Smith, S.B., Krebs, E.G., Walsh, K.A., and Titani, K. (1984)
    Guanosine cyclic 3′,5′-phosphate dependent protein kinase, a chimeric protein homol-
    ogous with two separate protein families. *Biochemistry 23*, 4207–4212.
Teichberg, V.I., and Changeux, J.-P. (1977) Evidence for protein phosphorylation and de-
    phosphorylation in membrane fragments isolated from the electric organs of *Electro-
    phoricus electricus*. *FEBS Lett. 74*, 76.
Teichberg, V.I., Sobel, A., and Changeux, J.P. (1977) In vitro phosphorylation of the acetyl-
    choline receptor. *Nature 267*, 540–542.
Theurkauf, W.E., and Vallee, R.B. (1982) Molecular characterization of the cAMP-dependent
    protein kinase bound to microtubule-associated protein 2. *J. Biol. Chem. 257*, 3284–
    3290.
Ueda, T. and Greengard, P. (1977) Adenosine 3′:5′-monophosphate-regulated phosphoprotein
    system of neuronal membranes. I. Solubilization, purification, and some properties of
    an endogenous phosphoprotein. *J. Biol. Chem. 252*, 5155–5163.
Ueda, T., Greengard, P., Berzins, K., Cohen, R.S., Blomberg, F., Grab. D.J., and Siekevitz,
    P. (1979) Subcellular distribution in cerebral cortex of two proteins phosphorylated by
    a cAMP-dependent protein kinase. *J. Cell. Biol. 83*, 308–319.
Ueda, T., Maeno, H., and Greengard, P. (1973) Regulation of endogenous phosphorylation
    of specific proteins in synaptic membrane fractions from rat brain by adenosine 3′:5′-
    monophosphate, *J. Biol. Chem. 248*, 8295–8305.
Vallee, R.B., DiBartolomeis, M.J., and Theurkauf, W.E. (1981) A protein kinase bound to
    the projection portion of MAP 2 (microtubule-associated protein 2). *J. Cell Biol. 90*,
    568–576.
Walaas, S.I., Nairn, A.C., and Greengard, P. (1983a) Regional distribution of calcium- and
    cyclic AMP-regulated protein phosphorylation systems in mammalian brain. I. Partic-
    ulate systems. *J. Neurosci. 3*, 291–301.
Walaas, S.I., Nairn, A.C., and Greengard, P. (1983b) Regional distribution of calcium- and
    cyclic AMP-regulated protein phosphorylation systems in mammalian brain. II. Soluble
    systems. *J. Neurosci. 3*, 302–311.
Walsh, D.A., Perkins, J.P., and Krebs, E.G. (1968) An adenosine 3′:5′-monophosphate-de-
    pendent protein kinase from rabbit skeletal muscle. *J. Biol. Chem. 243*, 3763–3774.
Walsh, P.A., Ashby, C.D., Gonzalez, C., Calkins, D., Fischer, E., and Krebs, E.G. (1971)

Purification and characterization of a protein kinase inhibitor of adenosine 3':5'-monophosphate-dependent protein kinases. *J. Biol. Chem. 246*, 1977–1985.

Walsh, P.A., Dabrowska, R., Hinkins, S., and Hartshorne, D.J. (1982) Calcium-independent myosin light chain kinase of smooth muscle preparation by limited chymotryptic digestion of the calcium ion dependent enzyme, purification, and characterization. *Biochemistry 21*, 1919–1923.

Walter, U. (1981) Distribution of cyclic GMP-dependent protein kinase in various rat tissues and cell lines determined by a sensitive and specific radioimmunoassay. *Eur. J. Biochem. 118*, 339–346.

Walter, U. and Greengard, P. (1981) Cyclic AMP-dependent and cyclic GMP-dependent protein kinases of nervous tissue. *Curr. Top. Cell. Reg. 19*, 219–256.

Walter, U., Kanof, P., Schulman H., and Greengard, P. (1978) Adenosine 3':5'-monophosphate receptor proteins in mammalian brain. *J. Biol. Chem. 253*, 6275–6280.

Walter, U., Uno, I., A.Y.-C., Liu, and Greengard, P. (1977) Identification, characterization and quantitative measurement of cyclic AMP receptor proteins in cytosol of various tissues using a photoaffinity ligand. *J. Biol. Chem. 252*, 6494–6500.

Wise, B.C., Guidotti, A., and Costa, E. (1983) Phosphorylation induces a decrease in the biological activity of the protein inhibitor (GABA-modulin) of γ-aminobutyric acid binding sites. *Proc. Natl. Acad. Sci. USA 80*, 886–890.

Yamauchi, T. and Fujisawa, H. (1981) A calmodulin-dependent protein that is involved in the activation of tryptophan 5, monooxygenase is specifically distributed in brain tissues. *FEBS Lett. 129*, 117–119.

5

Phosphorylation of Purified Ion Channel Proteins

RICHARD L. HUGANIR

Recent studies, many of which are described in this volume, have provided direct evidence that protein phosphorylation plays a role in modulating the activity of voltage-dependent potassium and calcium channels. But it has not been possible to determine whether or not the ion channels are directly phosphorylated since these particular channels have not been chemically identified. It may be that protein phosphorylation regulates modulator proteins or enzymes which, in turn, regulate the activity of the ion channel.

In contrast, two ion channels that have been purified and extensively characterized biochemically, the nicotinic acetylcholine receptor and the voltage-dependent sodium channel, are both known to be directly phosphorylated by multiple protein kinases, though the role of this phosphorylation in the regulation of their function is not known. In addition, recent studies have demonstrated that a purified preparation of the calcium channel antagonist receptor, which may be a component of the voltage-dependent calcium channel, is phosphorylated by cyclic AMP-dependent protein kinase. This chapter discusses the biochemical details of the phosphorylation of these three identified ion channels.

THE NICOTINIC ACETYLCHOLINE RECEPTOR

The nicotinic acetylcholine receptor is a neurotransmitter-regulated ion channel that mediates the depolarization of the postsynaptic membrane of nicotinic cholinergic synapses. Acetylcholine released from the presynaptic nerve terminal binds to the nicotinic acetylcholine receptor in the postsynaptic membrane. This causes the rapid opening of an ion channel that is permeable to sodium and potassium and other cations. The resulting depolarization of the membrane may trigger an action potential in the postsynaptic cell. The relative ease of electrophysiological studies at the neuromuscular junction as well as the abundance of the nicotinic acetylcholine receptor in the electric organs of electric fish have made this receptor the most completely characterized neurotransmitter receptor and ion channel in biology today. The acetyl-

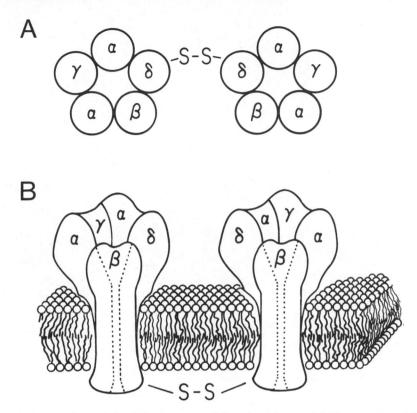

Fig. 5.1. Schematic models of the structure of the nicotinic acetylcholine receptor. (A) Arrangement of the five subunits around the central pit, as viewed from above the plane of the membrane; (B) cross section of the receptor in the plane of the membrane.

choline receptor has provided an excellent model system for the study of the structure, function, and regulation of membrane receptors and ion channels (Changeux, 1984).

Postsynaptic membranes highly enriched in the nicotinic acetylcholine receptor can be isolated from the electric organs of *Electrophorus electricus* and *Torpedo* and from mammalian skeletal muscle (Changeux, 1984). The nicotinic receptor can be solubilized from these postsynaptic membrane preparations and has been purified to homogeneity. The purified receptor is an M_r–255,000 pentameric complex that consists of four types of subunits, $\alpha(M_r$–40,000), $\beta(M_r$–50,000), $\gamma(M_r$–60,000) and $\delta(M_r$–65,000) in the stoichiometry of $\alpha_2\beta\gamma\delta$ (Reynolds & Karlin, 1979). The purified receptor is biologically functional when reconstituted into phospholipid vesicles, and it displays all the known biological properties of the nicotinic acetylcholine receptor in the native membrane (Anholt, 1981; Huganir & Racker, 1982; Tank et al., 1983). Although the four subunits are distinct and are encoded by different genes, they are highly homologous in amino acid sequence and structure. Each subunit spans the membrane and it has been proposed that the five subunits are arranged in a pentameric rosette around a central ion channel (Figure 5.1). In addition, based on an

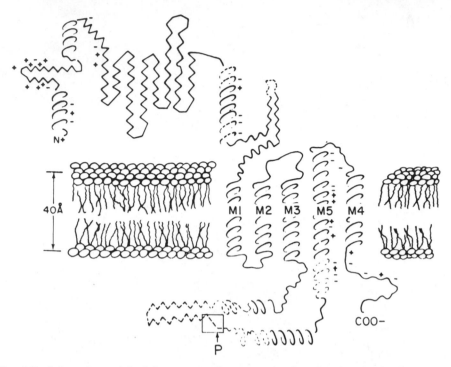

Fig. 5.2. Schematic model of the transmembrane topography of each subunit of the acetyl-choline receptor. P indicates the area of each subunit that is proposed to be phosphorylated by the various protein kinases (Adapted from Finer-Moore and Stroud, 1984).

analysis of the amino acid sequence of each subunit for hydrophobic and hydrophilic regions, models have been proposed for the transmembrane structure of each subunit (Noda et al., 1983b; Claudio et al., 1983; Devillers-Thiery et al., 1983). Each subunit has a large extracellular N-terminal region and four hydrophobic transmembrane segments (M_1–M_4) (Figure 5.2). A fifth transmembrane segment has recently been proposed (Finer-Moore & Stroud, 1984) to form an amphipathic α-helix (M_5). The hydrophobic half of the amphipathic α-helix is thought to face the membrane while the hydrophilic half lines the ion channel wall. Each subunit would thus contribute one amphipathic α-helix to form the pore of the ion channel.

Phosphorylation of the Nicotinic Acetylcholine Receptor

Gordon et al. (1977a, 1979) and Teichberg and Changeux (1977) first demonstrated that postsynaptic membranes enriched in the nicotinic acetylcholine receptor contain endogenous protein kinase and protein phosphatase activity. The protein kinase was subsequently shown to phosphorylate the nicotinic acetylcholine receptor. Early studies indicated that the γ and δ subunits are phosphorylated, and indirect evidence suggested that the α and β subunits are phosphorylated (Gordon et al., 1977b; Saitoh & Changeux, 1980, 1981; Smilowitz et al., 1981; Davis et al., 1982). It was not possible to demonstrate the regulation of this protein phosphorylation by cyclic AMP, cyclic GMP, calcium, or calcium/calmodulin in these studies. In general, it has been

SUBUNIT SPECIFICITY

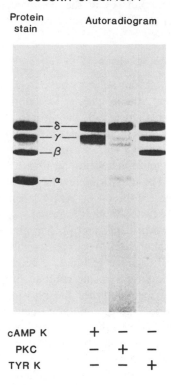

cAMP K	+	−	−
PKC	−	+	−
TYR K	−	−	+

Fig. 5.3. Subunit specificity of the three different protein kinases that phosphorylate the nicotinic acetylcholine receptor: polyacrylamide gel electrophoresis of acetylcholine receptor purified after phosphorylation by cyclic AMP-dependent protein kinase (cAMP); protein kinase C (PKC); tyrosine-specific protein kinase (TYR K).

difficult to study the regulation of phosphorylation of the acetylcholine receptor by second messengers because of the extremely active proteases present in *Torpedo* electroplax (Huganir & Racker, 1980).

Phosphorylation by Different Kinases

Recent studies have shown that the isolated postsynaptic membranes contain at least four different protein kinases: cyclic AMP-dependent protein kinase, calcium/calmodulin-dependent protein kinase II, protein kinase C, and a tyrosine-specific protein kinase (Smilowitz et al., 1981; Huganir & Greengard, 1983; Huganir et al., 1983, 1984). They have revealed that three of the endogenous protein kinases phosphorylate the nicotinic acetylcholine receptor in isolated postsynaptic membranes. The cyclic AMP-dependent protein kinase phosphorylates the γ and δ subunits, protein kinase C phosphorylates and δ and α subunits and the tyrosine-specific protein kinase phosphorylates and β, γ, and δ subunits (Figure 5.3). In addition, studies using purified cyclic AMP-dependent protein kinase, protein kinase C, tyrosine-specific protein kinases and purified nicotinic acetylcholine receptor have demonstrated that these kinases phosphorylate the purified receptor with the same subunit specificity as the endogenous protein kinases in the postsynaptic membrane (Huganir & Greengard, 1983; Zavoico et al., 1984; Huganir et al., 1983, 1984).

Phosphorylation Sites on the Subunits

The amino acid sequences of all four subunits have been examined for possible phosphorylation sites for the three protein kinases. Locations for all seven phosphorylation sites have been proposed (Figure 5.4), taking into account (1) the specificity of the three protein kinases for the subunits of the receptor (2) peptide maps of the phosphorylated subunits, and (3) the known primary amino acid sequence preferences of cyclic AMP-dependent protein kinase, protein kinase C, and tyrosine-specific protein kinases (see Chapter 4). The two serine residues proposed as the phosphorylation sites on the γ and δ subunits for the cyclic AMP-dependent protein kinase are preceded by three γ-subunit and two δ-subunit arginine residues, characteristic of other known substrates for cyclic AMP-dependent protein kinase. The two serine residues that are proposed to be phosphorylated by protein kinase C on the α and δ subunits are surrounded by lysine and arginine residues, characteristic of other known substrates for protein kinase. The three tyrosine residues proposed to be the phosphorylation sites on the β, γ, and δ subunits for the tyrosine-specific protein kinase are preceded by acidic amino acids such as glutamic acid or aspartic acid residues, a known characteristic of other known substrates for tyrosine-specific protein kinases.

The amino acid sequences immediately surrounding the phosphorylation sites on the various subunits are highly conserved (Noda et al., 1983a; Nef et al., 1984; LaPolla et al., 1984). This conservation of the phosphorylation sites in different species suggests that phosphorylation is an important regulatory mechanism in receptor function. All of the proposed phosphorylation sites are located on a common region of each of the subunits, with the three phosphorylation sites on the δ subunit being within 20 amino acids of each other (see Figure 5.4). This suggests that phosphorylation of the acetylcholine receptor by these three protein kinases may regulate the same property of the receptor. The phosphorylation sites are located on the major intracellular loop between M_3 and M_5 in the theoretical models of the structure of the receptor subunits (see Figure 5.2).

Physiological Significance

The physiological significance of the phosphorylation of the nicotinic acetylcholine receptor is unknown. It is clear that phosphorylation-dephosphorylation is not necessary for the opening and closing of the ion channel because functional purified receptor preparations are active in the absence of ATP (Huganir & Racker, 1982) and have no detectable protein kinase activity. One might speculate that phosphorylation of the major intracellular loop, adjacent to the membrane-spanning region (M_5) thought to form the ion channel, might regulate the conducting properties of the ion channel. Alternatively, phosphorylation of these areas of the subunits may regulate the interaction of the subunits with cytoskeletal elements and affect the localization of the receptor in the membrane.

In embryonic muscle and in denervated muscle the acetylcholine receptor is α-SUBUNIT

358
ARG – ARG – SER – SER(P) – SER – VAL – GLY – TYR – ILE – SER – LYS – ALA – GLN – GLU – TYR(P) – PHE – ASN – ILE – LYS – SER(P) – ARG
378

γ-SUBUNIT

350
ARG – ARG – ARG – SER – SER(P) – PHE – GLY – ILE – MET – ILE – LYS – ALA – GLU – GLU – TYR(P) – ILE – LEU – LYS – LYS – PRO – ARG
370

β-SUBUNIT

340
SER – PRO – ASP – SER – LYS – PRO – THR – ILE – ILE – SER – ARG – ALA – ASP – ASP – GLU – TYR(P) – PHE – ILE – ARG – LYS – PRO
360

α-SUBUNIT

314
LYS – ILE – PHE – ILE – ASP – THR – ILE – PRO – ASN – VAL – MET – PHE – PHE – SER – THR – MET – LYS – ARG – ALA – SER(P) – LYS
334

Fig. 5.4. Proposed locations of the phosphorylated amino acid residues on the α, β, γ and δ subunits of the nicotinic acetylcholine receptor. SER(P) and TYR(P) represent the amino acid residues that are phosphorylated. The kinases and their proposed phosphorylation sites are cyclic AMP-dependent protein kinase (γ subunit, Ser-354; δ subunit, Ser-361), protein kinase C (α subunit, SER-333; δ subunit, SER 377) and the tyrosine-specific protein kinase (β subunit, TYR-355; γ-subunit, TYR-364; δ subunit, TYR-372). The amino acids are numbered according to Noda et al. (1982, 1983b,c).

evenly distributed over the surface of the membrane and is mobile in the plane of the membrane. In contrast, in adult muscle the acetylcholine receptor is highly localized directly beneath the innervating neuron in the postjunctional folds where it can reach a surface density of $20,000/\mu m^2$ (Changeux et al., 1984). The molecular mechanism that regulates clustering of the receptor at the synapse is unknown; however, the properties of the adult muscle junctional receptor and the embryonic or denervated muscle extrajunctional receptor are known to differ in their ion channel properties, antigenic properties, isoelectric points, and metabolic stability (Katz & Miledi, 1972; Brockes et al., 1975; Weinberg & Hall, 1979). It has been suggested that some of these differences may be due to phosphorylation of the receptor. Saitoh and Changeux (1981) have reported that the acetylcholine receptors from the electric organs of neonatal and adult *Torpedo marmorata* differ in their thermal stability and isoelectric points. They reported that treatment of the mature form of the acetylcholine receptor with alkaline phosphatase shifts its isoelectric point to the isoelectric point of the immature form and decreases its thermal stability to that of the immature form. These results suggest that the differences between the mature and immature form of the receptor may be accounted for by a higher state of phosphorylation of the mature form.

Anthony et al. (1984) have recently examined the role of tyrosine-specific phosphorylation in the regulation of receptor clustering in chick myotubes. They have transformed chick myoblasts with the Rous sarcoma virus and have shown that after transformation, the receptors in the chick myotubes fail to cluster spontaneously and no longer respond to factors that induce clustering. The researchers demonstrated that this effect is due to the SRC gene product $pp60^{vsrc}$ of the virus, which is a tyrosine kinase (Anthony et al., 1984). These results, in combination with the identification of tyrosine phosphorylation of the nicotinic acetylcholine receptor in postsynaptic membranes (Huganir et al., 1984), suggest that tyrosine phosphorylation of the receptor may be involved in regulating receptor clustering.

Recent results have shown that agents that activate protein kinase C, such as phorbol esters, reduce acetylcholine sensitivity and increase the rate of desensitization of the nicotinic acetylcholine receptor in cultured myotubes (Eusebi et al., 1985). In addition, forskolin, an activator of adenylate cyclase, has recently been shown to promote a striking increase in the rate of acetylcholine receptor desensitization in intact rat soleus muscle and in primary muscle cell cultures (Middleton, Jaramillo & Schuetze, 1986).

Finally, a recent study has provided direct evidence that phosphorylation of the nicotinic acetylcholine receptor by cAMP-dependent protein kinase increases the rate of desensitization of the receptor. The nicotinic acetylcholine receptor was directly phosphorylated by cAMP-dependent protein kinase and then reconstituted into phospholipid vesicles. The ion transport properties of the purified phosphorylated receptor were then measured in the millisecond time range. Phosphorylation of the receptor was found to have no effect on the activation of the receptor by acetylcholine; however, it clearly increased the rate of desensitization of the receptor (Huganir, Delcour, Greengard, & Hess, 1986).

These results provide strong evidence that protein phosphorylation of the nicotinic acetylcholine receptor by cAMP-dependent protein kinase and protein kinase C increases the rate of desensitization of the receptor and may play a major role in the regulation of synaptic transmission at nicotinic cholinergic synapses.

THE VOLTAGE-DEPENDENT SODIUM CHANNEL

The voltage-dependent sodium channel mediates the depolarization of the membrane that occurs during the rising phase of the action potential in many excitable cells such as nerve, skeletal muscle, and heart (see Chapter 2). The sodium channel has been purified from the electric organs of *Electrophoricus electricus,* rat brain, and skeletal muscle (Miller et al., 1983; Barchi, 1983; Hartshorne & Catterall, 1984). All of these preparations of purified sodium channel have a major polypeptide of M_r–250,000, which has been designated the α subunit. In addition, the preparations from brain contain two smaller polypeptides of M_r–39,000 (β) and M_r–37,000 (β_1) and those from skeletal muscle contain two polypeptides of M_r–45,000 and M_r–38,000.

These purified preparations have been shown to display most of the physiological properties of the native sodium channel when they are reconstituted into phospholipid vesicles (Weigele & Barchi, 1982; Talvenheimo et al., 1982; Rosenberg et al., 1984a, b; Hartshorne et al., 1985). In addition, nucleic acid sequence coding for the α subunit of the sodium channel from *Electrophoricus electricus* has been cloned recently, and the complete amino acid sequence has been deduced from this sequence (Noda et al., 1984). From the analysis of the amino acid sequence of the α subunit for hydrophobic and hydrophilic regions, a model has been proposed for the transmembrane structure of the α subunit. The voltage-dependent sodium channel is the first voltage-dependent ion channel to be chemically isolated, and it has served as an excellent model system for the study of the structure, function, and regulation of voltage-dependent ion channels.

Phosphorylation of the Voltage-Dependent Sodium Channel

Partially purified preparations of the voltage-dependent sodium channel from brain contain a cyclic AMP-dependent protein kinase that has been demonstrated to selectively phosphorylate the α subunit of the sodium channel (Costa et al., 1982). Studies using purified preparations of the catalytic subunit of cyclic AMP-dependent protein kinase and purified sodium channel have demonstrated that this enzyme phosphorylates the α subunit on four different phosphorylation sites (Costa et al., 1982). More recent experiments have shown that the α subunit is phosphorylated in synaptic membrane preparations by exogenously added cyclic AMP-dependent protein kinase at four different phosphorylation sites (Costa & Catterall, 1984a). Moreover, it was demonstrated that these same phosphorylation sites are phosphorylated in intact synaptosomes in the presence of 8-bromo-cyclic AMP by the endogenous cyclic AMP-dependent protein kinase in the intact synaptosomes (Costa & Catterall, 1984a).

The α subunit of the purified sodium channel was also recently demonstrated to be phosphorylated at four phosphorylation sites by a purified preparation of protein kinase C (Costa & Catterall, 1984b). In addition, the α subunit of the sodium channel can be phosphorylated in isolated synaptic membranes by exogenous protein kinase C. Two of the sites phosphorylated by protein kinase C appear to be identical to the cyclic AMP-dependent protein kinase phosphorylation sites, whereas the other two sites appear to be unique to protein kinase C (Costa & Catterall, 1984b).

Physiological Significance

The functional significance of the phosphorylation of the voltage-dependent sodium channel is not known. As with the nicotinic acetylcholine receptor, the phosphorylation of the sodium channel does not mediate the opening and closing of the ion channel. However, it may regulate other properties of the channel such as the mean channel open time or the inactivation kinetics. Treatment of intact synaptosomes with 8-bromo-cyclic AMP has been reported to cause a small inhibition of the ^{22}Sodium influx mediated by the sodium channel (Costa & Catterall, 1984a). This could reflect a shift in the voltage dependence of activation, a decrease in the number of channels, or a decrease in the single channel conductance of the sodium channel. It has also been shown that the sodium channel is immobilized in muscle membrane and selectively localized near the neuromuscular junction (Stuhmer & Almers, 1982; Beam et al., 1985). Phosphorylation of the sodium channel may therefore possibly regulate the interaction of the channel with the cytoskeleton, and thereby regulate its mobility and localization near the neuromuscular junction. Further experimentation will be required to establish unequivocally a role of protein phosphorylation in the regulation of sodium channel properties.

THE VOLTAGE-DEPENDENT CALCIUM CHANNEL

There appear to be several different types of voltage-dependent calcium channels that mediate the voltage-dependent influx of calcium into excitable cells (Miller, 1985; see Chapter 11). The development of high-affinity probes such as the dihydropyridines nitrendipine, and nimodipine has permitted preliminary biochemical characterization of one class of voltage-dependent calcium channels that bind these agents. Radiation inactivation of [^{3}H]-nitrendipine-binding sites in smooth muscle membranes indicates that the voltage-dependent calcium channel in these membranes has a native molecular weight of 278,000 (Venter et al., 1983). In addition, an affinity label analog of the dihydropyridine nitrendipine inhibits the calcium channel in smooth muscle and covalently labels an M_r–45,000 and an M_r–35,000 protein (Venter et al., 1983). High-intensity ultraviolet irradiation of [^{3}H]-nitrendipine itself in the presence of isolated cardiac membranes photoaffinity labels an M_r–32,000 protein (Campbell et al., 1984). Recent studies have shown that a [^{3}H]-nitrendipine-binding component can be solubilized with nonionic detergent from rat brain and transverse tubule membranes from skeletal muscle (Curtis & Catterall, 1983). The solubilized [^{3}H]-nitrendipine-binding component has been purified from transverse tubules, and this purified preparation consists of three polypeptides, designated α (M_r–130,000), β

(M_r–50,000), and γ (M_r–33,000) (Curtis & Catterall, 1984). These proteins are thought to be components of a voltage-dependent calcium channel.

Phosphorylation of the Voltage-Dependent Calcium Channel

In contrast to the nicotinic acetylcholine receptor and the voltage-dependent sodium channel, the modulation by neurotransmitters and by cyclic AMP and cyclic AMP-dependent protein kinase of a voltage-dependent calcium channel has been well characterized in cardiac muscle (Reuter, 1983; see Chapter 11). β-adrenergic stimulation of cardiac muscle has been shown to enhance calcium conductance in these cells, and this modulation is mediated by cyclic AMP and by cyclic AMP-dependent protein phosphorylation (Osterrieder et al., 1982). It has therefore been presumed for some time that cyclic AMP-dependent protein kinase phosphorylates the voltage-dependent calcium channel or some related modulator protein. However, only recently has it been possible to analyze biochemically the phosphorylation of the calcium channel itself. Recent results have demonstrated that the catalytic subunit of cyclic AMP-dependent protein kinase phosphorylates the α and β subunits of the purified nitrendipine-binding component from transverse tubule membranes (Curtis & Catterall, 1985). In addition, the purified catalytic subunit appears to phosphorylate the β subunit in intact transverse tubule membranes. Although the effects of these phosphorylations on calcium channel function have not yet been investigated, these results suggest that phosphorylation of the β, and possibly the α, subunit could be involved in the modulation of calcium channel activity by neurotransmitters and hormones.

CONCLUSIONS

With the increasing number of ion channel proteins that have been biochemically isolated and identified, it is becoming possible to analyze the phosphorylation of the ion channel proteins at the biochemical level. With knowledge of structure and function relationships of various ion channels, it is hoped that how the addition of phosphate to certain areas of an ion channel modulates its activity will eventually be understood at a molecular level.

REFERENCES

Agnew, W.S. (1984) Voltage-regulated sodium channel molecules. *Anu. Rev. Physiol. 46*, 517–530.

Anholt, R. (1981) Reconstitution of acetylcholine receptors in model membranes *TIBS 6*, 288–291.

Anthony, D.T., Scheutze, S.M., and Rubin, L.L. (1984) Transformation by Rous sarcoma virus prevents acetylcholine receptor clustering on cultured chicken muscle fibers. *Proc. Natl. Acad. Sci. USA 81*, 2265–2269.

Barchi, R.L. (1983) Protein components of the purified sodium channel from rat skeletal muscle sarcolemma. *J. Neurochem. 40*, 1377–1385.

Beam, K.G., Caldwell, J.H., and Campbell, D.T. (1985) Na channels in skeletal muscle concentrated near the neuromuscular junction. *Nature 313*, 588–590.

Brockes, J.P., Berg, D.K., and Hall, Z.W. (1975) The biochemical properties and regulation of acetylcholine receptors in normal and denervated muscle. *Cold Spring Harbor Symp. Quant. Biol. 40*, 253–262.

Burgoyne, R.D. (1983) Regulation of the muscarinic acetylcholine receptor: Effects of phosphorylating conditions on agonist and antagonist binding. *J. Neurochem. 40*, 324–331.

Campbell, K.P., Lipshutz, G.M., and Denney, G.H. (1984) Direct photoaffinity labeling of the high affinity nitrendipine-binding site in subcellular membrane fractions isolated from canine myocardium. *J. Biol. Chem. 259*, 5384–5387.

Catterall, W.A. (1984) The molecular basis of neuronal excitability. *Science 223*, 653–661.

Changeux, J.-P. (1981) The acetylcholine receptor. An allosteric membrane protein. *Harvey Lecture Series 75*, 85–255.

Changeux, J.-P., Devillers-Thiery, A., and Chemouilli, P. (1984) Acetylcholine receptor: An allosteric protein. *Science 225*, 1335–1345.

Claudio, T., Ballivert, M., Patrick, J., and Heinemann, S. (1983) Nucleotide and deduced amino acid sequences of *Torpedo californica* aceytlcholine receptor α-subunit. *Proc. Natl. Acad. Sci. USA 80*, 1111–1115.

Costa, M.R.C., Casnellie, J.E., and Catterall, W.A. (1982) Selective phosphorylation of the alpha subunit of the sodium channel by cAMP-dependent protein kinase. *J. Biol. Chem. 257*, 7918–7921.

Costa, M.R.C. and Catterall, W.A. (1984a) Cyclic AMP-dependent phosphorylation of the a-subunit of the sodium channel in synaptic nerve ending particles. *J. Biol. Chem. 259*, 8210–8218.

Costa, M.R. and Catterall, W.A. (1984b) Phosphorylation in the a subunit of the sodium channel by protein kinase C. *Cell. Mol. Neurobiol. 4*, 291–297.

Curtis, B.M. and Catterall, W.A. (1983) Solubilization of the calcium antagonist receptor from rat brain. *J. Biol. Chem. 258*, 7280–7283.

Curtis, B.M. and Catterall, W.A. (1984) Purification of the calcium antagonist receptor of the voltage-sensitive calcium channel from skeletal muscle transverse tubules. *Biochemistry 23*, 2113.

Curtis, B.M. and Catterall, W.A. (1985) Phosphorylation of the calcium antagonist receptor of the voltage-sensitive calcium channel by cAMP-dependent protein kinase. *Proc. Natl. Acad. Sci. USA 82*, 2528–2532.

Davis, C.G., Gordon, A.S., and Diamond, I. (1982) Specificity and localization of the acetylcholine receptor kinase. *Proc. Natl. Acad. Sci. USA 79*, 3666–3670.

Devillers-Thiery, A., Giraudat, J., Bentaboulet, M., and Changeux, J.P. (1983) Complete mRNA coding sequence of the acetylcholine binding a-subunit of *Torpedo marmorata* acetylcholine receptor: A model for the transmembrane organization of polypeptide chain. *Proc. Natl. Acad. Sci. USA, 80*, 2067–2071.

Eusebi, F.M. Molinaro and Zani, B.M. (1985) Agents that activate protein kinase C reduce acetylcholine sensitivity in cultured myotubes. *J. Cell Biol. 100*, 1339–1342.

Finer-Moore, J. and Stroud, R.M. (1984) Amphipathic analysis and possible formation of the ion channel in an acetylcholine receptor. *Proc. Natl. Acad. Sci. 81*, 155–159.

Gordon, A.S., Davis, C.G., and Diamond, I. (1977a) Phosphorylation of membrane proteins at a cholinergic synapse. *Proc. Natl. Acad. Sci. USA 74*, 263–267.

Gordon, A.S., Davis, C.G., Milfay, D., and Diamond, I. (1977b) Phosphorylation of acetylcholine receptor by endogenous membrane protein kinase in receptor-enriched membranes of *Torpedo californica*. *Nature 267*, 539–540.

Gordon, A.S., Milfay, D. Davis, C.G., and Diamond, I. (1979) Protein phosphatase activity in acetylcholine receptor-enriched membranes. *Biochem. Biophys. Res. Commun. 87*, 876–883.

Hartshorne, R.P. and Catterall, W.A. (1984) The sodium channel from rat brain: Purification and subunit composition. *J. Biol. Chem. 259*, 1667–1675.

Hartshorne, R.P., Keller, B.U., Talvenheimo, J.A., Catterall, W.A., and Montal, M. (1985) Functional reconstitution of the purified brain sodium channel in planar lipid bilayers. *Proc. Natl. Acad. Sci. USA 82*, 240–244.

Huganir, R.L., Delcour, A., Greengard, P., and Hess, G. (1986) Regulation of desensitization of the nicotinic acetylcholine receptor by protein phosphorylation. *Nature, 321*, 774–776.

Huganir, R.L., Albert, K.A., and Greengard, P. (1983) Phosphorylation of the nicotinic acetylcholine receptor by Ca/phospholipid-dependent protein kinase, and comparison with its phosphorylation by cAMP-dependent protein kinase. *Soc. Neurosci. Abstr. 9*, 578.

Huganir, R.L. and Greengard, P. (1983) cAMP-dependent protein kinase phosphorylates the nicotinic acetylcholine receptor. *Proc. Natl. Acad. Sci. USA 80*, 1130–1134.

Huganir, R.L., Miles, K., and Greengard, P. (1984) Phosphorylation of the nicotinic acetylcholine receptor by an endogenous tyrosine-specific protein kinase. *Proc. Natl. Acad. Sci. USA 81*, 6963–6972.

Huganir, R.L. and Racker, E. (1980) Endogenous and exogenous proteolysis of the acetylcholine receptor from *Torpedo californica*. *J. Supramolecular Structure 14*, 13–19.

Huganir, R.L. and Racker, E. (1982) Properties of proteoliposomes reconstituted with acetylcholine receptor from *Torpedo californica*. *J. Biol. Chem. 257*, 9372–9378.

Katz, B. and Miledi, R. (1972) The statistical nature of the acetylcholine potential and its molecular components. *J. Physiol. 224*, 665.

LaPolla, R.J., Mayne, K.M., and Davidson, N. (1984) Isolation and characterization of cDNA clone for the complete protein coding region of the δ subunit of the mouse acetylcholine receptor. *Proc. Natl. Acad. Sci. USA 81*, 7970–7974.

Merlie, J.P., Changeux, J.P., and Gros, F. (1978) Skeletal muscle acetylcholine receptor: Purification, characterization, and turnover in muscle cell cultures. *J. Biol. Chem. 253*, 2882.

Middleton, P., Jaramillo, F., and Schuetze, S.M. (1980) Forskolin increases the rate of acetylcholine receptor desensitization at rat soleus endplate. *Proc. Natl. Acad. Sci. USA*, in press.

Miller, J.A., Agnew, W.S., and Levinson, S.R. (1983) Principal glycopeptide of the tetrodotoxin/saxitoxin binding protein from *Electrophorus electricus:* Isolation and partial chemical and physical characterization. *Biochemistry 22*, 462–470.

Miller, R.J. (1985) How many types of calcium channels exist in neurones? *Trends in Neurosci. 8*, 45–47.

Nef, P., Mauron, A., Stalder, R., Alliod, C., and Ballivet, M. (1984) Structure, linkage, and sequence of the two genes encoding the α and δ subunits of the nicotinic acetylcholine receptor. *Proc. Natl. Acad. Sci. USA 81*, 7975–7979.

Noda, M, Furutani, Y., Takahashi, H., Toyosato, M., Tanabe, T., Shimizu, S., Kikyotani, S., Kayano, T., Hirose, T. Inayama, S., and Numa, S. (1983a) Cloning and sequence analysis of calf cDNA and human genomic DNA encoding α-subunit precursor of muscle actylcholine receptor. *Nature 305*, 818–823.

Noda, M., Takahashi, H., Tanabe, T., Toyosato, M., Furutani, Y., Hirose, T., Asai, M., Inayama, S., Miyata, T., and Numa, S. (1982) Primary structure of α subunit precursor of *Torpedo californica* acetylcholine receptor deduced from cDNA sequence. *Nature 299*, 793–797.

Noda, M., Takahashi, H., Tanabe, T., Toyosato, M., Kikyotani, S., Furutani, Y., Hirose, T., Takashima, H., Inayama, S., Miyata, T., and Numa, S. (1983b) Structural homology of *Torpedo californica* acetylcholine receptor subunits. *Nature 302*, 528–532.

Noda, M., Takahashi, H., Tanabe, T., Toyosato, M., Kikyotani, S., Hirose, T., Asai, M., Takashima, H., Inayama, S., Miyate, T., and Numa, S. (1983c) Primary structures of β- and α-subunit precursors of *Torpedo californica* acetylcholine receptor deduced from cDNA sequence. *Nature 301*, 251–255.

Noda, M., Shimizu, S., Tanabe, T., Takai, T., Kayano, T., Ikeda, T., Takahashi, H., Nakayama, H., Kanaoka, Y., Minamino, N., Kangawa, K., Matsuo, H., Raftery, M.A., Hirose, T., Inayama, S., Hayashida, H., Miyata, T., and Numa, S. (1984) Primary structure of *Electrophorus electicus* sodium channel deduced from cDNA sequence. *Nature 312*, 121–127.

Osterrieder, W. Brum, B., Hescheler, J., Trautwein, W., Flockerzi, V., and Hofman, F. (1982) Injection of subunits of cyclic AMP-dependent protein kinase into cardiac myocytes modulates Ca current. *Nature 298*, 576–578.

Reuter, H. (1983) Calcium channel modulation by neurotransmitters, enzymes, and drugs. *Nature 301*, 569–574.

Reynolds, J.A. and Karlin, A. (1979) Molecular weight in detergent solution of acetylcholine receptor from *Torpedo californica*. *Biochemistry 17*, 2035.

Rosenberg, R.L., Tomiko, S.A., and Agnew, W.S. (1984a) Reconstitution of neurotoxin-modulated ion transport by the voltage-regulated sodium channel isolated from the electroplax of *Electrophorus electricus*. *Proc. Natl. Acad. Sci. USA 81*, 1239–1243.

Rosenberg, R.L., Tomiko, S.A., and Agnew, W.S. (1984b) Single-channel properties of the reconstituted voltage-regulated Na channel isolated from the elctroplax of *Electrophorus electricus*. *Proc. Natl. Acad. Sci. USA 81*, 5594–5598.

Saitoh, T. and Changeux, J.-P. (1980) Phosphorylation in vitro of membrane fragments from *Torpedo marmorata* electric organ. Effect on membrane solubilization by detergents. *Eur. J. Biochem. 105*, 51–62.

Saitoh, T. and Changeux, J.-P. (1981) Change in the state of phosphorylation of acetylcholine receptor during maturation of the electromotor synapse in *Torpedo marmorata* electric organ. *Proc. Natl. Acad. Sci. USA 78*, 443k0–4434.

Smilowitz, H., Hadjian, R.A., Dwyer, J., and Feinstein, M.B. (1981) Regulation of acetylcholine receptor phosphorylation by calcium and calmodulin. *Proc. Natl. Acad. Sci. USA 78*, 4708–4712.

Stuhmer, W. and Almers, W. (1982) Photobleaching through the glass micropipettes: Sodium channels without lateral mobility in the sarcolemma of frog skeletal muscle. *Proc. Natl. Acad. Sci. USA 79*, 946–950.

Talvenheimo, J.A., Tamkun, M.M., and Catterall, W.A. (1982) Reconstitution of neurotoxin-stimulated sodium transport by the voltage-sensitive sodium channel purified from rat brain. *J. Biol. Chem. 257*, 11868–11871.

Tank, D.W., Huganir, R.L., Greengard, P., and Webb, W.W. (1983) Patch-recorded single-channel currents of the purified and reconstituted *Torpedo* acetylcholine receptor. *Proc. Natl. Acad. Sci. USA 80*, 5129–5133.

Teichberg, V.I. and Changeux, J.-P. (1977) Evidence for protein phosphorylation and dephosphorylation in membrane fragments isolated from the electric organs of *Electrophoricus electricus*. *FEBS Lett. 74*, 76.

Teichberg, V.I., Sobel, A., and Changeux, J.P. (1977) In vitro phosphorylation of the acetylcholine receptor. *Nature 267*, 540–542.

Venter, J.C., Fraser, C.M., Schabert, J.S., Jung, C.Y., Bolger, G., and Triggle, D.J. (1983) Molecular properties of the slow inward calcium channel. *J. Biol. Chem. 258*, 9344–9348.

Weigele. J.B. and Barchi, R.L. (1982) Functional reconstitution of the purified sodium channel protein from rat sarcolemma. *Proc. Natl. Acad. Sci. USA 79*, 3651–3655.

Weinberg, C.B. and Hall, Z.W. (1979) Antibodies from patients with myasthenia gravis recognize determinants unique to extrajunctional acetylcholine receptors. *Proc. Natl. Acad. Sci. USA 76*, 504–506.

Zavoico, G.B., Comerci, C., Subers, E., Egan, J.J., Huang, C.-K., Feinstein, M.B., and Smilowitz, H. (1984) cAMP, not Ca/calmodulin, regulates the phosphorylation of acetylcholine receptor in *Torpedo californica* electroplax. *Biochim. et Biophys. Acta 770*, 225–229.

6

The Control of
Rhythmic Neuronal Firing

JACK A. BENSON
WILLIAM B. ADAMS

Several different types of neurons and neuronal networks, when isolated from phasic inputs originating elsewhere in the nervous system, can display regular, periodic output. This activity ranges from a simple rhythm of bursts of action potentials alternating with silent intervals, as in the molluscan bursting neurons (Adams & Benson, 1985), to the complex rhythmic patterns exhibited by multiply-connected neurons, as in the lobster stomatogastric ganglion (Selverston et al., 1976). Among the many aspects of these systems that have been investigated, two points of special interest stand out:

1. Burst generation and rhythmicity are endogenous properties of the neuron or network. In other words, the periodic generation of bursts of action potentials arises from processes at work within the system and requires no phasic input from other parts of the nervous system. Some systems, such as the lobster stomatogastric ganglion, do require a tonic input to maintain their rhythmic output (Russell & Hartline, 1978; Raper, 1979). Others, such as the molluscan neuronal bursters, typically remain rhythmically active in isolated ganglia for hours without phasic or tonic input (Strumwasser, 1965; Alving, 1968).

2. When interconnections with other parts of the nervous system are intact, the endogenous rhythmic activity can be modified greatly by input from neurons that synapse onto the bursting system or release neurohormones in its vicinity (Parnas et al., 1974; Nagy & Dickinson, 1983). In extreme cases, the endogenously bursting system may be rendered silent, or its activity may be changed to such an extent that a periodic influence is hard to detect in the output (Stinnakre & Tauc, 1969). This alteration of the endogenous activity by extrinsic influences constitutes modulation, and it is by this means that the endogenously active elements of the nervous system adapt their activity appropriately in response to changes in the animal's environment.

APLYSIA NEURON R15

In this chapter, we examine some aspects of the modulation of endogenous bursting activity in the identified neuron R15, which is located in the abdominal ganglion of

100

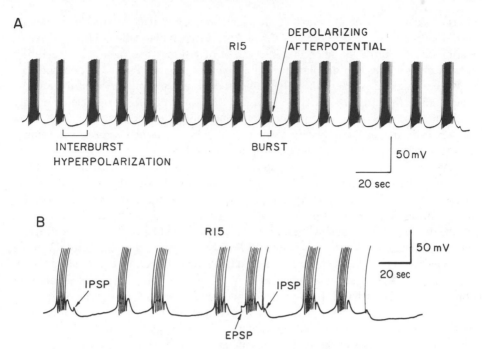

Fig. 6.1. Bursting in neuron R15. (A) The abominal ganglion was removed from the animal and superfused with *Aplysia* saline. Neuron R15 was impaled with a microelectrode to measure its endogenous activity. Note the regular, rhythmic activity, composed of bursts of action potentials separated by interburst hyperpolarizations. Each burst ends with a characteristic depolarizing afterpotential *(arrow)*. (B) Recording from a semiintact preparation. (Courtesy of J.D. Roth, K. Lukowiak, and R.W. Berry.) Note the irregular bursting pattern and the presence of synaptic potentials *(arrows)*.

the opisthobranch mollusc *Aplysia* (Frazier et al., 1967). Although R15 appears to play a role in osmoregulation and water balance, it must be admitted that its function is not fully understood. Despite this, R15 is the most thoroughly studied endogenous burster, and one of the most extensively investigated of all identified neurons (Adams & Benson, 1985). In the following pages we will discuss some of the characteristic electrical properties of R15, particularly those which underlie R15's modulation by serotonin, dopamine, and synaptic input. We will show that some of the membrane characteristics and voltage-dependent ionic currents involved in burst generation in R15 are also an intrinsic part of the modulatory mechanism. In other words, some individual ion currents have dual functions, taking part in both the generation of the burst cycle and its modulation by external input.

To understand the generation and modulation of activity in R15, it is necessary to look first at the burst cycle itself. Figure 6.1A shows the rhythmic burst pattern typically recorded from R15 in an isolated abdominal ganglion. The burst consists of a train of action potentials whose frequency increases until midburst and then decreases. At the end of the burst is a characteristic slow depolarizing afterpotential (arrow in Figure 6.1A) followed by the interburst hyperpolarization. The hyperpolarization decays during the interburst interval, at first slowly and then at an increasing rate, leading finally to a depolarizing inflection that triggers the first action potential of the next burst. Several of the calcium-dependent ion currents that contribute to the generation of bursting are described in Figure 8.8 of Chapter 8. This cycle of activity is endogenous to the neuron and does not require input, either tonic or phasic, from elsewhere in the nervous system (Strumwasser, 1965; Alving; 1968). Such input, however, can greatly modify the bursting pattern.

When the central nervous system is intact, R15 is bombarded by a variety of spontaneous synaptic inputs that interrupt the bursting activity (Figure 6.1B). Some of these excitatory and inhibitory synaptic inputs can be measured with an electrode in the soma and are evident in the interburst intervals in Figure 6.1B *(arrows)*. As a result, the bursts are of unequal duration and are separated by prolonged and irregular interburst intervals. Although synapses that alter the membrane conductance in the neuropil may not have such large direct modulatory effects on the somal activity, they may modulate the responsiveness of the neuron to other synaptic inputs as a consequence of the change in membrane conductance in the synaptic region.

Although spontaneous synaptic activity is difficult to study, experimental stimulation of some of the nerves leading to the abdominal ganglion can activate synaptic inputs to R15, which induce long-lasting inhibition of rhythmic activity. Such stimulation may silence the cell for as long as 3 hours, after which the normal bursting cycle gradually resumes (Parnas & Strumwasser, 1974). Application of serotonin ($10^{-5}M$) or dopamine ($10^{-4}M$) can also reduce the frequency of and finally stop bursting (Ascher, 1972; Drummond et al., 1980). Some of the ionic and molecular mechanisms underlying these modulatory effects will be discussed later in this chapter.

SIGNIFICANCE OF THE STEADY-STATE CURRENT VOLTAGE RELATIONSHIP

Examination of the steady-state I-V relation in R15 below the threshold for action potential generation provides an understanding of the mechanisms involving particular ion currents in the generation and modulation of bursting. As will be shown later, the characteristics of this I-V relation allow various functionally similar forms of inhibition to be achieved by means of different ionic mechanisms. This means that different inputs to R15 can act by separate mechanisms to produce qualitatively similar modulatory effects but, for example, with different time courses for these inputs.

If the membrane voltage is voltage clamped (see Chapter 2) at a number of voltages for long periods of time, or swept very slowly over a range of voltages, then plotting the measured current against the corresponding voltage yields the steady-state I-V curve. The shape of an I-V curve reflects all the conductance pathways that are active at each voltage and can be quite complex in some cells. Before discussing the experimentally observed I-V curve of R15, it is worthwhile to consider some simpler, theoretical I-V curves, the electrical circuits from which they arise, and what the curves can tell us about the stability of these circuits.

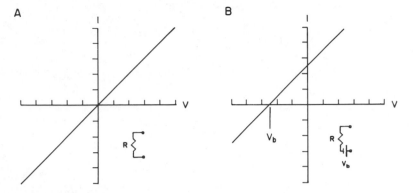

Fig. 6.2. I-V curves from simple electrical elements. In Figures 6.2 to 6.9 the abscissa plots the membrane voltage, with the more positive voltages to the right; the voltages are measured from inside the cell with respect to the outside or bathing medium. The ordinate plots the membrane current, with the more positive current upwards; positive (outward) currents represent a net flow of current across the cell membrane from inside to outside. (A) The I-V curve measured by "voltage-clamping" a resistor is a straight line that passes through the origin and has a slope $G = 1/R$. (B) The I-V curve of a resistor-battery combination is also a straight line with slope $G = 1/R$, but the line passes through the zero-current axis at the battery voltage, that is, at the "equilibrium potential."

Theoretical I-V Curves

Figures 6.2 to 6.4 illustrate the I-V curves that result from relatively simple combinations of conductance pathways. In Figure 6.2A the cell membrane is represented as a linear resistor, that is, a constant conductance at all membrane voltages. The resulting I-V curve is a straight line and the slope of the line ($\Delta I/\Delta V$) is equal to the conductance ($G = 1/R$) of the resistor. The line passes through the origin because, with no current flowing ($I = 0$), the voltage must equal zero. In Figure 6.2B, a battery is added in series with the resistor. (This combination is often used as a simplified representation of an individual ion conductance pathway, where the battery voltage represents the equilibrium potential for the ion in question.) The I-V curve is again a straight line with slope $G = 1/R$, but now it passes through the zero-current axis at the battery voltage. The current through such a pathway is given by

$$I = G(V - V_b)$$

where V_b is the battery voltage. With no current flowing, the voltage will be equal to V_b and, since the I-V curve passes through the axis with positive slope, the voltage will be stable at that value. Any perturbation that tends to move the voltage in the positive (depolarizing) direction would cause a positive (outward or hyperpolarizing) current to flow and bring the voltage back to V_b. Similarly, a perturbation in the negative (hyperpolarizing) direction would cause a negative (inward or depolarizing) current to flow, which also tends to bring the voltage back to V_b. In simple terms, this negative feedback causes the system to be stable at the voltage at which the I-V curve crosses the zero-current axis with a positive slope. In contrast, when a nega-

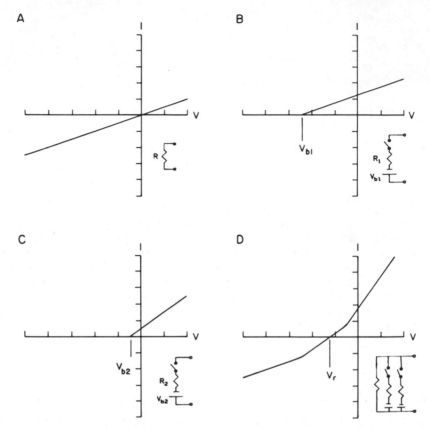

Fig. 6.3. I-V curves from combinations of simple electrical elements. A resistor and two resistor-battery-switch combinations are used to model three independent pathways. (A) A resistor models a conductance pathway that has a constant conductance at all voltages. (B, C) Resistor-battery-switch combinations model two conductance pathways that turn on (the switches close) when the voltage is more positive than the battery voltage. Different resistors and battery voltages are used for the two pathways. (D) The three conductance pathways in A, B, and C are connected in parallel. The current that flows through the parallel combination is the sum of the currents that flow through the individual pathways. Note the increases in slope as the switch-controlled pathways turn on with more positive voltage.

tively sloping I-V curve intersects the zero-current axis, the system is in an unstable state.

In general, different conductance pathways in a cell membrane can be modeled as the parallel combination of several conductance pathways, and the net current flow through the membrane will be the sum of the current flows through each of these individual conductance pathways. Figure 6.3 illustrates the I-V curve that would result from three conductance pathways. One of the pathways (Figure 6.3A) has a constant conductance, so that its I-V curve is a straight line passing through the origin (this might represent a "leak" conductance). Each of the other two conductance pathways (Figure 6.3B and C) is modeled with a battery, a resistor, and a switch that closes when the voltage is more positive than the battery voltage. (These are intended to represent in a simple fashion conductance pathways activated by depolarization.) The I-V curves for each of these two pathways consist of two straight-line segments: where $V < V_b$, the current is zero; where $V > V_b$, the line has a slope $1/R$ and intersects the zero-current axis at V_b. When all three conductance pathways are combined (Figure 6.3D), the resulting I-V curve consists of three straight-line segments. The slope, and hence the conductance, is smallest over that range of voltages in which only pathway 1 is active, and the slope increases successively with more positive voltages as pathways 2 and 3 are activated. The I-V curve passes through the zero-current axis with positive slope at voltage V_r (r for resting poten-tial). V_r can be calculated from R, R_1, and V_{b1} since pathway 2 is not active at that voltage.

Of course, ion conductance pathways in cell membranes do not turn on as sharply as the switches used for the illustrations in Figure 6.3 (see, e.g., the activation curves for various ion currents in Chapter 2). A more realistic approximation of the variation of conductance with voltage in a cell membrane is shown in Figure 6.4A. Here the conductance increases gradually with voltage between -80 and $+20$ mV. If this conductance is combined with a battery and the battery voltage is chosen to be more negative than the voltages required to activate the variable conductance, positive or *outward* current will be produced upon activation, and the I-V curve for the pathway will have the shape shown in Figure 6.4B. Combining such a conductance pathway with a simple resistor of resistance R gives rise to the I-V curve illustrated in Figure 6.4C. At very negative voltages the variable conductance is not activated and the slope of the I-V curve is approximately $1/R$. As the voltage is made more positive, the variable conductance activates and the I-V curve looks similar to the one shown in Figure 6.3D. The conductance in Figure 6.4C activates gradually with voltage, however, so there are no sharp corners in the I-V curve. The resting potential (V_r) cannot be calculated easily but can be seen in Figure 6.4C to be near -30 mV.

A very different picture emerges if the battery voltage is made more positive than the activation range (see Figure 6.4D and E). The current through the variable conductance pathway (Figure 6.4D) is close to zero at very negative voltages and begins to flow *inward* (negative current) as the conductance is activated by more positive voltages. Combining this variable conductance pathway with a linear resistor produces the I-V curve in Figure 6.4E. At very negative voltages the slope of the I-V curve is again approximately $1/R$. But as the voltage is made more positive, and the variable conductance is activated, the net current becomes more negative. The result is a region of "negative slope conductance" or, by tradition, "negative slope resistance" (NSR). A second important feature of Figure 6.4E is that the I-V curve crosses the zero-current axis only at a positive voltage, well above the action poten-tial threshold. At negative voltages it lies below the zero-current axis, producing a continuous flow of inward or depolarizing current. If a cell with this I-V curve were released from voltage clamp, the inward current would drive the membrane voltage to the action potential threshold, and the cell would no longer be in a steady state but would fire action potentials repetitively. In other words, because of the interven-tion of the action potentials, the cell would have no stable resting potential. Such an

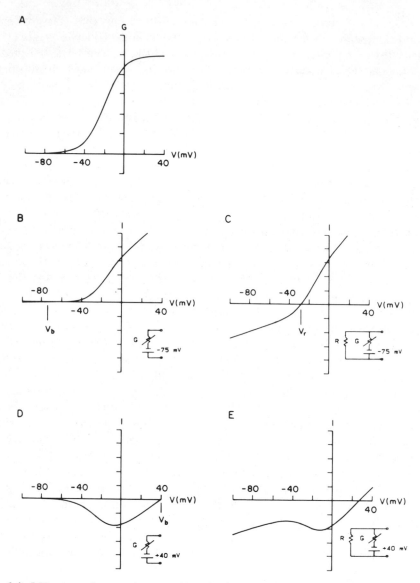

Fig. 6.4. I-V curves from pathways with voltage-dependent conductances. (A) A conductance-voltage plot for a conductance that activates gradually between −80 and +20 mV; (B) I-V curve for a variable conductance as in A, in series with a battery with a voltage of −75 mV; (C) I-V curve for a linear resistor in parallel with the variable conductance pathway illustrated in B; (D) I-V curve for a variable conductance as in A, in series with a battery with a voltage of +40 mV; (E) I-V curve for a linear resistor in parallel with the variable conductance pathway illustrated in D. Note the region of negative slope resistance between −45 and −15 mV.

106

I-V curve is a characteristic of endogenously active neurons such as R15 which, of course, have no stable resting potential when exhibiting their rhythmic cycle (Wilson & Wachtel, 1974). Additional currents, activated by the burst and hyperpolarizing in direction, terminate the burst. These currents are not reflected in the subthreshold I-V curve.

Steady-State Current-Voltage Relationship in Neuron R15

The steady-state I-V curve of R15 is illustrated in Figure 6.5. At membrane potentials more negative than about -85 mV, the curve is linear. At more positive potentials, however, the slope becomes less steep, a phenomenon known as anomalous rectification (Katz, 1949). This expression is synonymous with inward rectification (see Chapter 2). In the case of R15, anomalous rectification arises from two sources. First, the potassium conductance that provides much of the membrane current at very negative potentials (more negative than -80 mV, the linear region of the I-V curve) is itself anomalously rectifying, displaying an ability to pass large inward but only small outward potassium current (Benson & Levitan, 1983). This current, $I_{K(r)}$ (see Chapter 2), plays an important role in the modulation of R15's activity. A second source of anomalous rectification in R15 is the voltage-dependent activation of an inward current. Activation of this current begins at -80 to -60 mV and increases up to -30 to -10 mV (Smith et al., 1975). As for the I-V curve of the model system in Figure 6.4E, the I-V curve of R15 in this range of potentials can be described as a region of NSR, and the current responsible for the NSR is designated I_{NSR} (Adams & Benson, 1985). Although both $I_{K(r)}$ and I_{NSR} are comparatively small, they have pronounced influences on bursting activity. Furthermore, I_{NSR} not only modulates bursting activity but is an important component of the endogenous bursting mechanism itself (Adams & Benson, 1985).

The somal membrane of R15, like that of other molluscan neurons, contains a large number of conductance pathways (see Chapter 2), including at least four distinct pathways for potassium and probably two each for sodium and calcium (Adams & Benson, 1985). However, some of these pathways are activated only during or as a result of action potential generation, and one other pathway (A-current) is inactivated under steady-state conditions (see Chapter 2). In the range of membrane potentials between the action potential threshold and the most negative voltages encountered during generation of bursting activity (i.e., the maximum interburst hyperpolarization), the steady-state I-V curve (Figure 6.5) can be reconstructed by the summation of only three currents, together with a small linear leak current. One of these currents is the delayed rectifying potassium current $I_{K(v)}$ (Figure 6.6A). It has an I-V curve similar to that illustrated in Figure 6.4B, with a reversal potential near E_K, -75mV, and activation at potentials positive to -70 mV. In addition, $I_{K(r)}$ (Figure 6.6B) and I_{NSR} (Figure 6.6C) contribute as described earlier. Finally, a residual, voltage-independent linear leak component (Figure 6.6D) can be detected, for example, at very hyperpolarized potentials when the anomalous rectifier is blocked completely by a potassium channel blocker such as cesium (Benson & Levitan, 1983). The summation of $I_{K(v)}$, $I_{K(r)}$, I_{NSR}, and I_{leak} is plotted in Figure 6.6E (I_{mem}). Note

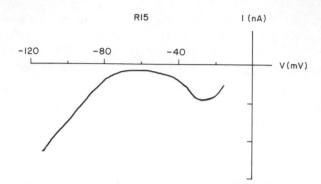

Fig. 6.5. Steady-state I-V curve for neuron R15. The abdominal ganglion was removed from the animal and cell R15 was impaled with two microelectrodes for voltage clamping. The membrane potential was slowly swept through a range of voltages (abscissa); the current flow through the cell membrane is plotted on the ordinate as a function of membrane potential. Note the close approach of the I-V curve to the zero-current axis between −70 and −50 mV and the negative resistance region between −50 and −30 mV. (Data provided by Edwin S. Levitan.)

the resemblance of this reconstructed curve to the measured I-V curve in Figure 6.5. At potentials more negative than about −80 mV the predominant current is $I_{K(r)}$. Between −80 and −40 mV the I-V curve reflects primarily the contributions of $I_{K(r)}$ and I_{NSR}, with I_{NSR} becoming more important with depolarization. At still more depolarized potentials, $I_{K(v)}$ becomes increasingly large, and above −20 mV the faster and much larger action potential currents (not shown) begin to appear.

MODULATION OF THE ACTIVITY OF R15

Although the I-V curve in Figure 6.5 has been referred to as a steady-state I-V curve, it is a steady-state that is imposed by the voltage clamp, not one produced by the cell itself. This can be inferred from the observation that, for all voltages up to and including the threshold for action potential generation (usually −30 to −20mV in this cell), the I-V curve lies below the zero-current axis. As explained earlier, for a cell to be stable in the absence of any externally applied current, its I-V curve must pass through the zero-current axis with positive slope. It should be noted from Figure 6.5 that the I-V curve of R15 approaches the zero-current axis at potentials between −80 and −60 mV. Thus, a small increase in *net* outward current, produced by either an increase in outward potassium current or a decrease in an inward current, could shift the I-V curve to cross the zero-current axis at a potential below the action potential threshold, thereby stabilizing the membrane potential. Experimental observations have shown that this, in fact, is the common strategy for inhibitory modulation of neuron R15 by serotonin, dopamine, and particular synaptic inputs. We can now discuss the different mechanisms by which this common strategy is achieved.

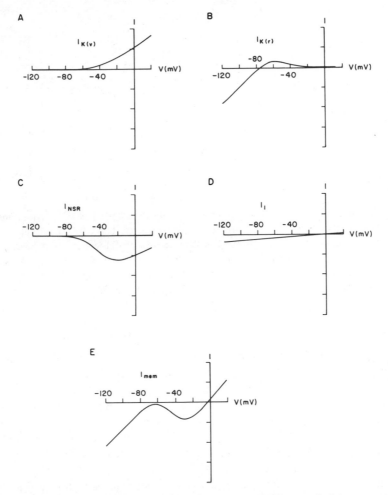

Fig. 6.6. Reconstruction of the I-V curve of neuron R15. Three underlying currents—$I_{K(v)}$ (A), $I_{K(r)}$ (B), and I_{NSR} (C)—together with a linear leak current I_1 (D), are summed together to reconstruct the total steady-state membrane current, I_{mem} (E). Compare the I-V curve in E with the measured I-V curve in Figure 6.5.

Theoretical Considerations

Figure 6.7 illustrates how changes in $I_{K(r)}$ and I_{NSR} would alter the shape of the I-V curve to give rise to a stable resting potential for the cell. In both graphs, the control I-V curves are identical to that in Figure 6.6E. In Figure 6.7A, $I_{K(r)}$ is increased by 50 and 100%. With a 50% increase in $I_{K(r)}$, the I-V curve just intersects the zero-current axis. With a 100% increase, however, the I-V curve crosses the axis with a positive slope to produce a stable resting potential of about -70 mV. Notice, however, that the I-V curve recrosses the axis at about -60 mV and then remains below

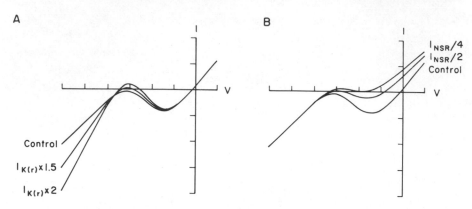

Fig. 6.7. Modulation of conductances: theoretical considerations. Changes in the underlying currents produce corresponding changes in the reconstructed I-V curve for total membrane current. In both graphs, the control curve is the reconstructed I-V curve that was shown in Figure 6.6E. (A) $I_{K(r)}$ is increased by 50% ($I_{K(r)} \times 1.5$) and by 100% ($I_{K(r)} \times 2$). The slopes of the I-V curves increase at negative potentials and the curves intersect the zero-current axis. (B) I_{NSR} is decreased by 50% ($I_{NSR}/2$) and by 75% ($I_{NSR}/4$). The depth of the NSR is reduced and the curves intersect the zero-current axis.

the axis. Thus, if some current were injected to push the membrane potential "over the hump" the cell would repetitively fire action potentials.

In Figure 6.7B, I_{NSR} is decreased by 50 and 75%. Both of these actions give rise to a stable resting potential by causing the I-V curve to cross the axis with positive slope at about -70 mV. With a 50% reduction of I_{NSR} it would again be possible to start the cell firing by nudging the membrane potential "over the hump" in the I-V curve, but with a 75% reduction the I-V curve lies above the zero-current axis at all potentials positive to -70 mV and the cell would be stably silent.

In the previous paragraphs we have shown how an increase in $I_{K(r)}$ or a decrease in I_{NSR} leads to hyperpolarization and ultimately to stabilization of R15's membrane potential. We now can address the question of whether these alterations can be induced by putative transmitters and by synaptic inputs onto R15. In fact, application to R15 of serotonin increases $I_{K(r)}$, and application of dopamine decreases I_{NSR}. Stimulation of the branchial nerve, which contains axons presynaptic to R15, also gives rise to changes in the I-V curve in a manner that indicates both an increase in $I_{K(r)}$ and a decrease in I_{NSR}. These effects will now be considered in more detail.

Modulation by Serotonin

The application of serotonin to R15 results in a hyperpolarization of slow onset and long duration (Drummond et al., 1980), and at $10^{-5}M$, serotonin can often inhibit bursting entirely. The ionic mechanism of this response is an increase in $I_{K(r)}$ (Benson & Levitan, 1983) as illustrated theoretically in Figure 6.7A. Under experimental conditions, $I_{K(r)}$ is partially activated even in the absence of serotonin. Although this current rectifies, it is an imperfect rectifier and it contributes a small outward current at membrane potentials from 5 to 35 mV more positive than E_K (see Chapter 2). This is important because it is in this range of potentials that $I_{K(r)}$ exerts its modulatory effects on the burst pattern (under physiological conditions the membrane voltage is never negative to E_K). Figure 6.8 shows how a small increase in the outward $I_{K(r)}$ brings the I-V curve closer to the zero-current axis. At low serotonin concentrations, activation of $I_{K(r)}$ produces a net decrease in total (inward) membrane current over the range of membrane voltages traversed during the interburst phase of the burst cycle, making the interburst hyperpolarization greater (Figure 6.8). At high serotonin concentrations, the net membrane current can often be reduced to zero by the increase in outward $I_{K(r)}$. The neuron is thereby rendered silent and stable at the hyperpolarized membrane voltage at which the I-V curve crosses the zero-current axis with a positive slope (usually -75 to -65 mV) (Drummond et al., 1980).

Modulation by Dopamine

Ascher (1972) showed that R15 is hyperpolarized, often for many minutes, when exposed to dopamine. Figure 6.8 shows that when dopamine is applied to a voltage-clamped R15, it has the effect of reducing the magnitude of the NSR of the I-V curve (Boisson & Gola, 1976; Wilson & Wachtel, 1978). In contrast to serotonin, which increases $I_{K(r)}$, dopamine reduces I_{NSR}. After application of dopamine, the I-V curve passes through the zero-current axis with a positive slope at a membrane potential below threshold for the voltage-dependent action potential currents. As with serotonin, this means that the membrane potential stabilizes at the potential at which the I-V curve crosses the axis. This is observed experimentally (see Figure 6.8), and the neuron remains silent as long as dopamine is applied. It should be noted that I_{NSR} is not simply a "synaptic" current but is voltage dependent and plays an important role in burst generation (Adams & Levitan, 1985; Kramer & Zucker, 1985). Dopamine thus acts not by hyperpolarizing the neuron in the manner of a classic inhibitory postsynaptic potential but by modulating one of the more important burst currents.

Modulation by Synaptic Stimulation

Parnas and Strumwasser (1974) showed that stimulation of the branchial nerve gives rise to a long-lasting inhibition of the bursting activity of R15 (see Figure 6.8). At least two distinct ionic mechanisms contribute to this inhibition, an increase in $I_{K(r)}$ and a decrease in I_{NSR} (Adams et al., 1980). These two components can be separated in time as well as by pharmacological treatments. The responses of $I_{K(r)}$ to serotonin and to stimulation of the nerve appear to be the same, and if serotonin is applied first, then subsequent nerve stimulation no longer activates $I_{K(r)}$ but only produces a decrease in I_{NSR}. Is serotonin the transmitter for this input? At the moment sufficient data on which to base a decision are not available. No serotonergic neurons are known to be presynaptic to R15, and therefore it cannot be assumed that serotonin is one of the synaptic transmitters, even though its action mimics one ionic component of the synaptic response.

A similar question arises regarding dopamine. Both dopamine and the other component of the synaptic input exert their effects by reducing I_{NSR}, and after appli-

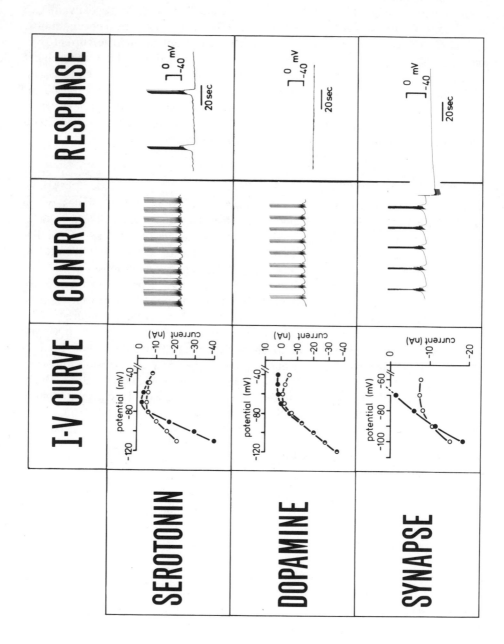

cation of dopamine, subsequent nerve stimulation does not alter I_{NSR} but only produces an increase in $I_{K(r)}$ (Adams et al., 1980). In this case, however, an answer to the question of the identity of the physiological transmitter is suggested by pharmacological experiments. Compounds such as d-lysergic acid diethylamide (d-LSD) and dihydroergotamine, which block the effects of dopamine and the dopamine-like agonists, do not block the inhibitory synaptic input (Ascher, 1972; Adams et al., 1978; Gospe & Wilson, 1982). Although the interpretation of these results is complicated by the observation that d-LSD and dihydroergotamine are also partial serotonin agonists when applied to R15 (Drummond et al., 1980), the results suggest that dopamine may not be the neurotransmitter. Perhaps just as interesting is the possibility that the channels for I_{NSR} might be controlled by two distinct populations of receptors, those for dopamine and those for the so far unidentified endogenous neurotransmitter.

MOLECULAR MECHANISM OF THE MODULATION BY SEROTONIN

The increase in $I_{K(r)}$ caused by the application of serotonin to the cell body of R15 is slow in onset and outlasts the period of application. These characteristics are typical features of physiological responses mediated by a second messenger. In other words, the receptor, in this case for serotonin, is physically separated from the K^+ channels mediating $I_{K(r)}$, and a metabolic process of some kind is required to form a link between the two (see Chapter 1). In the case of R15, the link is the chain of events that begins with the activation of adenylate cyclase and the production of cyclic AMP. The latter, through one or more steps of cyclic AMP-dependent protein phosphorylation, activates the channel (see Chapter 4).

The serotonin-induced hyperpolarizing response of R15 is one of the few neuronal responses in which all of the necessary criteria (Robison et al., 1971; Greengard, 1976) have been fulfilled to assign definitively the role of second messenger to cyclic AMP. The evidence implicating cyclic AMP as a second messenger has come from a variety of physiological, biochemical, and pharmacological experiments and can be summarized as follows:

Fig. 6.8. Modulation of conductances: experimental results. Neuron R15 was voltage clamped as described in Figure 6.5. The left column shows the control I-V curves with open symbols and the experimental I-V curves with filled symbols. *(Top)* Addition of 10 μM serotonin to the bathing medium increases the slope of the I-V curve at negative potentials and decreases the net inward current by increasing $I_{K(r)}$. *(Middle)* Addition of 100 μM dopamine to the bathing medium reduces the depth of the NSR and causes a net outward current flow at potentials positive to -70 mV by decreasing I_{NSR}. Note that the horizontal axis is drawn above the zero current level for purposes of clarity. *(Bottom)* Stimulation of the branchial nerve both increases the slope at negative potentials and reduces the depth of the NSR. In all three cases the modulation of membrane current results in hyperpolarization of the nonvoltage-clamped cell. (Compare the traces in the middle and right columns).

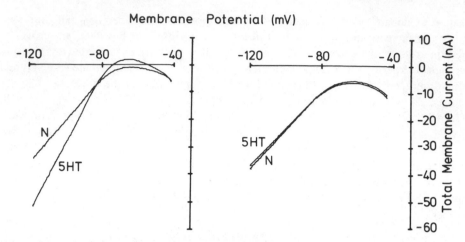

Fig. 6.9. Protein kinase inhibitor blocks the serotonin response. The serotonin response was measured under voltage clamp before (A) and shortly after (B) injection of the cell with PKI. The serotonin response was completely inhibited, whereas the dopamine response was unaffected in the same cell (not shown). Modified from Adams and Levitan (1982).

1. Serotonin hyperpolarizes R15 by activating the anomalously rectifying potassium current (Benson & Levitan, 1983). As far as is known, this current is not activated by any other transmitter. [It should be noted, however, that there is evidence that serotonin and cyclic AMP both modulate other ion currents in R15 (Ewald & Eckert, 1983; Connor & Hockberger, 1984; Lotshaw et al, 1986)].

2. Serotonin activates an adenylate cyclase in the somal membrane of R15 (Levitan, 1978) and this cyclase is linked to a receptor specific for serotonin. Pharmacological analysis of the serotonin receptors in isolated membranes shows that the serotonin receptor mediating the hyperpolarization of R15 is indistinguishable from the serotonin receptor associated with the adenylate cyclase (Drummond et al., 1980; Levitan & Drummond, 1980). This means that the same serotonin receptor mediates hyperpolarization and increases intracellular cyclic AMP. Inhibition of the adenylate cyclase by injection of the GDP analog GDPβS blocks the action of serotonin (Lemos & Levitan, 1984).

3. Increased intracellular cyclic AMP hyperpolarizes R15 and does so by activating $I_{K(r)}$, the same current that serotonin activates. The hyperpolarization is obtained no matter which of the following means is used to increase intracellular cyclic AMP:

a. Extracellular application or intracellular injection of phosphodiesterase-resistant cyclic AMP analogs (Treistman & Levitan, 1976a; Drummond et al., 1980).

b. Application of phosphodiesterase inhibitors. These compounds prevent or reduce the breakdown of cyclic AMP, thereby causing an increase in cyclic AMP that mimics or enhances the effect of serotonin (Treistman & Levitan, 1976a; Drummond et al., 1980).

c. Intraneuronal injection of the guanosine triphosphate (GTP) analog guanylylimidodiphosphate, an activator of adenylate cyclase (Treistman & Levitan, 1976b; Lemos & Levitan, 1984).

4. It has been proposed that cyclic AMP acts exclusively by activation of cyclic AMP-dependent protein kinases (see Chapter 4). Protein kinase inhibitor (PKI), the naturally occurring, heat-stable, 10,000-dalton protein that binds with high affinity to the active catalytic subunit of cyclic AMP-dependent protein kinase and inhibits its phosphorylating activity, also inhibits the *Aplysia* catalytic subunit (Adams & Levitan, 1982). Injection of PKI into R15 completely inhibits the serotonin response (Figure 6.9) but has no effect on the cyclic AMP-independent dopamine response (Adams & Levitan, 1982).

Taking all these lines of evidence together leaves little room for doubt that cyclic AMP mediates the hyperpolarization of R15 that is produced by serotonin and that this mediation requires cyclic AMP-dependent protein phosphorylation.

CONCLUSION

The cell bodies of molluscan bursting neurons, such as R15, possess a far greater abundance of conductance pathways than do squid axons (Adams & Benson, 1985). Some of these currents account for the complex action potential waveforms observed in the cell bodies. Other currents, which may be orders of magnitude smaller than the action potential currents, play critical roles in determining the characteristics of the rhythmic activity of the cell. The reason that very small currents can have such large effects is because they are active at membrane potentials where the larger currents are not; thus, they are responsible for the characteristics of the subthreshold I-V curve. The interplay of these small currents, reflected in part by changes in the shape of the I-V curve, determines whether or not, and with what time course, the membrane potential reaches threshold for activation of the larger currents. There seems to be ample teleological justification for the differences between axons and cell bodies in the molluscs. Axons are all-or-none conductors of information from one location to another, whereas the cell bodies are integrators of information from many sources. The cell body (or cell body–axon hillock) must "decide" whether or not to generate an action potential for subsequent transmission by the axon. This decision is based on a delicate balance of the many modulatory inputs with, in the case of R15, signals generated endogenously by the cell body itself.

In this chapter, we have discussed two mechanisms by which the endogenous rhythmic activity of neuron R15 can be modulated by input from elsewhere in the nervous system. The membrane currents $I_{K(r)}$ and I_{NSR} are major contributors to the net membrane current at potentials below the threshold for action potential generation. As a result, they play an important role in shaping the pattern of rhythmic activity in the cell. The modulation of these currents, by serotonin and dopamine and by synaptic input, provides sensitive mechanisms for modulation of the burst activity of the cell. However, in addition to the modulatory effects described in this chapter, numerous synaptic inputs onto R15 act by means of classic synaptic currents. These synaptic inputs do not alter the burst currents directly but rather influence activity purely by their depolarizing or hyperpolarizing actions. As with most other central neurons, R15 integrates the effects of its various synaptic inputs in order to produce an appropriate output. Because it is endogenously and rhythmically active, modulatory input is integrated not only topologically, as in silent neurons, but also by interaction with the periodic variations in the membrane potential and by direct effects on the currents underlying this periodic activity.

REFERENCES

Adams, W.B. and Benson, J.A. (1985) The generation and modulation of endogenous rhythmicity in the Aplysia bursting pacemaker neurone R15. Prog. Biophys. Molec. Biol. 46, 1–49.

Adams, W.B., Drummond, A.H., and Levitan, I.B. (1978) Dopamine currents in cell R15 of Aplysia. Experientia 34, 921.

Adams, W.B. and Levitan, I.B. (1982) Intracellular injection of protein kinase inhibitor blocks the serotonin-induced increase in K^+ conductance in Aplysia neuron R15. Proc. Natl. Acad. Sci. USA 79, 3877–3880.

Adams, W.B. and Levitan, I.B. (1985) Voltage and ion dependences of the slow currents which mediate bursting in Aplysia neurone R15. J. Physiol., London 360, 69–93.

Adams, W.B., Parnas, I., and Levitan, I.B. (1980) Mechanism of long-lasting synaptic inhibition in Aplysia neuron R15. J. Neurophysiol. 44, 1148–1160.

Alving, B.O. (1980) Spontaneous activity in isolated somata of Aplysia pacemaker neurons. J. Gen. Physiol. 51, 29–45.

Anderson, W.W. and Barker, D.L. (1981) Synaptic mechanisms that generate network oscillations in the absence of discrete postsynaptic potentials. J. Exp. Zool. 216, 187–191.

Ascher, P. (1972) Inhibitory and excitatory effects of dopamine on Aplysia neurones. J. Physiol., London 225, 173–209.

Benson, J.A. and Cooke, I.M. (1984) Driver potentials and the organization of rhythmic bursting in crustacean ganglia. Trends Neurosci. 7, 85–91.

Benson, J.A. and Levitan, I.B. (1983) Serotonin increases an anomalously rectifying K^+ current in Aplysia neuron R15. Proc. Natl. Acad. Sci. USA 80, 3522–3525.

Boisson, M. and Gola, M. (1976) Current-voltage relations in ILD- or dopamine-stabilized bursting neurone in Aplysia. Comp. Biochem. Physiol. 54C, 109–113.

Connor, J.A. and Hockberger, P. (1984) A novel membrane sodium current induced by injection of cyclic nucleotides into gastropod neurones. J. Physiol., London 354, 139–162.

Drummond, A.H., Benson, J.A., and Levitan, I.B. (1980) Serotonin-induced hyperpolarization of an identified Aplysia neuron is mediated by cyclic AMP. Proc. Natl. Acad. Sci. USA 77, 5013–5017.

Drummond, A.H., Bucher, F., and Levitan, I.B. (1980) Distribution of serotonin and dopamine receptors in Aplysia tissues; analysis by [³H]LSD binding and adenylate cyclase stimulation. Brain Res. 184, 163–177.

Ewald, D. and Eckert, R. (1983) Cyclic AMP enhances calcium-dependent potassium current in Aplysia neurons. Cell Molec. Neurobiol. 3, 345–353.

Frazier, W.T., Kandel, E.R., Kupfermann, I., Waziri, R., and Coggeshall, R.E. (1967) Morphological and functional properties of identified neurons in the abdominal ganglion of Aplysia californica. J. Neurophysiol. 30, 1288–1351.

Gospe, S.M. and Wilson, W.A. (1982) Burst-firing inhibition of cell R15 in Aplysia califor-

nica: Pharmacological studies of the effects of tyramine, phenethylamine and amphetamine. *Comp. Biochem. Physiol. 71C,* 249–254.

Greengard, P. (1976) Possible role for cyclic nucleotides and phosphorylated membrane proteins in postsynaptic actions of neurotransmitters. *Nature 260,* 101–108.

Hermann, A. and Gorman, A.L.F. (1979) External and internal effects of tetraethylammonium on voltage-dependent and Ca-dependent K^+ current components in molluscan pacemaker neurons. *Neurosci. Lett. 12,* 87–92.

Katz, B. (1949) Les constantes electriques de la membrane du muscle. *Archs. Sci. Physiol. 3,* 285–300.

Kramer, R.H. and Zucker R.S. (1985) Calcium-induced inactivation of calcium current causes the interburst hyperpolarization of *Aplysia* bursting pacemaker neurones. *J. Physiol., London. 362,* 131–160.

Kupfermann, I. and Weiss, K.R. (1976) Water regulation by a presumptive hormone contained in identified neurosecretory cell R15 of *Aplysia. J. Gen. Physiol. 67,* 113–123.

Lemos, J.R. and Levitan, I.B. (1984) Intracellular injection of guanyl nucleotides alters the serontonin-induced increase in potassium conductance in *Aplysia* neuron R15. *J. Gen. Physiol. 83,* 269–285.

Levitan, I.B. (1978) Adenylate cyclase in isolated *Helix* and *Aplysia* neuronal cell bodies: Stimulation by serotonin and peptide-containing extract. *Brain Res. 154,* 404–408.

Levitan, I.B. and Drummond, A.H. (1980) Neuronal serotonin receptors and cyclic AMP: Biochemical, pharmacological and electrophysiological analysis. In *Neurotransmitters and Their Receptors* (eds. U.Z. Littauer et al.), pp. 163–176, John Wiley & Sons, London.

Lotshaw, D.P., Levitan, E.S., and Levitan, I.B. (1986) Fine tuning of neuronal electrical activity: modulation of several ion channels by intracellular messengers in a single identified nerve cell. *J. Exptl. Biol.,* in press.

Nagy, F. and Dickinson, P.S. (1983) Control of a central pattern generator by an identified modulatory interneurone in Crustacea. I. Modulation of the pyloric motor output. *J. Exp. Biol. 105,* 33–58.

Neher, E. and Lux, H.D. (1972) Differential action of TEA^+ on two K^+-current components of a molluscan neurone. *Pflugers Arch. 336,* 87–100.

Parnas, I., Armstrong, D., and Strumwasser, F. (1974) Prolonged excitatory and inhibitory synaptic modulation of a bursting pacemaker neuron. *J. Neurophysiol. 37,* 594–608.

Parnas, I. and Strumwasser, F. (1974) Mechanisms of long-lasting inhibition of a bursting pacemaker neuron. *J. Neurophysiol. 37,* 609–620.

Raper, J.A. (1979) Nonimpulse-mediated synaptic transmission during the generation of a cyclic motor program. *Science 205,* 304–306.

Robison, A., Butcher, R., and Sutherland, E. (1971) *Cyclic AMP.* Academic Press, New York.

Roth, J.D., Lukowiak, K., and Berry, R.W. (1984) Long-lasting inhibition of neuron R15 of *Aplysia:* Role of the interneuron II network. *Comp. Biochem. Physiol. 78A,* 83–89.

Russell, D.F. (1979) CNS control of pattern generators in the lobster stomatogastric ganglion. *Brain Res. 177,* 598–602.

Russell, D.F. and Hartline, D.K. (1978) Bursting neural networks: A re-examination. *Science 200.* 453–456.

Selverston, A.I., Russell, D.F., Miller, J.P., and King, D.G. (1976) The stomatogastric nervous system: Structure and function of a small neural network. *Prog. Neurobiol. 7,* 215–290.

Smith, T.G., Barker, J.L., and Gainer, H. (1975) Requirements for bursting pacemaker potential activity in molluscan neurones. *Nature 253,* 450–452.

Stinnakre, J. and Tauc, L. (1969) Central neuronal response to the activation of osmoreceptors in the osphradium of *Aplysia. J. Exp. Biol. 51*, 347–361.

Strumwasser, F. (1965) The demonstration and manipulation of a circadian rhythm in a single neuron. In *Circadian Clocks* (ed. J. Aschoff), pp. 442–462, North-Holland Publishing Co., Amsterdam.

Treistman, S.N. and Levitan, I.B. (1976a) Alteration of electrical activity in molluscan neurones by cyclic nucleotides and peptide factors. *Nature 261*, 62–64.

Treistman, S.N. and Levitan, I.B. (1976b) Intraneuronal guanylylimidodiphosphate injection mimics long-term synaptic hyperpolarization in *Aplysia. Proc. Natl. Acad. Sci. USA 73*, 4689–4692.

Wilson, W.A. and Wachtel, H. (1974) Negative resistance characteristic essential for the maintenance of slow oscillations in bursting neurons. *Science 186*, 932–934.

Wilson, W.A. and Wachtel, H. (1978) Prolonged inhibition in burst firing neurons: Synaptic inactivation of the slow regenerative inward current. *Science 202*, 772–775.

Woodson, P.B.J. and Schlapfer, W.T. (1979) The amplitude of post-tetanic potentiation of the EPSP RC1-R15 in *Aplysia* is modulated by environmental parameters. *Brain Res. 173*, 225–242.

7

Potassium Currents That Regulate Action Potentials and Repetitive Firing

JUDITH A. STRONG
LEONARD K. KACZMAREK

One of the themes that runs through this volume is the remarkable diversity in the properties of potassium channels in neuronal membranes. During their development, neurons select different combinations of potassium channels that allow them to generate specific forms of spontaneous and evoked electrical activity (Hille, 1984). Furthermore, in the mature nervous system, stimuli that modulate the properties of one or more of a neuron's potassium channels can transform and "fine tune" the properties of that cell in very specific ways. Such transformations allow sensory information to be encoded, stored, and integrated and allow different patterns of motor output to be generated.

All potassium channels, when open, will tend to hyperpolarize the cell membrane toward E_K. In the simplest case, the opening of a potassium channel would therefore be expected to hyperpolarize the cell and hence reduce membrane excitability. The functional role of a given potassium channel, however, depends on its voltage dependence, its kinetic properties, and its sensitivity to chemical modulation.

This chapter examines the roles of two types of potassium channels, delayed rectifier channels and A-current channels (see Chapter 2), and explains how modulation of the ionic conductances mediated by these channels alters the electrical behavior of neurons. These topics will be illustrated with the example of the bag cell neurons of *Aplysia*. In response to stimulation, these neurons undergo a sequence of long-lasting changes in their electrical properties, which allows them to act as a biological "switch" to trigger a series of behaviors used in reproduction.

Another topic introduced in this chapter, and covered in more detail in Chapter 11, is the modulation of the voltage-dependent calcium current in the bag cell neurons. The modulation of the calcium current has effects that superficially resemble those seen when a voltage-dependent potassium current is modulated. As will be shown, however, the effects on the calcium and the potassium currents are brought about through very different intracellular mechanisms.

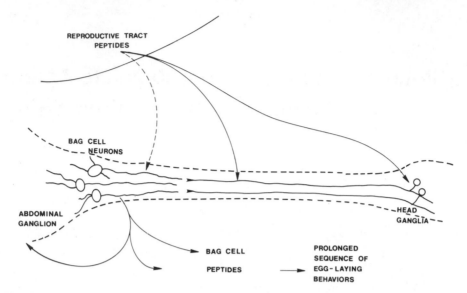

Fig. 7.1. Schematic drawing of the bag cell neuronal system. One cluster of bag cell neurons within the abdominal ganglion is depicted. The pleuroabdominal connective nerves that join the abdominal ganglion to the head ganglia may be stimulated to trigger afterdischarge in the bag cell neurons. Afterdischarges may also be induced by application of peptides from the reproductive tract.

THE BAG CELL NEURONS

The peptidergic bag cell neurons are found in two symmetrical clusters of 200 to 400 neurons each in the abdominal ganglion (Kupfermann & Kandel, 1970). They are anatomically isolated from other neurons in the abdominal ganglion (Figure 7.1) and appear to be homogeneous in their biochemical and electrophysiological properties. For this reason, and because they undergo very prolonged changes in excitability that can be directly related to alterations in the behavior of the animal, these neurons have proved to be a model system for the investigation of biochemical mechanisms that regulate neuronal excitability.

In their resting state, the cells have high membrane potentials, are electrically silent, and will fire only a few action potentials in response to injection of a constant depolarizing current. However, in response to the application of peptides from the reproductive tract or to brief (5- to 10-sec) electrical stimulation of an afferent input from the head ganglia, these neurons depolarize and enter a prolonged period of spontaneous activity termed an afterdischarge (Kupfermann & Kandel, 1970; Heller et al. 1980). This afterdischarge represents a profound transformation of the cells' electrical properties, during which the cells acquire the ability to fire repetitively and their action potentials undergo significant increases in height and width. The individual neurons in a cluster are electrically coupled and, during the afterdischarge, fire in complete synchrony.

An afterdischarge usually lasts about 30 minutes, and during this time, the cells

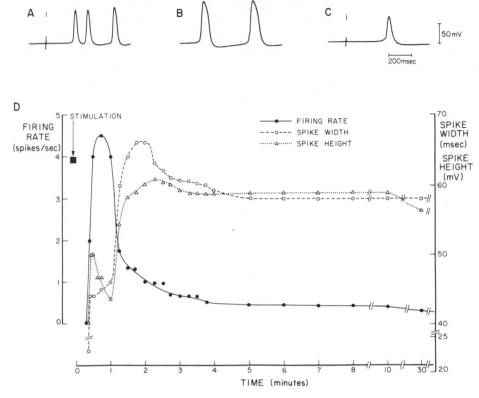

Fig. 7.2. The onset of afterdischarge in bag cell neurons. (A) Action potentials at the very onset of an afterdischarge; (B) action potentials enhanced in height and width 10 minutes after the onset of afterdischarge; (C) action potentials in the refractory period that follows afterdischarge; (D) firing rate and action potential height and width during the onset of an afterdischarge (Kaczmarek et al., 1982).

release several neuroactive peptides. These peptides act on other neurons in the nervous system as well as on peripheral targets to bring about a series of fixed behaviors, lasting several hours, that constitute egg-laying behavior (Strumwasser et al., 1980). The increase in amplitude of their action potentials, which occurs during the first 2 minutes of the afterdischarge, serves to enhance calcium entry during the discharge and, therefore, aids in the secretion of the peptides (Figure 7.2). Following an afterdischarge the bag cell neurons enter a prolonged inhibited state that lasts many hours. During this inhibited state, stimulation can no longer trigger a long-lasting afterdischarge (see last section).

At the onset of the afterdischarge, cyclic AMP levels in the bag cell neurons become elevated (Kaczmarek et al., 1978), and increases in phosphorylation of proteins that are substrates for cyclic AMP dependent-protein kinase *in vitro* can be observed (Jennings et al., 1982). The increase in cyclic AMP produces several important changes in the properties of these neurons, including increases in synthesis of peptides that are released during the discharge (Bruehl & Berry, 1985). One important set of changes induced by the activation of the cyclic AMP-dependent protein kinase that is dealt with here is its effect on the properties of specific ion channels. Analogs of cyclic AMP, or agents that elevate cyclic AMP levels, when applied to clusters of bag cell neurons in the abdominal ganglion, trigger the characteristic afterdischarges of these neurons. Moreover, the duration of an afterdischarge may be significantly prolonged by phosphodiesterase inhibitors, which slow the catabolism of cyclic AMP to 5'-AMP (Kaczmarek et al., 1978).

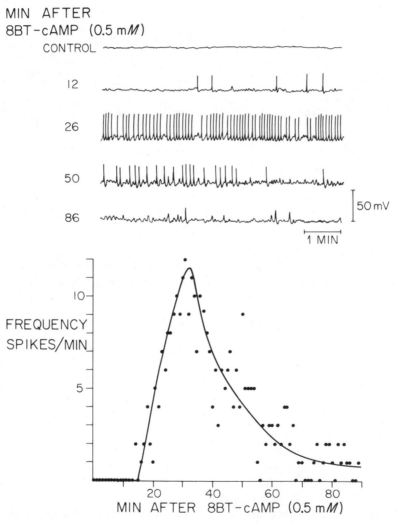

Fig. 7.3. Onset of discharge in an isolated bag cell neuron in cell culture. The upper chart tracings show the onset of discharge following exposure of an isolated bag cell neuron to the cyclic AMP analog 8-benzylthio-cyclic AMP. The lower graph plots the frequency of firing following addition of 8-benzylthio-cyclic AMP (Kaczmarek & Strumwasser, 1981).

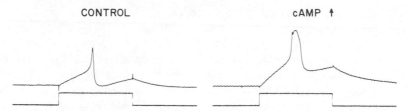

Fig. 7.4. Enhancement of action potentials by cyclic AMP. Action potentials were evoked in an isolated bag cell neuron by a depolarizing current pulse *(lower traces)* before and after elevation of cellular cyclic AMP levels using forskolin and theophylline (Kaczmarek & Kauer, 1983).

INVESTIGATION OF MECHANISMS OF NEUROMODULATION IN ISOLATED NEURONS

To study the modulation of electrical activity in a neuron, it is essential to use as simple a preparation as is feasible. In particular the interactions among different types of neurons in a nervous system may make the interpretation of many types of pharmacological experiments somewhat ambiguous. One approach that can be taken with some types of neurons is to study their electrical properties in primary cell culture where interactions with other cells are eliminated. This approach has been used for the bag cell neurons, which retain many of their morphological and electrical characteristics in cell culture.

Isolated cultured bag cell neurons generally show no spontaneous activity. However, in response to cyclic AMP analogs or to activation of adenylate cyclase by forskolin, several changes take place in their electrical properties. The height and width of the cells' action potentials are enhanced. Subthreshold oscillations of membrane potential occur shortly after exposure to cyclic AMP analogs, and these may reach threshold and thus generate repetitive discharge. In addition, the input resistance of the cell membrane is increased (Kaczmarek & Strumwasser, 1981). The effects of cyclic AMP on action potentials and on spontaneous firing are shown in Figures 7.3 and 7.4. These effects are qualitatively similar to those observed with intact clusters of bag cell neurons in the abdominal ganglion, although there are some quantitative differences in duration of discharge and firing rate.

Evidence that these changes in excitability are related to the activation of cyclic AMP-dependent protein kinase has come from experiments using the catalytic subunit of this enzyme as well as the protein kinase inhibitor protein (PKI) (see Chapter 4). Intracellular injections of purified catalytic subunit of cyclic AMP-dependent protein kinase induce changes in action potential shape, input resistance, and membrane oscillations that are similar to those induced by cyclic AMP (Kaczmarek et al., 1980). Moreover, intracellular injections of the specific PKI that binds to and inhibits the endogenous catalytic subunit prevent and reverse the electrical effects of elevations of cyclic AMP (Kaczmarek et al., 1984).

MODULATION OF VOLTAGE-DEPENDENT
POTASSIUM CHANNELS

Ionic currents in the cultured bag cell neurons have been characterized using both a two-microelectrode voltage clamp technique and the whole cell patch clamp technique (see Chapter 2). Like other neurons, the bag cell neurons contain a number of distinct currents including sodium current, calcium current, delayed potassium current, calcium-activated potassium currents, and A-current (Kaczmarek & Strumwasser, 1984; Strong, 1984; Strong & Kaczmarek, 1985). This section provides a general discussion of the properties of the A-current and delayed rectifier current, followed by a description of how elevations in cyclic AMP levels produce changes in the properties of these currents in the bag cell neurons.

Properties of A-Current

The A-current, or transient outward current, was first discovered in marine eggs; it occurs in many excitable tissues, although it is often lacking in axons (Hagiwara et al., 1961; Rogawski, 1985). A major difference between the A-current and the channels that contribute to delayed rectification is their voltage dependence. As described in Chapter 2, the A-current is largely inactivated when the membrane potential of a cell is held positive to -60 mV. To visualize this current in voltage clamp recordings, the membrane potential must first be set to a more negative potential to remove this steady-state inactivation.

In those neurons that have rather negative resting potentials and are not spontaneously active, much of the A-current is not inactivated at the resting potential. In these cells, the current functions to reduce the cells' responsiveness to brief excitations such as brief synaptic currents. To elicit an action potential, a depolarizing input must last long enough to cause inactivation of the A-current. This effect is illustrated in Figure 7.5 for the response of a hypothetical model neuron to a sustained depolarization. The figure shows both the voltage response of the cell to the depolarizing current and the time course of the conductance of the A-current. The kinetic parameters (which bear a suspicious resemblance to those of bag cell neurons) have been chosen so that the time constant for the inactivation of the A-current, after the cell is depolarized, is relatively slow (150 msec). At the onset of the stimulus, the cell membrane depolarizes; the A-current begins to activate at the same time. This current acts to prevent further depolarization of the membrane potential and can result, as shown, in a transient hyperpolarizing "notch" close to the time of maximal activation of the current. The A-current then starts to inactivate and the membrane slowly depolarizes toward threshold. In the example shown, a single action potential is triggered after a delay of almost 300 msec. A clear experimental example of how the A-current can act in this way, ensuring that only a sustained synaptic input will cause a neuron to fire, has been described for the motorneurons that control the inking response of *Aplysia* (Byrne, 1980). (It is interesting to note that this effect of A-current on firing in response to a sustained depolarization is directly opposite to that of the M-current, which allows action potentials to be generated early but not late during a depolarizing stimulus. See Chapter 11.)

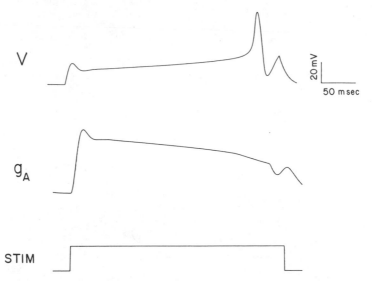

Fig. 7.5. Effect of slowly inactivating A-current on response of a neuron to depolarization. Simulations of membrane voltage (V) and conductance of A-current channels on depolarization of a model neuron by a stimulating current pulse. Time constant of inactivation of A-current = 150 msec.

Because the A-current is activated at potentials that are subthreshold for triggering action potentials, it can also play a role in determining the frequency of repetitive firing in neurons that are spontaneously active or that fire repetitively in response to tonic depolarization (Connor & Stevens, 1971a; Connor, 1978). This is illustrated in Figure 7.6, which shows a simulation of the same model neuron as in Figure 7.5 but with a much more rapid rate of inactivation of the A-current (time constant = 20 msec). Following the onset of the depolarizing stimulus, the A-current activates as before but rapidly inactivates so that the cell depolarizes to threshold very soon after the onset of the stimulus. The A-current continues to inactivate during the action potential. However, the hyperpolarization following the action potential allows the A-current to partly recover from inactivation. The current therefore turns on again while the cell depolarizes toward the threshold for a second action potential. The cycle of activation and inactivation is repeated throughout the stimulus. Activation is maximal during the interval between action potentials and contributes to the regulation of the firing rate.

The quantitative parameters of the A-current, especially of its kinetics, may vary considerably between different types of neurons (Connor, 1978; Serrano, 1982; see also Aghajanian, 1985). Probably these variations represent adaptations for controlling different physiological functions. A comparison of Figures 7.5 and 7.6 shows that a difference in the kinetics of the A-current, particularly in the rate of inactivation, can result in a significant change in a neuron's electrical responses. Such a change in the kinetics of the A-current can also occur within a single cell type and,

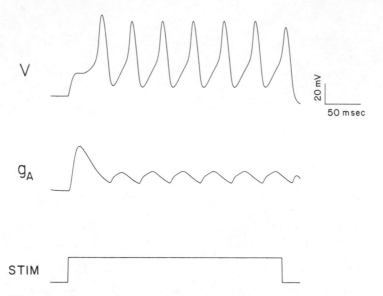

Fig. 7.6. Effect of rapidly inactivating A-current on response of a neuron to depolarization. Simulations of membrane voltage (V) and conductance of A-current channels on depolarization of a neuron by a stimulus current pulse. Time constant of inactivation of A-current = 20 msec.

as described in the next section, occurs in the bag cell neurons in response to agents which increase the intracellular concentration of cyclic AMP.

Modulation of A-Current in the Bag Cell Neurons

Following exposure of isolated bag cell neurons to membrane permeant cyclic AMP analogs (Kaczmarek & Strumwasser, 1984), or to the adenylate cyclase activator forskolin and a phosphodiesterase inhibitor (Strong, 1984), the amplitude of the A-current is reduced. This reduction in amplitude is accompanied by a marked increase in the rate at which the current inactivates during a depolarizing pulse. Figure 7.7 shows the A-current evoked by stepping the membrane potential from −90 to −25 mV before and after elevation of cellular cyclic AMP levels with forskolin.

The rate of inactivation increases at all potentials, but the largest effect is seen at potentials more positive than −50 mV, that is, in the region in which the A-current is normally activated. In this range of membrane potentials, elevations of cyclic AMP speed the rate of inactivation by approximately fivefold. Figure 7.7 also shows an analysis of the alteration in the kinetics of the A-current, which indicates that the change in the A-current amplitude can be explained by the increase in the rate of inactivation and suggests that no change occurs in the number of active A-channels in the membrane.

On the left side of Figure 7.7, the inactivating phase of the A-current has been fitted with a single exponential curve with the form

$$I(\text{control}) = A \exp(-t/\tau 1)$$

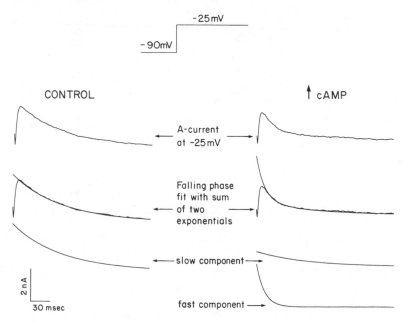

7.7. Effect of elevation of cyclic AMP on the rate of inactivation of A-current in an isolated bag cell neuron. The upper curves show A-current traces before and after elevation of cyclic AMP levels using forskolin and theophylline. In the lower traces, the inactivating phase of the A-current has been fit by exponential curves (Strong, 1984).

where t is time after the onset of the depolarizarion, $\tau 1$ is the time constant for the rate of inactivation, and A is the amplitude of the current extrapolated to $t = 0$. The center panel on the left shows that the falling phase of current can readily be fit with this single exponential with a time constant $\tau 1 = 76$ msec. The lowest panel on the left shows the fitted curve alone.

After elevations of cyclic AMP, the falling phase can no longer be fit by a single exponential. As shown on the righthand side of Figure 7.7, it can be fit readily with the sum of two exponential curves

$$I(\text{cAMP}) = A \exp(-t/\tau 1) + B \exp(-t/\tau 2)$$

where $\tau 1$ is the same time constant as that of the control while $\tau 2$ is the time constant of a much more rapidly inactivating component. Again, A and B are the amplitudes of these two components extrapolated to $t = 0$.

Following an elevation of cyclic AMP levels in a cell, the relative amplitudes of these two components change, although the time constants themselves do not alter. This is illustrated in Figure 7.8, in which the amplitudes of the two components are shown as a function of time after exposure of the cell to forskolin. The figure shows that, although the relative amplitudes of A and B change with time, their sum remains constant. The simplest interpretation of such a result is that the number of channels that carry the A-current is not altered by cyclic AMP but the relative proportion of channels that inactivate with the rapid time constant is markedly increased by cyclic

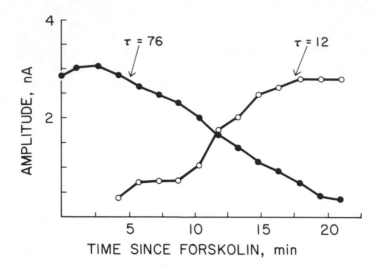

Fig. 7.8. Time course of the change in amplitudes of the rapidly and slowly inactivating components of A-current after elevation of cyclic AMP. Inactivating phase of A-current in an isolated bag cell neurons was fit with time constants 76 msec (slow component) and 12 msec (rapid component) at various times after elevation of cyclic AMP levels using forskolin (Strong, 1984).

AMP. Such an increase in the rate of inactivation causes the inactivation process to overlap considerably with activation and explains the reduction of peak A-current following cyclic AMP elevation (see Figure 7.7). Other parameters of the A-current, including the kinetics of its activation and the steady-state voltage dependence of activation and inactivation, are unaffected by cyclic AMP (Strong, 1984).

As discussed above, the A-current influences the interstimulus interval in repetitively firing cells and determines the latency with which action potentials are evoked following a depolarizing stimulus. In isolated bag cell neurons the change in firing pattern seen after elevation of cyclic AMP levels is indeed similar to the simulated change in firing pattern seen in a model neuron when the rate of inactivation of A-current is increased (see Figures 7.5 and 7.6). The more rapid inactivation of the A-current, and the resultant reduction in peak A-current, may therefore function *in vivo* to transform the bag cell neurons from cells that are incapable of firing repetitively into ones that can fire repetitively for more than 30 minutes during the afterdischarge.

The modification of the A-current cannot, however, explain all of the changes in the properties of the bag cell neurons upon synaptic stimulation or elevation of intracellular cyclic AMP concentrations. In particular, it cannot explain the marked enhancement that occurs in the width of the action potentials. Such broadening of action potentials occurs even when the membrane potential of the cell is maintained at a positive value, which ensures that the A-current is almost entirely inactivated (see Figure 7.4). The way an elevation in cyclic AMP actually influences the action potentials in the bag cell neurons is through its effects on the delayed potassium currents.

Properties of Delayed Potassium Currents

First described in giant axons of the squid by Hodgkin and Huxley (1952), delayed potassium current (delayed rectification) has been found in all excitable cells studied with the single exception of mammalian node of Ranvier. As described in Chapter 2, delayed potassium currents constitute a heterogenous class of channels whose main function is to repolarize the action potential. The pharmacological and kinetic properties of delayed outward currents differ from species to species and may also differ from cell to cell in a given animal (Hille, 1984). In some instances, as will be described, several different components of delayed potassium current may coexist in a single cell.

Modulation of Delayed Potassium Currents in the Bag Cell Neurons

In the above studies, the A-current could be examined in isolation from other currents because of its distinctive activation at more negative potentials. Depolarization to more positive potentials (i.e., above 0 mV) elicits a number of currents that are not as readily isolated from one another. To study the electrophysiological effects of cyclic AMP in these more positive voltage regions, the whole cell patch clamp technique, which permits experimental control of small intracellular ions (see Chapter 2), has been used.

Using this technique, the calcium-activated potassium current can be blocked by dialysis with intracellular solutions containing the calcium chelator, EGTA (20 mM) thus unmasking delayed voltage-dependent potassium current. In the bag cell neurons, this delayed rectifying potassium current consists of two kinetically distinct components (Strong & Kaczmarek, 1985). One component, I_{K1}, resembles the delayed rectifier found in axons. It does not inactivate during 100-msec depolarizations (but will inactivate during much longer depolarizations). The second component of delayed current, I_{K2}, is distinguished from I_{K1} by its faster kinetic properties and by the fact that it partially inactivates during 100-msec depolarizations.

Figure 7.9 shows how these two components may be differentiated from one another during a depolarization. In the control, the membrane potential has been stepped from -50 mV to $+30$ mV for varying periods of time after which the membrane potential is repolarized to -50 mV. The currents observed immediately after repolarization are shown, in enlarged form, underneath the plot of total current. These currents that are observed on repolarization are termed "tail currents"; they represent current flowing through potassium channels, opened by the prior depolarization, that have not yet closed. At -50 mV these channels begin to close and their rate of closing can be measured and fitted by theoretical curves. Such tail currents provide two pieces of information. First, the amplitude of the tail current immediately following repolarization gives an indication of the amount of potassium current activated during the depolarization. Second, the rate of decay of the tail currents gives an index of the rate at which the potassium channels close. In cases in which a single class of potassium channel is believed to exist, as in the squid giant axon, the rate of decay can be fit by a single exponential (Hodgkin & Huxley, 1952). As

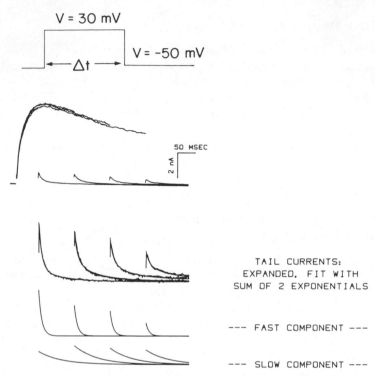

Fig. 7.9. Tail currents of delayed potassium currents. The upper trace shows superimposed traces of delayed voltage-dependent potassium currents in an internally dialyzed neuron. The tail currents observed on repolarization from +30 to −50 mV are shown below, together with the exponential curves that fit the tail currents (Strong & Kaczmarek, 1985).

is shown in Figure 7.9, the decay of the tail currents in the bag cell neurons cannot be fit by a single exponential but displays two distinct phases of decay, each of which can be represented by a single exponential. The different tail currents, measured by repolarizing the membrane at different times, show that these two components also inactivate at different rates during a depolarization. The component that is fit by a small time constant (fast component, I_{K2}) progressively diminishes in amplitude throughout the 300-msec pulse. The slower component (I_{K1}) does not inactivate during the pulse.

Several lines of evidence suggest that these two components of outward current are likely to represent the activity of different species of ion channels in the membrane of bag cell neurons, although the possibility that there is only one species of delayed potassium channel with fiendishly complex kinetics cannot be ruled out (Strong & Kaczmarek, 1985). An elevation of cyclic AMP in the bag cell neurons brings about a significant diminution in these delayed potassium currents (Figure 7.10). Cyclic AMP does not, however, affect the two components in the same way. An analysis of tail currents, using the method illustrated in Figure 7.9 indicates that elevations of cyclic AMP simply reduce the amplitude of the slower component, I_{K1},

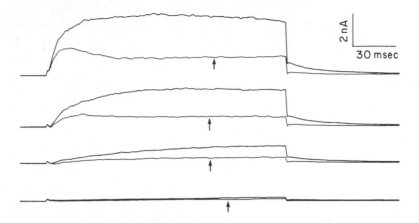

→ FORSKOLIN / THEOPHYLLINE

Fig. 7.10. Diminution of delayed potassium currents by cyclic AMP. Delayed potassium currents were evoked in an isolated internally dialyzed bag cell neuron by stepping the membrane potential form −60 mV to the indicated potentials. The lower trace in each case is the current observed after elevation of cyclic AMP levels using forskolin (Strong & Kaczmarek, 1985).

with no apparent change in its kinetic behavior. However, elevation of cyclic AMP levels produces an increase in the rate at which component I_{K2} inactivates, an effect that is similar to that seen with the A-current. This increased rate of inactivation can be seen as the pronounced "sag" in the delayed current in the lower current traces in Figure 7.10.

Both I_{K1} and I_{K2} play a role in repolarization of the action potential. Because of its inactivation however, I_{K2} would not be expected to play a major role when neurons are firing rapidly. The reduction of these currents by cyclic AMP may underlie the marked enhancement of action potential width seen during an afterdischarge *in vivo*. Such modulation of the shape of the action potential, a hallmark of many modulatory transmitters, would in turn be expected to have several important functional consequences. The most immediate result of broadening the action potential may be an enhancement of calcium influx and transmitter release. The influx of calcium that occurs during an action potential in a neuronal cell body may also contribute to metabolic processes, such as those regulating protein synthesis.

PROTEIN KINASE C AND THE REGULATION OF CALCIUM CURRENT

In addition to the cyclic AMP-dependent protein kinase system, the bag cell neurons may also use the inositol trisphosphate/diacyglycerol-protein kinase C system (see Chapter 4) to regulate their excitability. Protein kinase C is present in membrane

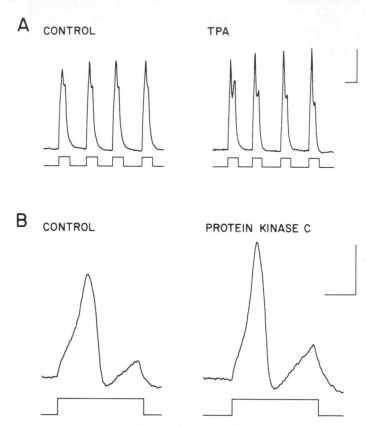

Fig. 7.11. Enhancement of calcium action potentials by a phorbol ester and protein kinase C. (A) Action potentials evoked in an isolated bag cell neuron by four consecutive depolarizing current pulses before and after exposure of the cell to 10 nM TPA; (B) on a more expanded time scale, the enhancement of action potentials in an isolated bag cell neuron by direct microinjection of protein kinase C (Calibration bars: 20 mV, 200 msec) (DeRiemer et al., 1985b).

fractions prepared from the bag cell neurons and, as in other tissues, may be activated by phorbol esters, agents that mimic the action of the membrane-soluble second messenger, diacylglycerol (DeRiemer et al., 1985a). When isolated bag cell neurons in cell culture are exposed to an active phorbol ester such as 12-*O*-tetradecanoyl-13-phorbol acetate (TPA), their action potentials can be observed to increase in height (Figure 7.11). As is also shown in Figure 7.11, this enhancement of action potentials can be mimicked by direct microinjection of protein kinase C itself into isolated neurons. In contrast to the effects of cyclic AMP described earlier, TPA and protein kinase C induce little change in the width of the action potentials (DeRiemer et al., 1985b).

Can this effect also be explained by some effect on the voltage-dependent potassium currents? Voltage clamp experiments have revealed that it cannot. Using the whole cell patch clamp technique, no effects of TPA can be observed on either the delayed voltage-dependent potassium currents or the A-current. However, the inward calcium current, measured in voltage-clamped, internally dialyzed neurons, is markedly enhanced by TPA application (DeRiemer et al., 1985b). Because in these neurons the calcium current is a major contributor to the rising phase of action potentials, this effect can account for the enhancement of the action potentials. A further account of this effect is given in Chapter 11, which deals with modulation of calcium currents.

SPECIFICITY OF THE EFFECTS OF PROTEIN KINASE SYSTEMS ON THE PROPERTIES OF DIFFERENT ION CHANNELS

It is likely that the cyclic AMP system and the protein kinase C system act together to transform the firing pattern and shape of action potentials in the bag cell neurons following stimulation. Interestingly, these two second messenger systems have a similar effect on the action potentials of these neurons but by very different mechanisms; the cyclic AMP system enhances action potentials by the depression of the delayed potassium currents whereas the protein kinase C system increases the calcium current.

Whether or not the specific changes in the kinetics and amplitudes of the voltage-dependent potassium and calcium currents described previously can explain all of the transitions in excitability these neurons undergo is not clear. Certainly, additional second messenger systems may modulate the activity of ion channels in these cells during their prolonged transitions in excitability.

One important comment about the roles of different kinase systems must be made. As yet uncharacterized systems of protein kinases may exist within neurons. These may have substrate specifities that are either similar to those of the known kinases or may display greater specificity toward certain ion channels, for example, the different classes of potassium channels. The potential role that such kinases might play in neuromodulation is not known. Knowing that a channel is modulated by the cyclic AMP-dependent protein kinase does not therefore guarantee that it is not also modulated by other systems during physiological activity.

OTHER MECHANISMS FOR MODULATION OF EXCITABILITY IN THE BAG CELL NEURONS

We have seen that the ion channels of the bag cell neurons are subject to a high degree of modulation by different second messenger systems. This is part of how the cells change their properties to cause the release of their peptides and therefore trigger a sequence of motor acts. However, to carry out the full repertoire of changes needed to control these behaviors, the bag cell neurons may also avail themselves of some other regulatory mechanisms (see Chapter 1). Two such processes that may modulate the properties of these neurons are (1) changes in the rate of synthesis of their neuroactive peptides and (2) longer-term regulation of their response to cyclic

AMP while the behaviors that have been triggered are in progress. A brief account of these processes is given to emphasize the degree of plasticity that one neuronal type may generate to carry out its normal physiological role.

Autoreceptor-Mediated Peptide Actions

The onset of an afterdischarge in the bag cell neurons is associated with changes in the phosphorylation state of proteins (Jennings et al., 1982). Changes in some phosphoprotein substrates within these cells must be directly or indirectly responsible for the changes in the properties of the ion channels. Evidence suggests, however, that the roles of the major phosphoprotein substrates within the bag cell neurons may be related to peptide synthesis and processing (Kaczmarek et al., 1986). Both depolarization and elevation of cyclic AMP levels have been shown to increase the rate of synthesis of the precursor protein to the peptides released by these neurons (Berry & Arch, 1981; Bruehl & Berry, 1985). Such regulation of peptide synthesis may be more than a "housekeeping" function; evidence exists that at least one of the bag cell peptides has both electrical and biochemical actions on the bag cell neurons themselves (Rothman et al., 1983; Kauer & Kaczmarek, 1985a). The state of peptide synthesis, processing, and release may therefore directly affect their excitability. The role that such processes play in neuromodulation is still largely unexplored.

Prolonged Period of Inhibition Prevents
Spontaneous Activity during Triggered Behaviors

At the end of a normal afterdischarge, which usually lasts about 30 minutes, the cells enter a second state during which normal stimulation generally fails to trigger an afterdischarge and even intense stimulation can generate only short, low-frequency discharges. This has been termed the refractory period and it is believed to prevent further discharges in the cells while the sequence of egg-laying behaviors initiated by the bag cell peptides is in progress. Recovery from the refractory period occurs gradually over 10 to 20 hours (Kaczmarek & Kauer, 1983).

During the refractory period elevations of cyclic AMP also fail to trigger or prolong afterdischarges (Kauer & Kaczmarek, 1985b). The cellular mechanism of this very prolonged inhibition of activity and loss of response to cyclic AMP is not known. Evidence indicates, however, that calcium entry during the afterdischarge plays a role in generating this refractory period (Kaczmarek & Kauer, 1983).

CONCLUSIONS

To carry out their biological role as a sophisticated switch, which triggers a series of prolonged behaviors, the bag cell neurons undergo a series of changes in their cellular and electrical properties. They provide a powerful example of how intracellular biochemical reactions are used to transform the excitability of a neuron. It has been seen that at least four distinct ionic conductances are modulated in these neurons by two different second messenger-protein kinase systems. Modulation of both the amplitude and the kinetics of these currents has been observed; it occurs in ways that are consistent with the transformation of the electrical properties of these neurons when they are stimulated.

A full understanding of the prolonged nature of the transitions in excitability that are observed in these and other neurons whose properties must change over periods of many hours, or even days, may require investigation not only of direct effects of second messenger systems on specific ion channels, but also of the diverse mechanisms that regulate the expression of the second messenger responses themselves.

REFERENCES

Aghajanian, G.K. (1985) Modulation of a transient outward current in serotonergic neurones by adrenoceptors. *Nature 315*, 501–503.

Berridge, M.J. (1984) Inositol triphosphate and diacylglycerol as second messengers. *Biochem J. 220*, 345–360.

Berry, R.W. and Arch, S. (1981) Activation of neurosecretory cells enhances their synthesis of secretory protein. *Brain Res. 215*, 115–123.

Bruehl, C.L. and Berry, R.W. (1985) Regulation of synthesis of the neurosecretory egg-laying hormone of *Aplysia:* Antagonistic roles of calcium and cyclic adenosine 3',5'-monophosphate. *J. Neurosci. 5*, 1233–1238.

Byrne, J.H. (1980) Analysis of ionic conductance mechanisms in motor cells mediating inking behavior in *Aplysia californica. J. Neurophysiol. 43*, 630–650.

Connor, J.A. (1978) Slow repetitive activity from fast conductance changes in neurons. *Fed. Proc. 37*, 2139–2145.

Connor, J.A. and Stevens, C.F. (1971a) Predictions of repetitive firing behavior from voltage clamp data on an isolated neurone soma. *J. Physiol. 213*, 31–53.

Connor, J.A. and Stevens, C.F. (1971b) Voltage clamp studies of a transient outward membrane current in gastropod neural somata. *J. Physiol 213*, 21–30.

DeRiemer, S.A., Greengard, P., and Kaczmarek, L.K. (1985a) Calcium/diacylglycerol/phosphatidyl serine dependent protein phosphorylation in the *Aplysia* nervous system. *J. Neurosci. 5*, 2672–2676.

DeRiemer, S.A., Strong, J.A., Albert, K.A., Greengard, P., and Kaczmarek, L.K. (1985b) Enhancement of calcium current in *Aplysia* neurones by phorbol ester and protein kinase C. *Nature 313*, 313–315.

Dudek, F.E. and Blankenship, J.E. (1977) Neuroendocrine cells of *Aplysia brasiliana*. II. Bag cell prepotentials and potentiation. *J. Neurophysiol. 40*, 1312–1324.

Hagiwara, S., Kusano, K. and Saito, N. (1961) Membrane changes of *Onchidium* nerve cell in potassium-rich media. *J. Physiol. 155*, 470–489.

Hamill, O.P., Marty, A., Neher, E., Sakmann, B., and Sigworth, F.J. (1981) Improved patch-clamp techniques for high-resolution current recording from cells and cell-free membrane patches. *Pflugers Arch. 391*, 85–100.

Heller, E., Kaczmarek, L.K., Hunkapiller, M.W., Hood, L.E., and Strumwasser, F. (1980) Purification and primary structure of two neuroactive peptides that cause bag cell afterdischarge and egg-laying in *Aplysia. Proc. Natl. Acad. Sci. USA 77*, 2328–2332.

Hille, B. (1984) *Ionic Channels of Excitable Membranes*. Sinauer Assoc., Sunderland, MA.

Hodgkin, A.L. and Huxley A.F., (1952) The components of membrane conductance in the giant axon of *Loligo. J. Physiol. 116*, 473–496.

Jennings, K.R., Kaczmarek, L.K., Hewick, R.M., Dreyer, W.J., and Strumwasser, F. (1982) Protein phosphorylation during afterdischarge in peptidergic neurons of *Aplysia. J. Neurosci. 2*, 158–168.

Kaczmarek, L.K., Jennings, K., and Strumwasser, F. (1978) neurotransmitter modulation, phosphodiesterase inhibitor effects, and cAMP correlates of afterdischarge in peptidergic neurites. *Proc. Natl. Acad. Sci. USA 75*, 5200–5204.

Kaczmarek, L.K., Jennings, K.R., Strumwasser, F., Nairn, A.C., Walter, U., Wilson, F.D., and Greengard, P. (1980) Microinjection of catalytic subunit of cyclic AMP-dependent protein kinase enhances calcium action potentials of bag cell neurons in cell culture. *Proc. Natl. Acad. Sci. USA 77*, 7487–7491.

Kaczmarek, L.K., Jennings, K.R., and Strumwasser F. (1982) An early sodium and a late calcium phase in the afterdischarge of peptide secreting neurons of *Aplysia. Brain Res. 283*, 105–115.

Kaczmarek, L.K. and Kauer, J.A. (1983) Calcium entry causes a prolonged refractory period in peptidergic neurons of *Aplysia. J. Neurosci. 11*, 2230–2239.

Kaczmarek, L.K., Nairn, A.C., and Greengard, P. (1984) Microinjection of protein kinase inhibitor prevents enhancement of action potentials in peptidergic neurons of *Aplysia. Soc. Neurosci. Abstr. 10*, 895.

Kaczmarek, L.K., Strong, J.A., and Kauer, J.A. (1986) The role of protein kinases in the control of prolonged changes in neuronal excitability. *Prog. Brain Res.*, in press.

Kaczmarek, L.K. and Strumwasser, F. (1981) The expression of long lasting afterdischarge by isolated *Aplysia* bag cell neurons. *J. Neurosci 1*, 626–634.

Kaczmarek, L.K. and Strumwasser, F. (1984) A voltage clamp analysis of currents underlying cAMP-induced membrane modulation in isolated peptidergic neurons of *Aplysia. J. Neurophysiol. 52*, 340–349.

Kauer, J.A and Kaczmarek, L.K. (1985a) A neuropeptide autoreceptor mediates changes in neuronal excitability. *Soc. Neurosci. Abstr. 11*, 710.

Kauer, J.A and Kaczmarek, L.K. (1985b) Peptidergic neurons of *Aplysia* lose their response to cyclic adenosine 3':5'-monophosphate during a prolonged refractory period. *J. Neurosci. 5*, 1399–1345.

Kupfermann, I. and Kandel, E.R. (1970) Electrophysiological properties and functional interconnections of two symmetrical neurosecretory clusters (bag cells) in abdominal ganglion of *Aplysia. J. Neurophysiol. 33*, 865–876.

Nishizuka, Y. (1984) The role of protein kinase C in cell surface signal transduction and tumour promotion. *Nature 308*, 693–697.

Rogawski, M.A. (1985) The A-current: How ubiquitous a feature of excitable cells is it? *Trends in Neurosci. 8*, 214–219.

Rothman, B.S., Mayeri, E., Brown, R.O. Yuan, P., and Shively, J. (1983) Primary structure and neuronal effects of α-bag cell peptide, a second candidate neurotransmitter encoded by a single gene in bag cell neurons of *Aplysia. Proc. Natl. Acad. Sci. USA 80*, 5733–5757.

Scheller, R.H., Jackson, J.F., McAllister, L.B., Schwartz, J.H., Kandel, E.R., and Axel, R. (1982) A family of genes that code for ELH, a neuropeptide eliciting a stereotyped pattern of behavior in *Aplysia. Cell 28*, 707–719.

Seamon, K.B., Padgett, W., and Daly, J.W. (1981) Forskolin: Unique diterpene activator of adenylate cyclase in membranes and in intact cells. *Proc. Natl. Acad. Sci. USA 78*, 3363–3367.

Serrano, E.E. (1982) Variability in molluscan neuron soma currents. PhD thesis, Stanford University, Stanford, CA.

Strong, J.A. (1984) Modulation of potassium current kinetics in bag cell neurons of *Aplysia* by an activator of adenylate cyclase. *J. Neurosci. 4*, 2722–2783.

Strong, J.A. and Kaczmarek, L.K. (1985) Multiple components of delayed potassium current in peptidergic neurons of *Aplysia:* Modulation by an activator of adenylate cyclase. *J. Neurosci. 6*, 819–822.

Strumwasser, F.L., Kaczmarek, L.K., Chiu, A.Y., Heller, E., Jennings, K.R., and Viele, D.P. (1980) Peptides controlling behavior in *Aplysia*. In *Peptides: Integrators of Cell and Tissue Functions* (ed. F.E. Bloom), pp. 197–218. Raven Press, New York.

Thompson, S.H. and Aldrich, R.A. (1980) Membrane potassium channels. In *The Cell Surface and Neuronal Function* (eds. C.W. Cotman, G. Poste, and G.L. Nicolson), pp. 50–78. Elsevier/North Holland Biomedical Press, Amsterdam.

8

Ion Channels Regulated by Calcium

DOUGLAS A. EWALD
IRWIN B. LEVITAN

Excitable cells, in performing the various functions for which they are differentiated, must respond to many types of chemical and electrical signals from other cells. Converting this information into an appropriate physiological response often involves intracellular "messengers" whose concentration is sensitive to the extracellular signals and which are capable of regulating the response. It has been known since the beginning of modern electrophysiology that one such messenger is calcium. Two of the first uses of modern electrophysiological techniques were to demonstrate the singular importance of a transient increase in cytoplasmic concentration of calcium for the regulation of neurotransmitter release in neurons (Fatt & Katz, 1952) and of contraction in muscle cells (Huxley & Niedergerke, 1954). Since then many other physiological responses have been shown to be regulated by this intracellular signal (Campbell, 1983). This chapter is concerned with one aspect of this calcium regulatory system, the membrane currents that are modulated by intracellular calcium.

The intracellular concentration of calcium in neurons and muscle cells is very low ($\sim 0.1 \mu M$) in the resting state. This is because calcium channels, through which calcium enters the cytoplasm down its concentration gradient, are closed at normal resting potentials, and the small amount of calcium that does enter is well buffered or actively extruded (Baker, 1972). The physiological signals that can open voltage-dependent calcium channels and turn on calcium current (I_{Ca}) depend on depolarization of the membrane potential from its resting state (see Chapters 2 and 11). Depolarization can cause calcium to accumulate in the cytoplasm, especially near the inner surface of the plasma membrane, to concentrations ten to a hundred times its resting level (Gorman & Thomas, 1980). At these concentrations calcium binds to certain calcium-receptor proteins, such as calmodulin, and certain enzymes, such as protein kinase C, to regulate a physiological response (Rasmussen & Barrett, 1984).

It is well known that these calcium-regulated processes can also be modulated by various hormones and neurotransmitters and that this modulation involves an increase in the concentration of other intracellular messengers such as cyclic AMP (Rasmussen, 1981). For example, cyclic AMP mediates the noradrenergic modulation of cardiac pacemaker activity (see Chapter 11) and can modulate the release of neurotransmitters from synapses (Brunelli et al., 1976) and from neuromuscular junctions (Wilson; 1974). This situation of one intracellular messenger, cyclic AMP, modulating the regulation of physiological processes by another intracellular messenger, calcium, raises the question of the identity of the cellular sites at which these messenger systems interact. Because an important common step in all these calcium-regulated processes is the voltage-dependent entry of calcium into cells across their plasma membranes, it has long been suspected that the rise in intracellular cyclic AMP concentration associated with their modulation somehow affects the actual production of the calcium signal at the plasma membrane. Thus, we will first discuss the network of calcium-regulated currents, including the calcium current itself, that produce the calcium signal, and then consider the modulation of these currents by cyclic AMP mechanisms.

THREE IONIC CURRENTS REGULATED BY CALCIUM

Ionic currents across biological membranes are generated by the flow of ions down their electrochemical gradients through ion channels (see Chapter 3). Electrophysiological studies have shown that calcium can regulate at least three different ionic currents. Assuming, for the moment, that each ionic current is generated by a single type of channel, we can depict the actions of intracellular calcium on ion channels,

Fig. 8.1. Schematic diagram of the entry of calcium into neurons and its actions on the three types of ion channels that produce I_{Ca}, $I_{K(Ca)}$, and $I_{cation(Ca)}$. Depolarization-activated calcium channels allow calcium to enter the cytoplasm (see Chapter 11). The inward current (I_{Ca}) that flows as a result of activation of these channels causes further depolarization. When cytoplasmic calcium reaches micromolar concentration levels, it activates a channel type selective for potassium (a). The outward current that flows as a result of these channels being activated, $I_{K(Ca)}$, causes hyperpolarization. Cytoplasmic calcium also activates a channel type selective for both sodium and potassium (b), and the resulting inward current (at resting voltages), $I_{cation(Ca)}$, causes depolarization. Finally, cytoplasmic calcium inactivates the calcium channels through which it enters (c). This action of calcium, in concert with the hyperpolarization caused by $I_{K(Ca)}$, turns off I_{Ca}.

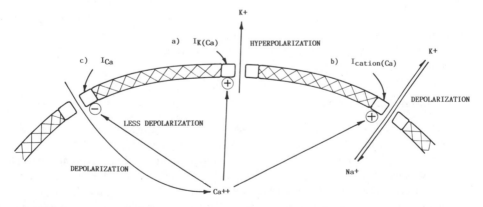

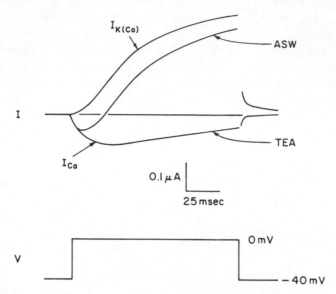

Fig. 8.2. Separation of I_{Ca} and $I_{K(Ca)}$ in a molluscan neuron. Neuron R15 of the *Aplysia* abdominal ganglion was voltage clamped at -40 mV in artificial seawater (ASW) with 45-μM TTX to block sodium current. A voltage clamp pulse to 0 mV for 150 msec *(bottom)* elicited the current marked ASW. After exposure to 200-mM TEA (replacing sodium) to block potassium currents, the same pulse produced the current marked TEA, which is I_{Ca} (see text). The difference between these two currents is the potassium current blocked by TEA, which, under these conditions, is $I_{K(Ca)}$ (see text) (from Eckert & Ewald, 1982).

as shown in Figure 8.1. One action of calcium is to activate a type of channel that is strictly selective for potassium (Figure 8.1A; Meech, 1978). The outward current, $I_{K(Ca)}$, which flows as a result of these channels opening, tends to repolarize the membrane potential toward the potassium reversal potential. Another action of calcium is to activate a type of channel that allows the flow of both sodium and potassium (Figure 8.1B; Kass et al., 1978). In the resting range of membrane potentials it carries a net inward current, $I_{cation(Ca)}$, which tends to depolarize the membrane toward the sodium plus potassium reversal potential. A third action of calcium is to inactivate the same depolarization-activated calcium channels through which it enters the cell (Figure 8.1C; Eckert & Tillotson, 1981), This inactivation of I_{Ca}, in conjunction with the repolarization produced by activation of $I_{K(Ca)}$, turns off the voltage-dependent entry of calcium.

Activation of $I_{K(Ca)}$ by Calcium

One can observe I_{Ca}, $I_{K(Ca)}$, and $I_{cation(Ca)}$ separately by treating voltage-clamped neurons with specific pharmacological agents and making judicious use of voltage clamp potential steps. Tetrodotoxin (TTX) is used to block sodium current so that the only inward currents are I_{Ca} and $I_{cation(Ca)}$. Trace (ASW) in Figure 8.2 is the current evoked by a step from -40 to 0 mV in a TTX-treated neuron R15 of *Aplysia*. It consists of first inward and then outward current. After exposure to tetraethylammonium (TEA),

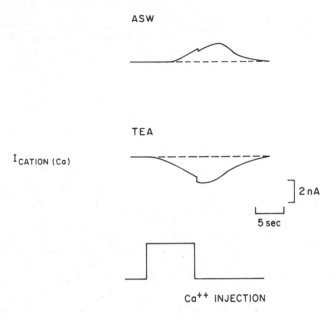

Fig. 8.3. Separation of $I_{cation(Ca)}$ from other currents in a molluscan neuron. A left-upper-quadrant neuron of the *Aplysia* abdominal ganglion was voltage clamped to -45 mV in ASW. An 8-sec iontophoretic injection of calcium caused the outward current shown in the upper trace. This is a mixture of $I_{cation(Ca)}$ and $I_{K(ca)}$. After exposure to 50-mM TEA, which blocks $I_{K(Ca)}$, the same calcium injection caused the inward current shown in the lower trace. This inward current $I_{cation(Ca)}$, allows the flow of both sodium and potassium and thus reverses at about -20 mV. Note that the end of the calcium injection is accompanied by artifacts in the current traces (from Kramer & Zucker, 1958a).

which blocks all potassium currents at this potential, the current is entirely inward (trace TEA).

Since the current is measured near the reversal potential of $I_{cation(Ca)}$, this inward current is entirely I_{Ca}. Notice that I_{Ca} reaches a peak early during the pulse and then gradually declines; as we will see below, this decline reflects calcium-dependent inactivation of I_{Ca}. The difference between trace ASW and trace TEA is thus the potassium current blocked by TEA. Under these conditions the potassium current is entirely $I_{K(Ca)}$, since other potassium currents are not activated at this combination of holding and pulse potentials (see Chapter 2). Thus, we have a clear picture of $I_{K(Ca)}$ in the absence of other currents.

Activation of $I_{cation(Ca)}$ by Calcium

The two calcium-activated currents can be experimentally separated from I_{Ca} by injecting calcium into a voltage-clamped neuron (Kramer & Zucker, 1985a). At holding potentials more depolarized than -50 mV, calcium injection evokes a net outward current, which is the sum of outward current carried by $I_{K(Ca)}$ and an inward current (Figure 8.3). When $I_{K(Ca)}$ is blocked by exposure to TEA, this inward current,

$I_{cation(Ca)}$, is revealed (Figure 8.3). First described in cardiac cells as the "transient inward current" (Kass et al., 1978), it allows the flow of both sodium and potassium and thus is an inward current at potentials more hyperpolarized than its reversal potential, about -20 mV. These two actions of calcium on $I_{cation(Ca)}$ and $I_{K(Ca)}$ create a stabilizing effect toward a membrane potential of about -50 mV. At more hyperpolarized potentials, the driving force for $I_{K(Ca)}$ is small compared with that for $I_{cation(Ca)}$, and calcium injection evokes a net inward current (predominantly $I_{cation(Ca)}$, causing depolarization. Conversely, at membrane potentials more depolarized then -50 mV, the driving force for $I_{cation(Ca)}$ is small compared with that for $I_{K(Ca)}$, and calcium injection evokes a net outward current (predominantly $I_{K(Ca)}$), causing hyperpolarization.

Inactivation of I_{Ca} by Calcium

As already noted, I_{Ca} reaches a peak and then decreases during a depolarizing pulse (see Figure 8.2), and it is thought that in some cells this reflects calcium-dependent inactivation of I_{Ca}. The intracellular calcium effect of decreasing I_{Ca} has been demonstrated in molluscan neurons in a variety of ways. I_{Ca}, during a depolarizing pulse, is decreased by calcium entry during a prior depolarization, and injection of the calcium chelator ethylene glycol-bis (β-amino ethyl ether) N, N, N', N'-tetraacetic acid (EGTA) prevents this decrease (Eckert & Tillotson, 1981). Furthermore, injection of calcium, but not magnesium, reversibly decreases I_{Ca} (Standen, 1981). In these experiments, however, isolation of I_{Ca} depends on blockage of potassium current by TEA or cesium, which might not be total; they therefore leave open the possibility of a calcium-activated outward current, such as $I_{K(Ca)}$, producing an apparent decrease in the inward I_{Ca}. The following experiment excludes this possibility.

The depolarized potentials needed for activation of I_{Ca} are far from the potassium reversal potential, so it is difficult to measure I_{Ca} in the absence of a large driving force for potassium flow. One way to circumvent this problem is to measure the calcium current that flows for a few milliseconds after the activating pulse is turned off ("tail" currents) at a potential where the potassium driving force is close to zero. This is achieved by increasing the external potassium concentration to bring the potassium reversal potential, E_K, close to the holding potential. Figure 8.4A shows a voltage-clamp pulse from a holding potential (-40 mV), near the new potassium reversal potential, to a potential where I_{Ca} is activated ($+20$ mV). During the pulse the potassium driving force ($V - E_K$) is about 60 mV, but when the pulse is turned off, the driving force on potassium drops to close to zero. The calcium driving force is large both during and after the pulse because the calcium reversal potential is $\sim +150$ mV. The calcium channels do not close instantaneously after the end of the pulse, but relax exponentially. During this time a brief, exponentially decaying calcium tail current can be measured at the holding potential where the potassium driving force is close to zero and virtually no potassium current can flow (Figure 8.4B). For this technique to be practical, the neurons are severed from their axons and the temperature is held at 12°C. Under these conditions the closing of the calcium channels after the end of the pulse is much slower than the time needed to change voltage at the end of the pulse. In addition, potassium current is blocked with

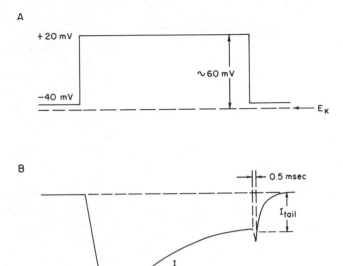

Fig. 8.4. An idealization of the tail current technique for measuring calcium current in the absence of potassium current. (A) The cell body of an axotomized molluscan neuron is voltage clamped at -40 mV in ASW with elevated potassium concentration. Extracellular potassium is increased so that the potassium reversal potential (E_K) approaches this holding potential and little or no potassium current will flow at the holding potential. During a 100-msec pulse to $+20$ mV, the driving force on potassium flow ($V - E_K$) is about 60 mV. At the end of the pulse the potassium driving force drops to close to zero mV. (B) Currents during and after the pulse. After the pulse ends, the calcium channels activated during the pulse do not close instantaneously but relax exponentially. During this time a brief, exponentially decaying calcium tail current (I_{tail}) can be measured at a potential where the potassium driving force is close to zero. The amplitude of the tail current is measured at a fixed time after the pulse ends (e.g., 0.5 msec).

TEA and sodium current is blocked with TTX, so that the current during the pulse is as close to a pure I_{Ca} as is possible with these pharmacological treatments.

Figure 8.5 shows calcium tail currents recorded under the conditions described above. The tail current labeled "V_1 off" followed a 7-msec pulse to $+20$ mV. A "prepulse" (200 msec, to $+10$ mV) given 1 sec before the 7-msec test pulse substantially reduces the amplitude of the tail current ("V_1 on"). The amplitude of the prepulse was varied to show that this long-lasting inactivation of the tail current amplitude is mediated by a long-lasting elevation of intracellular calcium concentration. Figure 8.6 shows that the most effective voltage range for producing inactivation is by prepulses of $+10$ to $+60$ mV (filled circles). This coincides with the voltage range of maximum calcium entry (Eckert & Tillotson, 1981). Furthermore, the inactivation by the prepulse is almost completely blocked by injecting the neuron with the calcium chelator EGTA (open circles in Figure 8.6) The voltage change

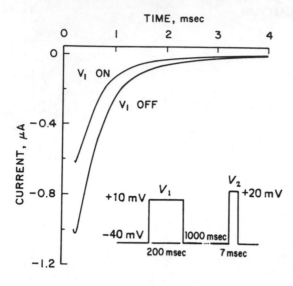

Fig. 8.5. Inactivation of calcium tail currents in an axotomized left-upper-quadrant neuron of the *Aplysia* abdominal ganglion. V_1 off is a calcium tail current recorded following a 7-msec voltage-clamp pulse to +20 mV (V_2 in inset) in the presence of 200-mM TEA and 45-μM TTX. A 200-msec prepulse to +10 mV (V_1 in inset), given 1 sec before the 7-msec test pulse, reduces the amplitude of the tail current by ~50% during its entire time course (V_1 on) (from Eckert & Ewald, 1983).

Fig. 8.6. Inactivation of calcium tail currents as a function of prepulse potential. Calcium tail currents were recorded as described in Figure 8.5 following a 10-msec voltage-clamp pulse to +10 mV (V_2 in inset). A 200-msec prepulse to various potentials (V_1 in inset) was given 1 sec before the 10-msec test pulse. The amplitude of the tail current was measured 0.5 msec after the end of the test pulses and plotted as a function of the prepulse potential *(filled circles)*. The maximum inactivation occurs with prepulse potentials between +10 and +60 mV. After injection of the calcium chelator EGTA, inactivation of I_{tail} by the prepulse is almost completely absent *(open circles)* (from Eckert & Ewald, 1983).

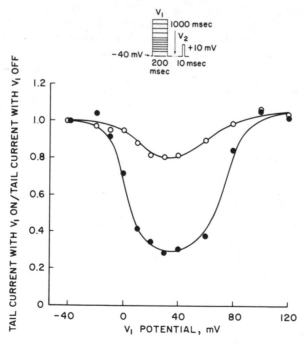

during the prepulse is exactly the same in the EGTA-injected neurons, but inactivation is greatly reduced, and thus little or none of the inactivation is voltage dependent. Rather, the inactivation of calcium channels in these neurons, measured in the absence of potassium flow, is strictly calcium dependent.

A FUNCTIONAL ROLE OF CALCIUM-REGULATED CURRENTS IN BURSTING ACTIVITY

Regulation of I_{Ca}, $I_{K(Ca)}$, and $I_{cation(Ca)}$ by calcium entry has been demonstrated in types of neurons with widely varied physiological activities and functions. A first step in determining the relative importance and coordination of these three actions of calcium in a particular physiological situation is to study their magnitudes and time courses. One of the most complete examples of this type of analysis is the bursting activity of certain *Aplysia* neurons. In these neurons an alternating cycle of depolarization and hyperpolarization gives rise to seconds-long bursts of action potentials with an interburst period of tens of seconds (Chapter 6). Figure 8.7 shows the currents measured immediately after voltage clamping one of these neurons (R15) to − 30 mV at various times during its burst cycle. A net inward current accompanies the bursting phase of the cycle and a net outward current accompanies the interburst hyperpolarization. Using the calcium indicator dye Arsenazo III, it has been shown that intracellular calcium builds up during the burst and gradually declines between bursts (Gorman & Thomas, 1980). The peak of calcium at the end of the burst and its gradual decline during the interburst interval, in concert with the gradual decline of the interburst itself, strongly suggest that the interburst hyperpolarization is calcium dependent. $I_{K(Ca)}$ is present in this neuron, and it was thought for more than a decade that this hyperpolarization results from activation of $I_{K(Ca)}$. However, it has been shown recently that the outward currents measured between bursts (as in Figure 8.7) are not sensitive to changes in extracellular potassium or to TEA, as is the $I_{K(Ca)}$ evoked by calcium injection (Adams & Levitan, 1985; Kramer & Zucker, 1985a,b). Thus, this outward current, which is responsible for the generation of the interburst hyperpolarization, is not $I_{K(Ca)}$. The only other mechanism for intracellular calcium to produce a net outward current is to inactivate a resting I_{Ca}. Therefore, the most reasonable model consistent with the data (Adams & Levitan, 1985; Kramer & Zucker, 1985b) is that the interburst hyperpolarization results from the calcium-dependent inactivation of a resting I_{Ca} by calcium accumulated intracellularly during the burst. This periodic inactivation of a resting inward current yields an apparent periodic outward current. By this model a new burst is initiated when intracellular calcium returns to its normal low level, so that I_{Ca} is no longer inactivated, and the membrane potential returns to a level of depolarization where I_{Ca} will flow again.

$I_{cation(Ca)}$ also contributes to bursting. The activation of $I_{cation(Ca)}$ by calcium during the burst phase of the cycle augments the voltage-dependent I_{Ca} and accelerates spiking frequency during the burst. It cannot play a significant role in the interburst hyperpolarization because its changes during this phase run counter to the observed changes in membrane potential. Finally, the activation of $I_{K(Ca)}$ is important during the burst phase of the cycle when it may serve to decrease spike frequency toward

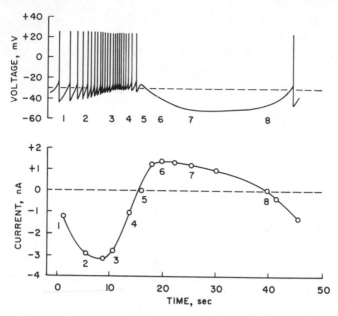

Fig. 8.7. Total membrane current recorded at various times during the bursting pacemaker cycle of neuron R15 of the *Aplysia* abdominal ganglion. The change in membrane potential during a single pacemaker cycle is shown in the top trace. In subsequent cycles the membrane was clamped to −30 mV *(dashed line in top trace)* at the times indicated by the numbers below the record. After each cycle during which the voltage clamp was activated, the cell was allowed to pass through a full cycle of activity in the nonvoltage clamp mode. *(Bottom)* A plot of the peak current at 1 sec after turning on the clamp. The total current is inward during the burst and outward between bursts (from Gorman, Hermann, & Thomas, 1982).

the end of the burst. It appears to play only a minor role in generating the interburst hyperpolarization, because it decays too quickly and the predominant outward current responsible for this phase is not a potassium current.

Figure 8.8 shows idealizations of these three calcium-sensitive currents during the burst cycle. Figure 8.8A shows the voltage changes of a single cycle of pacemaker activity. Figure 8.8B is an idealized plot of I_{Ca} during this cycle. If the voltage were clamped to a potential in the middle of this pacemaker range, a "resting" I_{Ca} would flow (1). A dashed line is drawn through the whole cycle at this level for reference. At more depolarized potentials during the burst this depolarization-activated inward current is increased above the resting level (2). Toward the end of the burst accumulation of intracellular calcium causes an inactivation of I_{Ca}. Inward I_{Ca} is then less than the resting level (3) and a net outward current relative to rest is measured during the interburst hyperpolarization. Inactivation subsides as intracellular calcium concentration is reduced by buffering and transport systems in the neuron's cytoplasm and membranes. I_{Ca} then returns to the resting level, which is unstable because of the presence of other depolarizing currents, and the next burst begins. Figure 8.8C shows an idealization of inward $I_{cation(Ca)}$ activated by calcium entry during the burst

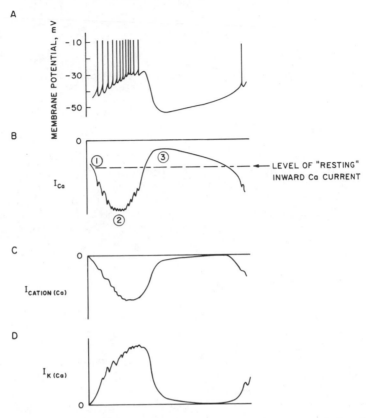

Fig. 8.8 Idealization of the time courses of calcium-regulated currents during the bursting pacemaker cycle of *Aplysia* neuron R15. Change in membrane potential (A) and idealizations of I_{Ca} (B), $I_{cation(Ca)}$ (C), and $I_{K(Ca)}$ (D) during a single pacemaker cycle. See the text for an explanation (based on Adams & Levitan, 1985; Kramer & Zucker, 1985b).

phase of the cycle. It augments the voltage-dependent I_{Ca} and accelerates the spiking frequency of the burst. Figure 8.8D shows an idealization of outward $I_{K(Ca)}$ during a burst cycle. It is generated by each spike of the burst and then decays very quickly at the end of the burst. Toward the end of the burst its effect may be to decrease the spike frequency.

SINGLE-CHANNEL RECORDINGS OF CALCIUM-REGULATED CHANNELS

The recent development by Neher, Sakmann, and colleagues of "gigaseal" recording techniques on small membrane patches (Hamill et al., 1981) has made it possible to study the single channel currents that underlie the macroscopic currents described above. In the "cell-attached" patch configuration (see Figure 2.10 in Chapter 2) the

3 μM Ca⁺⁺

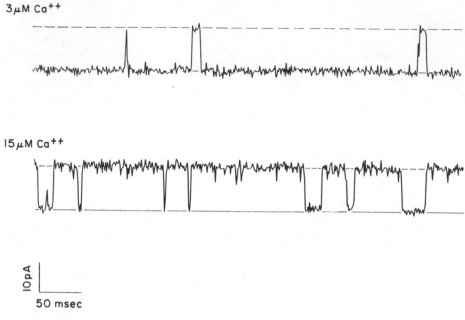

15 μM Ca⁺⁺

10 pA

50 msec

Fig. 8.9. Calcium dependence of the large conductance (~200 pS) calcium-activated potassium channel. This channel, derived from muscle T-tubule membrane, was incorporated into a planar phospholipid bilayer, as described in the text. The bilayer was voltage clamped at +80 mV and exposed to calcium/EGTA buffers having free calcium concentrations of $3 \mu M$ *(top trace)* and 15 μM *(bottom trace)*. Channel openings are observed as upward deflections of the current trace. The channel typically opens in bursts lasting tens to hundreds of milliseconds, with numerous closings of much shorter duration. The open probability is greatly increased by the fivefold increase in free calcium concentration (data courtesy of C. Miller).

ionic composition on the inside of the patch is under the control of the cell rather than the investigator, and this situation can impose constraints on the detailed characterization of some channel properties including unit conductance, ion dependence, kinetic behavior, and modulation. These properties can often be better characterized by detaching the patch from the neuron under conditions that expose the inner membrane surface—the detached or inside-out patch configuration (see Chapter 2).

Calcium-Activated Potassium Channels

Calcium-activated potassium channels have been favorite channels for study because of their interesting dual activation by both calcium and voltage. Two types of this channel have been found, one of which has an exceptionally large unit conductance (~200 pS). Figure 8.9 shows the activity of this channel derived from muscle T-tubule membrane after it has been incorporated into a phospholipid planar bilayer. In this technique a membrane vesicle preparation is reconstituted with exogenous phospholipid, and vesicles containing channels are fused with planar bilayers (80 to 200μ

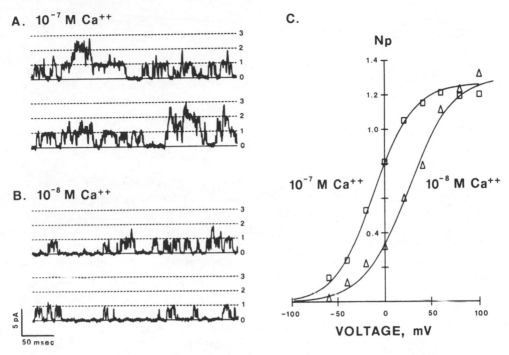

Fig. 8.10. Calcium and voltage dependence of the small conductance (~50 pS) calcium-activated potassium channel. (A) A detached patch of *Helix* neuron membrane exposed to a calcium/EGTA buffer having a free calcium concentration of 10^{-7} M. At least three potassium-selective channels exist in this patch. The dotted lines and numbers to the right of the traces indicate the number of open channels. The unitary current (2.4 pA) at this voltage (0 mV) corresponds to a unit conductance of ~20 pS. The maximal unit conductance, measured at higher potassium concentration, is ~50 pS. (B) Channel activity is decreased substantially when the same patch is exposed to a free calcium concentration of 10^{-8} M. (C) Channel activity is expressed in units of Np, where N is the number of active channels in the patch and p is the open probability of a single channel. The plot shows this analysis as a function of membrane voltage for both 10^{-7}-M *(squares)* and 10^{-8} M *(triangles)* free calcium concentration, each fitted with a Boltzmann curve. This tenfold change in free calcium concentration shifts the fitted curve by ~30 mV with little change in maximum Np and slope (from Ewald et al., 1985).

in diameter) formed across the opening between two chambers (see Chapter 2). The calcium sensitivity of this channel can vary over a rather wide range depending on its source. In this case it is closed almost all the time in 3-μM calcium and open almost all the time in 15-μM calcium (see also Chapter 3).

Another type of calcium-activated potassium channel is found in some molluscan neurons (Lux et al., 1981). In detached patches it has a maximal single channel conductance of ~50 pS and is more sensitive to calcium than the large calcium-activated potassium channel. Figure 8.10 shows channel activity in a detached patch from a *Helix* neuron. The patch contains at least three of these potassium channels.

Note that there is relatively little activity in the presence of 10^{-8}-M calcium (Figure 8.10B) compared with 10^{-7}-M calcium (Figure 8.10A). The channel activity in these patches is the sum of the openings of some number of identical channels. Because the exact number is uncertain, the activity is analyzed in terms of the dual variable, Np, which is the product of the number of channels N, and the open probability of a single channel, p. For the records shown (taken at 0 mV) Np was 0.8 in 10^{-7}-M calcium and 0.4 in 10^{-8}-M calcium. Np varies sigmoidally with voltage for each calcium concentration (Figure 8.10C). The curves that best fit the data for the two calcium concentrations have the same slope and maximum but are shifted by ~30 mV along the voltage axis.

One way of describing the interaction of calcium and voltage on the activity of this channel is to say that an increase in calcium concentration shifts the voltage activation curve to the left. If, instead, Np had been plotted as a function of calcium concentration for two different voltages, similar sigmoidal plots would have been obtained, and the interaction can be described by saying that depolarizing voltage shifts the calcium activation curve to the left. Thus, at this level of analysis the two forms of activation are indistinguishable (see also Figure 3.7). A more detailed kinetic analysis, in particular an analysis of the probability of closed intervals, can reveal the number of "states" a channel goes through preceding its opening. This type of analysis has been done on one type of gating of the large calcium-activated potassium channel, and it suggests that the voltage dependence of channel activity is due to the voltage dependence of calcium binding (see Chapter 3).

Calcium-Activated Monovalent Cation Channel

The properties of the calcium-activated monovalent cation channel, which underlies $I_{cation(Ca)}$, make it less amenable to the detailed kinetic analysis that has been possible, for instance, on the large calcium-activated potassium channel. Its unit conductance is only 20 pS; its activation is relatively insensitive to voltage; and, although it is activated by calcium, its probability of being open decreases with time at a constant concentration of calcium (Colquhoun et al., 1981). Its calcium dependence can be demonstrated in a detached patch by making rapid transitions between exposures to different calcium concentrations (Yellen, 1982). Figure 8.11 shows that the activity of this channel, seen when a patch of neuroblastoma membrane is exposed to 10^{-6}-M calcium, disappears reversibly when the calcium concentration is reduced to below 10^{-8}-M.

Calcium Channels

There are at least three distinct types of calcium channels, which differ from each other in both their activation as a function of voltage and their inactivation as a function of time (see Chapter 11). The dependence of inactivation on calcium concentration has not yet been demonstrated for any of the three types, as it has been for macroscopic calcium currents in molluscan neurons. However, under some conditions, the time course and voltage dependence of the inactivation of channel activ-

10^{-6} M Ca^{++}

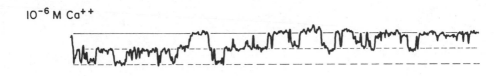

$< 10^{-8}$ M Ca^{++}

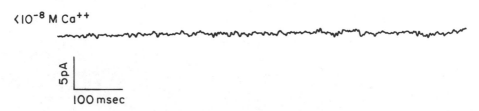

5pA

100 msec

Fig. 8.11. Calcium dependence of the calcium-activated monovalent cation channel. A detached patch of neuroblastoma cell membrane with sodium saline outside and potassium saline inside the patch pipette was exposed to 10^{-6}-M free calcium at -60 mV, and 2-pA inward current channels were observed *(top trace)*. Unlike calcium-activated potassium channels, these channels show little voltage dependence. Furthermore, both sodium and potassium can pass through these channels. Channel activity disappears when the free calcium concentration is reduced to $<10^{-8}$ M (5-mM EGTA with no added calcium, *bottom trace*) (from Yellen, 1982).

ity in cell-attached patches is consistent with this process being calcium dependent (Reuter et al., 1982).

MODULATION OF CALCIUM-REGULATED CURRENTS
BY CYCLIC AMP-DEPENDENT MECHANISMS

The gigaseal recording technique has provided a wealth of information about the ion channels underlying macroscopic currents. It also provides the opportunity to ask mechanistic questions about the changes in channel activity responsible for the modulation of these currents. What are the final crucial steps in the cascade of events that alters the functioning of these channels during their modulation? Do these alterations involve changes in the number of channels or their unit conductance or their kinetic behavior?

The most thoroughly studied pathway for the modulation of ionic currents involves the production of cyclic AMP from ATP by adenylate cyclase coupled to membrane receptors for various hormones and neurotransmitters. Cyclic AMP binds to the regulatory subunit of cyclic AMP-dependent protein kinase, releasing the catalytic subunit that catalyzes the phosphorylation of a wide variety of cytoplasmic and membrane proteins. Such phosphorylation can alter the functional properties of the proteins and thus modulate various physiological processes (see Chapter 4). At least

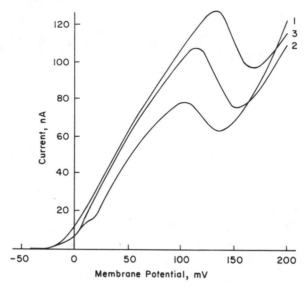

Fig. 8.12. Enhancement of $I_{K(Ca)}$ by intracellular perfusion of catalytic subunit of cAMP-dependent protein kinase. The currents shown here were obtained in an intracellularly perfused *Helix* neuron. In this technique a seal is formed between a perfusion pipette and the neuron membrane, and a low resistance pathway is opened through the membrane, allowing the neuron to be both voltage clamped and internally perfused (Kostyuk, 1982). The outward current activated by voltage clamp pulses to positive potentials consists of the delayed rectifier potassium current and $I_{K(Ca)}$. After obtaining the control trace (1) this neuron was perfused with 0.1-μM catalytic subunit. (ATP was included in the perfusion saline both before and during catalytic subunit perfusion.) Traces 2 and 3 were obtained 35 and 55 minutes after beginning catalytic subunit perfusion. Catalytic subunit causes an increase in outward current resulting from a selective increase in $I_{K(Ca)}$ (modified from DePeyer et al., 1982).

two of the currents discussed above—I_{Ca} and $I_{K(Ca)}$—are known to be modulated by this pathway. In cardiac muscle cells I_{Ca} is enhanced by norepinephrine and cyclic AMP and by intracellular injection of catalytic subunit (see Chapter 11). And in molluscan neurons $I_{K(Ca)}$ is enhanced by intracellular perfusion of catalytic subunit, *independent* of effects on I_{Ca} (DePeyer et al., 1982). The remainder of this chapter describes the latter result and more recent work focused on changes in the properties of the calcium-activated potassium channel that underlies $I_{K(Ca)}$.

In the intracellular perfusion technique a seal is formed between a perfusion pipette and the neuronal membrane, and a low resistance pathway is opened through the membrane, which allows experimental control of both membrane voltage and cytoplasmic contents (Kostyuk, 1982). In a perfused *Helix* neuron the outward current activated by voltage-clamp pulses to positive potentials consists of $I_{K(Ca)}$ and the delayed rectifier potassium current (see Figure 2.6 in Chapter 2). After internal perfusion of the neuron with 0.1-μM catalytic subunit there is a selective increase in the outward current (trace 1 is a control, and traces 2 and 3 in Figure 8.12 are 35 and

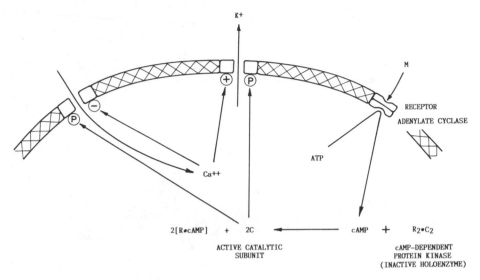

Fig. 8.13. Hypothetical model of a mechanism for the modulation of the calcium channel and the calcium-activated potassium channel by cyclic AMP-dependent phosphorylation. Modulators (M) interact with receptors coupled to adenylate cyclase *(right)*, which converts ATP to cyclic AMP (cAMP). Cyclic AMP binds to the regulatory subunit (R) of cAMP-dependent protein kinase releasing the catalytic subunit (C). Catalytic subunit can then phosphorylate the calcium channel *(left)* and the calcium-activated potassium channel *(top)* by transfer of the terminal phosphate of ATP. Phosphorylation of the channels alters their activity by mechanisms that remain to be determined. For the case of the calcium-activated potassium channel, a possible mechanism is enhancement of the calcium sensitivity of the channel.

55 minutes after catalytic subunit perfusion is begun), consistent with the possibility that phosphorylation selectively enhances $I_{K(Ca)}$ in these neurons.

An attractive hypothesis to explain the effects of catalytic subunit on $I_{K(Ca)}$ is that it is due to a direct phosphorylation of the calcium-activated potassium channel and that the properties of the phosphorylated channel are quite different from those of the nonphosphorylated channel. This hypothesis is schematized in Figure 8.13, which shows catalytic subunit interacting directly with the channels that underlie the macroscopic currents known to be modulated. But this hypothesis is tentative because the crucial phosphorylation site could instead, be on a nonchannel protein, which, when phosphorylated, would affect the functioning of the channel in some more indirect way (see Figure 1.6.B in Chapter 1). The single channel recording techniques described earlier can be used to determine whether or not the phosphorylation site is on the channel itself and to identify the changes in channel properties caused by phosphorylation that give rise to the changes observed in macroscopic currents. A change in macroscopic membrane current $I(=Npi)$ could be due to modulation of the number (N) of channels, of the open probability (p) of channels, or of the unit current (i) of the channel, or a combination of these. The results discussed below

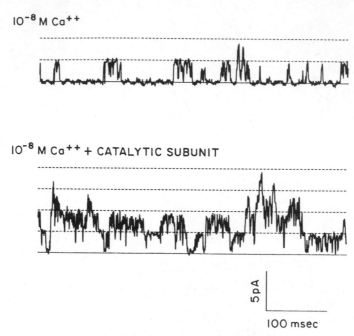

10^{-8} M Ca^{++}

10^{-8} M Ca^{++} + CATALYTIC SUBUNIT

5 pA

100 msec

Fig. 8.14. Increase in calcium-activated potassium channel activity caused by catalytic subunit in a detached membrane patch. *(Top)* Calcium-activated potassium channel activity in a detached patch of *Helix* neuron membrane exposed to 10^{-8}-M free calcium (same patch as shown in Figure 8.10); *(Bottom)* the channel activity increased abruptly to the level shown in this trace 50 sec after exposing the patch to 0.4-μM catalytic subunit (in 10^{-8}-M free calcium), and stayed at this heightened level for the remainder of the patch lifetime (5 minutes) (modified from Ewald et al., 1985).

suggest that the effects of catalytic subunit on $I_{K(Ca)}$ result from a change in the calcium-activated potassium channel's sensitivity to calcium (a change in p).

The effect of catalytic subunit on these channels has been examined with two methods. Using standard patch clamp techniques, detached inside-out patches that contain homogeneous populations of calcium-activated potassium channels can be obtained (see Figure 8.10). Exposing such patches to catalytic subunit causes an abrupt long-lasting change in channel activity without any change in the unit conductance of the channels (Figure 8.14). Because a large number of channels are present in these membrane patches, it is not yet clear whether this increase in activity is due to an increase in the open probability of channels already active (an increase in p) or to the appearance of new active channels (an increase in N).

The other method used to examine single calcium-activated potassium channels is to reconstitute channels into artificial phospholipid bilayers in either of two configurations. The first configuration is the planar bilayer described in the section on the large conductance calcium-activated potassium channel. In the other configuration, reconstituted phospholipid vesicles are allowed to form a monolayer surface, and the tip of a patch electrode is passed twice through the monolayer surface to form a

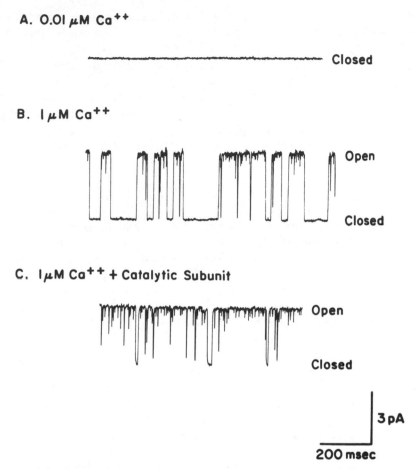

Fig. 8.15. Increase in calcium-activated potassium channel activity in a reconstituted phospholipid membrane. A crude membrane vesicle preparation from *Helix* neurons was reconstituted with exogenous phospholipid. The vesicles were allowed to form a monolayer surface, and the tip of a patch electrode was passed twice through this surface to form a bilayer membrane across the electrode tip (Wilmsen et al., 1983). This patch contained a single calcium-activated potassium channel that had a unitary conductance and calcium sensitivity similar to that of the channels seen in detached membrane patches. This bilayer channel is closed virtually all the time in 10^{-8}-M free calcium at 40 mV (A), but is open ~20% of the time when free calcium is raised to 10^{-6} M (B). There is a large increase in the open probability, p (fraction of time the channel is open), from 0.19 to 0.86 within 20 sec of beginning exposure to 0.1-μM catalytic subunit (in 10^{-6}-M free calcium) (C) (modified from Ewald et al., 1985).

bilayer membrane, containing a channel, across the electrode tip (Wilmsen et al., 1983). Single calcium-activated potassium channels, which are similar to those seen in detached patches, can be observed in such reconstituted membranes. The open probability of such single channels is increased dramatically following exposure to catalytic subunit (Figure 8.15). Because individual channels are effectively at infinite dilution in the artificial bilayer, it seems likely that only tightly bound regulatory components could remain associated with such reconstituted channels. Therefore, one important conclusion that can be drawn is that the phosphorylation site is on the channel protein itself or on some regulatory protein that is tightly bound to the channel. Furthermore, the voltage and calcium dependence of the increase in open probability caused by catalytic subunit are consistent with an increase in the channel's sensitivity to calcium. Thus, these single channel experiments strongly support the hypothesis that catalytic subunit phosphorylates a site, closely associated with the channel protein, which increases the calcium sensitivity of the channel.

CONCLUSIONS

Intracellular calcium is the signal for physiological processes of primary importance for neurons and muscle cells. As such, its entry into cells across the plasma membrane must be under tight feedback control. From studies on molluscan neurons we have learned much about how these control mechanisms operate. Depolarization of the membrane potential, which activates I_{Ca}, is the "on" switch for calcium entry. Calcium, once inside, limits further entry (1) indirectly by activating a current, $I_{K(Ca)}$, which hyperpolarizes the membrane potential and (2) directly by inactivating I_{Ca}. These two feedback mechanisms are the "off" switch for calcium entry. Calcium can also accentuate its own entry by activating a depolarizing current, $I_{cation(Ca)}$.

The bursting pacemaker activity of certain molluscan neurons provides an interesting example of how these calcium-regulated currents are coordinated in a real physiological situation. All the regulatory pathways are operating, but they are important at different phases of the burst cycle. It is the inactivation of I_{Ca} that is responsible for the timing of the bursts, and thus it is how these neurons handle intracellular calcium that determines the bursting frequency.

Modulation of this network of calcium-regulated currents involves another intracellular messenger—cyclic AMP. Cyclic AMP-dependent phosphorylation can affect two of these currents—I_{Ca} and $I_{K(Ca)}$. The advent of gigaseal recording techniques offers the opportunity to find out what changes in single channel activity underlie this modulation and whether or not the phosphorylation site is on the channel itself. The results on the calcium-activated potassium channel of molluscan neurons suggest that cyclic AMP-dependent phosphorylation increases this channel's sensitivity to calcium and that the phosphorylation site is closely associated with the channel protein.

REFERENCES

Adams, W.B. and Levitan, I.B. (1985) Voltage and ion dependences of the slow currents which mediate bursting in *Aplysia* neuron R15. *J. Physiol. 360*, 69–93.

Baker, P.F. (1972) Transport and metabolism of calcium ions in nerve. *Prog. Biophys. Molec. Biol. 24*, 177–223.

Brunelli, M., Castellucci, V,. and Kandel, E.R. (1976) Synaptic facilitation and behavioral sensitization in *Aplysia*: Possible role of serotonin and cyclic AMP. *Science 194* 1178–1181.

Campbell, A.K. (1983) *Intracellular Calcium: Its Universal Role as Regulator.* John Wiley & Sons, New York.

Chad, J., Eckert, R., and Ewald, D. (1984) Kinetics of calcium-dependent inactivation of calcium current in voltage-clamped neurons of *Aplysia californica. J. Physiol. 347,* 279–300.

Colquhoun, D., Neher, E., Reuter, H., and Stevens, C.F. (1981) Inward current channels activated by intracellular Ca^{++} in cultured cardiac cells. *Nature 294,* 752–754.

Coronado, R. and Latorre, R. (1983) Phospholipid bilayers made from monolayers on patch-clamp pipettes. *Biophys. J. 43,* 231–236.

DePeyer, J.E., Cachelin, A.B., Levitan, I.B. and Reuter, H. (1982) Ca^{++}-activated K^+ conductance in internally perfused snail neurons is enhanced by protein phosphorylation. *Proc. Natl. Acad. Sci. 79,* 4207–4211.

Eckert, R. and Ewald, D. (1982) Residual calcium ions depress activation of calcium-dependent current. *Science 216,* 730–733.

Eckert, R. and Ewald, D. (1983) Inactivation of calcium conductance characterized by tail current measurements in neurons of *Aplysia californica. J. Physiol. 345,* 549–565.

Eckert, R. and Tillotson, D. (1981) Calcium-mediated inactivation of calcium conductance in caesium-loaded giant neurons of *Aplysia californica. J. Physiol. 314,* 265–280.

Ewald, D., Williams, A., and Levitan, I.B. (1985) Modulation of single Ca^{++}-dependent K^+ channel activity by protein phosphorylation. *Nature 315,* 503–506.

Fatt, P. and Katz, B. (1952) Spontaneous subthreshold activity at motor nerve endings. *J. Physiol. 117,* 109–128.

Gorman, A.L.F., Hermann, A., and Thomas, M.V. (1982) Ionic requirements for membrane oscillations and their dependence on calcium concentration in a molluscan pace-maker neuron. *J. Physiol. 327,* 185–217.

Gorman, A.L.F. and Thomas, M.V. (1978) Changes in the intracellular concentration of calcium ions in a pace-maker neuron, measured with the mettalochromic indicator dye arsenazo III. *J. Physiol. 275,* 357–376.

Gorman, A.L.F. and Thomas, M.V. (1980) Intracellular calcium accumulation during depolarization in a molluscan neuron. *J Physiol. 308,* 259–285.

Hamill, O.P., Marty, A., Neher, E., Sakmann, B., and Sigworth, F.J. (1981) Improved patch-clamp techniques for high-resolution recording from cells and cell-free membrane patches. *Pflugers Arch. 391,* 85–100.

Huxley, A.F. and Niedergerke, R. (1954) Structural changes in striated muscle fibres. *Nature 173,* 971–973.

Kass, R.S., Tsien, R.S., and Weingart, R. (1978) Ionic basis of transient inward current induced by strophanthidin in cardiac purkinje fibres. *J. Physiol. 281,* 209–226.

Kostyuk, P.G. (1982) Intracellular perfusion of nerve cells and its effects on membrane currents. *Physiol. Rev. 64,* 435–454.

Kramer, R.H. and Zucker, R.S. (1985a) Calcium-dependent inward current in *Aplysia* bursting pacemaker neurons. *J. Physiol. 362,* 107–130.

Kramer, R.H. and Zucker, R.S. (1985b) Calcium-induced inactivations of calcium current causes the interburst hyperpolarization of *Aplysia* bursting neurons. *J. Physiol. 362,* 131–160.

Lux, H.D., Neher, E., and Marty, A. (1981) Single channel activity associated with the calcium-dependent outward current in *Helix pomatia. Pflugers Arch. 389,* 293–295.

Magleby, K.L. and Pallotta, B.S. (1983) Bursting kinetics of single calcium-activated potassium channels in cultured rat muscle. *J. Physiol. 344,* 605–623.

Meech, R.W. (1978) Calcium-dependent potassium activation in nervous tissues. *Annu. Rev. Biophy. Bioeng. 7*, 1–18.

Miller, C. (1983) Integral membrane channels: Studies in model membranes. *Physiol. Rev. 63*, 435–454.

Moczydlowski, E. and Latorre, R. (1983) Gating kinetics of Ca^{++}-activated K^+ channels from rat muscle incorporated into planar lipid bilayers: Evidence for two voltage-dependent Ca^{++} binding reactions. *J. Gen. Physiol. 82*, 511–542.

Osterrieder, W., Brum, G., Hescheler, J., and Trautwein, W. (1982) Injection of subunits of cyclic AMP-dependent protein kinase into cardiac myocytes modulates Ca^{++} current. *Nature 298*, 576–578.

Rasmussen, H. (1981) *Calcium and cAMP as Synarchic Messengers*. John Wiley & Sons, New York.

Rasmussen, H. and Barrett, P. (1984) Calcium messenger system: An integrated view. *Physiol. Rev. 64*, 938–984.

Reuter, H. (1974) Localization of beta adrenergic receptors, and effects of noradrenaline and cyclic nucleotides on action potentials, ionic currents and tension in mammalian cardiac muscle. *J. Physiol. 242*, 429–451.

Reuter, H., Stevens, C.F., Tsien, R.W., and Yellen, G. (1982) Properties of single calcium channels in cardiac cell culture. *Nature 297*, 501–504.

Standen, N.B. (1981) Calcium channel inactivation by intracellular calcium injection into *Helix* neurons. *Nature 293*, 158–159.

Tsien, R.W. (1973) Adrenaline-like effects of intracellular iontophoresis of cyclic AMP in cardiac purkinje fibres. *Nature New Biol. 245*, 120–122.

Tsien, R.W. (1983) Calcium channels in excitable cell membranes. *Annu. Rev. Physiol. 45*, 341–358.

Wilmsen, U., Methfessel, C., Hanke, W., and Boheim, G. (1983) Channel current fluctuation studies with solvent-free lipid bilayers using Neher-Sakmann pipettes. In *Physical Chemistry of Transmembrane Ion Motions*, pp. 479–485, Elsevier, New York.

Wilson, D.F. (1974) Effects of dibutyrl cyclic adenosine 3',5'-monophosphate, theophylline and aminophylline on neuromuscular transmission in the rat. *J. Pharmacol. Exp. Ther. 188*, 447–452.

Yellen, G. (1982) Single Ca^{++}-activated nonselective cation channels in neuroblastoma. *Nature 296*, 357–359.

9

The M-Current and Other Potassium Currents of Vertebrate Neurons

STEPHEN W. JONES
PAUL R. ADAMS

Until recently, our view of how vertebrate neurons integrate information was rather simple. Neurotransmitters acted to open channels in the postsynaptic membrane for a brief time (a few milliseconds). The effect of the transmitter depended on which ions passed through the channel—excitatory transmitters depolarized the cell by opening channels that, for example, passed both sodium and potassium, and inhibitory transmitters hyperpolarized the cell by opening channels for either chloride or potassium. The resulting voltage changes were then passively propagated from the synapses (on dendrites or the cell body) to the site of action potential initiation. If the summed voltage change reached threshold, the cell fired an action potential; if not, nothing further happened. This picture arose primarily from the classic work on neuromuscular junctions and spinal motoneurons by Katz, Eccles, and many others.

But there are synaptic potentials that act in qualitatively different ways. These include the slow excitatory postsynaptic potentials (EPSPs) that can be recorded from many vertebrate neurons. Neurotransmitters generally do not produce these slow EPSPs by acting directly to open channels—they act indirectly through second messengers to either open or *close* ion channels, or even do both. The channels involved often show strong voltage dependence, unlike classic synaptic channels. This means that it is necessary to examine the effects of the neurotransmitters quite carefully. By simply looking for a depolarization or a hyperpolarization one may completely miss a significant effect on the electrical behavior of a cell. In general, it is necessary first to define the normal active and passive membrane properties of the cell and then to look at the effects of the neurotransmitter on those properties. The most direct way to do this is to voltage clamp the cell and separate the different ionic conductances by their voltage dependence and pharmacology.

POTASSIUM CURRENTS IN VERTEBRATE NEURONS

As described earlier in this volume, potassium currents are major targets of modulatory neurotransmitter actions. This is a reasonable strategy since potassium currents

159

themselves can be thought of as modulatory. Sodium currents are required for initiation and propagation of the action potential. Because that is a necessary function of nearly all neurons, the sodium current is generally a robust phenomenon, rarely if ever directly affected by neurotransmitters. Modulation of calcium currents, by changing the intracellular calcium level, affects a very wide variety of cellular processes. The effect of modifying a potassium current, in contrast, can be quite specific. This is because of the sometimes bewildering array of potassium currents in a cell (see also Chapter 2) and the many functions potassium currents serve.

At this point, it may be useful to discuss briefly the potassium currents that have been described to date in vertebrate neurons. Many, although not all, of these were first found in invertebrate neurons. Not all cell types have all of these currents, and the relative importance of each current appears to vary from cell to cell. Several of these currents can be modulated by neurotransmitters; this also varies from cell to cell.

Delayed Rectifier

Currents with properties rather similar to the major voltage-dependent potassium current in squid giant axon have been observed in the axons and cell bodies of several vertebrate neurons. General characteristics include voltage-dependent activation over tens of milliseconds with a threshold positive to rest, a large maximal conductance, and slow inactivation. The delayed rectifier of vertebrate neurons is typically blocked by external tetraethylammonium (TEA) in the low millimolar range.

Calcium-Dependent Potassium Currents

It is important to note that, in many vertebrate neurons, there are two distinct potassium currents that can be activated by intracellular calcium. (Accordingly, the term $I_{K(Ca)}$, introduced in Chapter 2, is not appropriate, and a different nomenclature will be used here.) One of these calcium-dependent currents, often called I_C (not to be confused with I_{Ca}, the calcium current itself) is both calcium and voltage dependent, has a large single channel conductance, and can produce a large macroscopic current. The large conductance of the channel has made it a favorite of patch clampers, and its kinetics have been extensively studied in patches and in reconstituted membranes. Its strong voltage dependence causes it to turn off rapidly at the resting potential, at physiological concentrations of intracellular calcium. I_C is also blocked by millimolar concentrations of TEA. In bullfrog sympathetic neurons, it activates rapidly enough to repolarize the action potential (Adams et al., 1982c; MacDermott & Weight, 1982). Even though the bullfrog neurons have a perfectly good calcium current, removal of extracellular calcium causes a *broadening* of the action potential, because of blockade of I_C. I_C can be activated by neurotransmitters in several secretory cells, but this appears to be secondary to a rise in intracellular calcium, coming at least in part from intracellular stores (Petersen, 1984; Trautmann & Marty, 1984; Dubinsky & Oxford, 1985).

The second calcium-dependent potassium current has been less thoroughly characterized. In bullfrog sympathetic neurons, where it is called I_{AHP}, it is a small current with no obvious voltage dependence and is responsible for a slow (up to 1 sec) afterhyperpolarization (AHP) following a single action potential (Pennefather et al., 1985a). Many other neurons have TEA-resistant, calcium-sensitive AHPs, which may be due to I_{AHP}. I_{AHP} is relatively insensitive to TEA, but (unlike I_C) is sensitive to the bee venom toxin apamin at nanomolar concentrations in at least some preparations (Romey & Lazdunski, 1984; Pennefather et al., 1985a). Apamin-binding sites have been identified *in vitro* and may provide a means of biochemical isolation of this potassium channel (Hugues et al., 1982). It has not been proven that I_C and I_{AHP} flow through distinct channels, but their pharmacological differences make that likely. I_{AHP} is inhibited by neurotransmitter action in several neurons; this will be discussed in detail later. I_{AHP} is also blocked by *d*-tubocurarine, which is classically a neuromuscular blocking drug but also affects a variety of channels and receptors at somewhat higher concentrations.

A-Current

Some vertebrate cells have a transient potassium current, which is rapidly and completely inactivated at depolarized potentials. In many cells, the A-current is inactivated at rest, but inactivation can be removed during an AHP, allowing the A-current to be activated during a subsequent spike (see Chapter 7). 4-Aminopyridine (4-AP) blocks A-current in most preparations at millimolar or lower concentrations, and 4-AP is a powerful enhancer of neurotransmitter release (e.g., Heuser et al., 1979). There is some evidence that the A-current can be blocked by the action of neurotransmitters (Aghajanian, 1985; Dufy et al., 1983).

M-Current

The M-current (I_M) is the only one of these potassium currents not originally identified in invertebrate neurons. It is activated at more hyperpolarized potentials than the delayed rectifier, I_C, or A-current. It does not inactivate, so that it can be part of the resting potassium conductance of a cell. Although it is a relatively small current, its activation in the critical region between the resting potential and threshold for firing allows it to play an important role in limiting repetitive activity (Adams et al., 1982a). The M-current may be analogous to the serotonin-sensitive "S-current" of *Aplysia* sensory neurons, although some differences exist: The S-current is less voltage sensitive and is not blocked by barium (Klein et al., 1982; Siegelbaum et al., 1982). The M-current can be inhibited by several different neurotransmitters (see below).

Anomalous Rectifier

This quaintly named current is activated by *hyperpolarization*, unlike all the voltage-dependent conductances described previously. The anomalous rectifier appears to be the potassium conductance that determines the resting potential of skeletal muscle and possibly of some vertebrate neurons as well (Adrian, 1969; Stanfield et al., 1985). Anomalous rectifiers are inhibited by substance P in globus pallidus and by glutamate in retinal horizontal cells (Stanfield et al., 1985; Kaneko & Tachibana, 1985).

Leak

Almost all cells (neurons included) have large negative resting potentials and are much more permeable to potassium than to other cations at rest. This is often assumed to be due to the presence of voltage-*insensitive* "leakage" channels, which are predominantly permeable to potassium (e.g., in the Hodgkin and Huxley model). But there is little experimental evidence about the voltage dependence or other properties of the potassium channels open at rest. Most of the voltage-sensitive potassium currents described above are entirely closed at rest. M-current and the anomalous rectifier may contribute to the resting potential, but they are not present in all neurons. A few cells are depolarized (with an increase in resistance) when external calcium is removed, suggesting a resting I_{AHP}-like conductance. Amazingly, the nature of the resting potassium channels is unknown in the vast majority of cells. Since several neurotransmitters appear to close "resting" potassium channels, this is an important question.

SLOW EXCITATORY POTENTIALS IN BULLFROG SYMPATHETIC GANGLIA

Early Observations

The classic view is that autonomic ganglia are simple relays. Presynaptic stimulation leads directly to postsynaptic outputs, without further computation. At first glance, this appears to be particularly true for the large B cells of the caudal part of the paravertebral sympathetic chain in the bullfrog. Each B cell in the ganglion receives one major presynaptic input (plus occasional minor ones), and a single presynaptic action potential from the main input sets up a suprathreshold fast excitatory postsynaptic potential (EPSP). This is quite reminiscent of a vertebrate neuromuscular junction, even to the identity of the neurotransmitter (acetylcholine) and the receptor type (nicotinic). However, it has been known for several decades that sympathetic ganglia also show a variety of slow synaptic potentials in the second to minute time range. The mechanisms of these slow potentials have been quite controversial, and their role in information processing in the ganglia remains uncertain.

The B cells show two slow synaptic potentials—the slow EPSP and the late, slow EPSP (Figure 9.1). The slow EPSP results from the action of acetylcholine (ACh) on muscarinic receptors, and the late, slow EPSP results from the action of a peptide resembling luteinizing hormone-releasing hormone (LH-RH) (Jan et al., 1979, 1980). [Remarkably, these cells show three distinct EPSPs but no inhibitory postsynaptic potentials (IPSPs).] Both the slow and late, slow EPSP produce small (~10 mV) depolarizations, and generally do not themselves reach threshold for generation of action potentials. The voltage dependence of these EPSPs was unusual and variable from cell to cell (not to mention laboratory to laboratory). In most cases, the

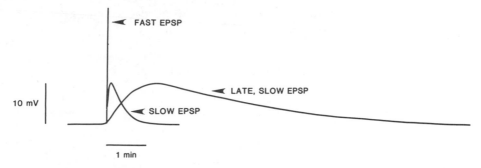

Fig. 9.1. Three EPSPs in bullfrog sympathetic neurons. A schematic diagram showing the time course and (approximate) amplitudes of EPSPs. Slow and late, slow EPSPs of this size require trains of presynaptic stimuli. The fast and slow EPSPs result from the release of ACh directly onto the cell; the late, slow EPSP results from release of an LH-RH-like peptide from high threshold (C fiber) inputs that do not form synapses directly on the B cells in the ganglion.

slow EPSPs did not show clear reversal potentials. Sometimes the conductance of the cell increased; sometimes it decreased. Clearly, the actions of the neurotransmitters were unusual (see review by Kuba & Koketsu, 1978). In retrospect, there were two problems: (1) the transmitters had more than one underlying effect and (2) the effects seen interacted with the intrinsic voltage-dependent conductances of the cell. Sorting all this out required knowledge of the voltage-dependent conductances, particularly the M-current.

M-Current

The B cells of bullfrog sympathetic ganglia are particularly favorable cells for voltage clamp studies. They are relatively large for vertebrate neurons (~50 μm in diameter), and they lack dendrites. All of the synaptic inputs are directly on the cell body. B cells have the usual array of voltage-dependent conductances: voltage-dependent sodium and calcium currents and all the potassium currents described earlier, except for the anomalous rectifier. The one surprise among the bullfrog ganglion currents was the M-current, which had not been described previously.

Separation of ionic currents is generally a difficult problem, even under voltage clamp, because several different currents may be turning on or off at any given time. Luckily, the M-current can be isolated quite easily over much of its voltage range, as it is activated at more hyperpolarized potentials than the other voltage-dependent currents in bullfrog sympathetic neurons. Figure 9.2 shows this: a small hyperpolarizing voltage step from a holding potential of −60 mV produces only a constant "leakage" current, but a small depolarizing step also elicits a slowly developing outward current resulting from slow activation of the M-current. Upon return to −60 mV, the M-current slowly turns off.

The M-current is kinetically quite simple. Its behavior can be described accurately by a model with only two states: open and closed. The transition between the

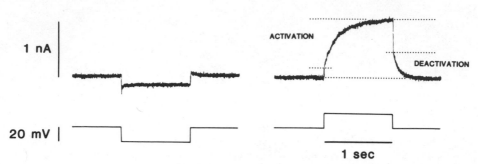

LEAK	M-CURRENT + LEAK

Fig. 9.2. The M-current. A 20-mV hyperpolarizing command from a holding potential of −60 mV produces a steady inward current, reflecting only the leakage conductance of the cell *(left)*. The input resistance (R = V/I = 20 mV/0.2 nA) is 100 $M\Omega$. A depolarizing command to −40 mV also activates a portion of the M-current, seen as the slowly developing outward current during the 1-sec step *(right)*.

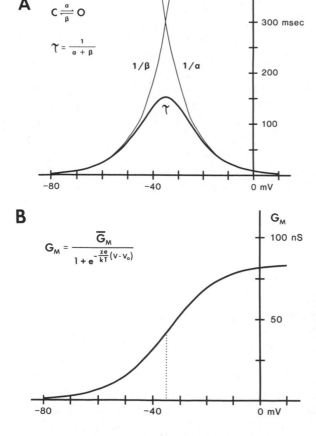

A

$$C \underset{\beta}{\overset{\alpha}{\rightleftharpoons}} O$$

$$\tau = \frac{1}{\alpha + \beta}$$

B

$$G_M = \frac{\bar{G}_M}{1 + e^{-\frac{ze}{kT}(V - V_o)}}$$

Fig. 9.3. Kinetics of the M-current. The model proposed by Adams et al. (1982a) is illustrated. (A) The time constant (τ) for the M-current as a function of voltage, showing that it is slowest at the voltage where it is half maximally activated (−35 mV). On the model, this is due to the voltage dependence of the rate constants for opening (α) and closing (β) of the M-current channel, shown as the lighter lines. (B) The steady-state M-current conductance (G_M, in nanosiemens, nS). Below −70 mV, the M-current is essentially all off; above 0 mV, it is essentially all turned on. The dotted line indicates the half maximal activation point (V_o).

states depends on the movement of a single charged particle within the hypothetical M-channel: the probability of the channel being open therefore depends on voltage, as the energy involved in moving a charged particle within the electrical field of the membrane depends on the voltage (see Chapter 3). The parameters for that model can be determined experimentally from two sorts of measurement—the fraction of the total M-current flowing at steady state at each voltage, and the time constant for opening or closing M-channels at each voltage (Figure 9.3). The major points are that half of the M-current channels are open at -35 mV, nearly all are closed below -60 mV, and the channels open and close relatively slowly (time constant about 100 msec) in the region between the resting potential and threshold for the action potential.

Muscarinic and Peptidergic Inhibitions of M-Current

For our purposes here, the important thing about the M-current is not its kinetics but its sensitivity to neurotransmitters. The most obvious and reproducible effect of muscarinic agonists, and also of certain analogs of LH-RH and of substance P, is a reduction of the M-current. Figure 9.4 illustrates this for substance P. The effects are a net inward current (due to turning *off* the *outward* M-current) in the M-current region, and a reduction in the *amplitude* of the slow relaxations observed when the M-current is turned on and off by pulses between -30 and -60 mV. The time course of the slow relaxations is not affected—that is, the effect of transmitters is not to change the intrinsic voltage sensitivity of the M-current but to reduce the maximal amount of M-current that can be activated. Note also that substance P causes no steady inward current at -60 mV, where nearly all of the M-current is turned off even in the absence of substance P. Other currents in these cells are insensitive, or much less sensitive, to neurotransmitters.

M-current and its inhibition are also reflected in the steady-state current-voltage relations of the cell (Figure 9.5). If the cell had no M-current, the steady-state I-V would be a straight line, reflecting only leakage conductance, in the region hyperpolarized to -30 mV (where delayed rectifier and other currents are mostly turned off). The M-current causes an upward curvature, or rectification, in the I-V beginning near -60 mV. Substance P, by inhibiting the M-current, reduces that rectification, making the steady-state I-V more nearly linear. The difference between the steady-state I-V curves with and without substance P is simply the current induced by substance P at each voltage (Figure 9.5B). If substance P inhibited a voltage-*insensitive* potassium conductance, the substance P-induced current would depend linearly on voltage, would be zero at the potassium equilibrium potential (E_K), and would reverse to an *outward* current hyperpolarized to E_K. The fact that the current induced by, for example, muscarinic agonists does not reverse was quite confusing in the days before the M-current was known and led some to believe that a potassium current might not be involved at all.

M-current inhibition by muscarinic agonists is prevented by low concentrations of muscarinic antagonists such as atropine and scopolamine, as expected for a classic muscarinic receptor. However, the M-current can also be inhibited by agonists for three other receptors, and those actions are not blocked by muscarinic antagonists.

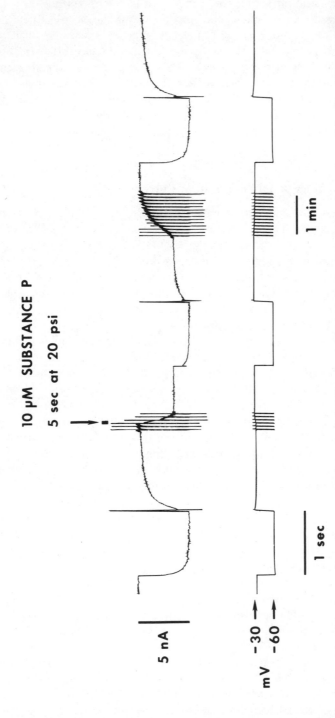

Fig. 9.4. Inhibition of the M-current by substance P. A bullfrog sympathetic neuron was voltage clamped to −30 mV, with 1-sec steps to −60 mV every 5 sec. Three fast records are shown: (*left*) control; (*middle*) at the peak effect of substance P, and (*right*) recovery. During the onset and recovery of the effect, the chart recorder was run 100 times slower to show the time course of the drug action. Substance P was applied to the cell by briefly applying positive pressure to a substance P-containing micropipette positioned near the cell.

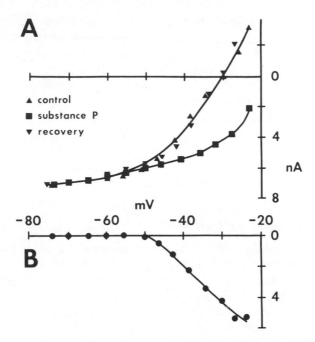

Fig. 9.5. The effect of substance P on steady-state current-voltage curves. (A) I-V relations before (▲), during (■), and after (▼) bath application of 10-μM substance P. The cell was held at −30 mV (zero current was defined as the steady-state current flowing at −30 mV in the control), with 1-sec steps to the indicated voltages. (B) The net current induced by substance P, from subtracting the control I-V curve from that observed in substance P. (Redrawn from Adams et al., 1983).

Jan et al. (1979) first found that LH-RH depolarized bullfrog sympathetic neurons, and Adams and Brown (1980) soon demonstrated M-current inhibition by LH-RH. The action of LH-RH appears to involve a specific receptor, as it is blocked by LH-RH analogs that were developed as antagonists of LH-RH receptors in mammalian pituitary. However, there are differences between LH-RH receptors in the bullfrog ganglion and those of either mammalian or frog pituitary—in particular, LH-RH acts at low, nanomolar concentrations in pituitary but at high, micromolar concentrations in the ganglion. This could be due in part to hydrolysis of the peptide or poor penetration into the ganglion, or both, but the rapid reversal of LH-RH action suggests that low-affinity binding is involved. One explanation for the difference is that the LH-RH like peptide in the bullfrog ganglion is not mammalian LH-RH (Eiden & Eskay, 1980). The endogenous peptide in the ganglion may be [Trp[7],Leu[8]]LH-RH, the LH-RH for teleost fish (Sherwood et al., 1983). Teleost LH-RH (T-LH-RH) is, in fact, about 20 times more potent than the mammalian form on the bullfrog ganglion (Jones, 1985).

Two more receptors also turn off M-current in B cells. These receptors are sensitive to neither muscarinic nor LH-RH antagonists. Substance P and several related peptides called tachykinins inhibit the M-current (Adams et al., 1983; Jones,

1985). One interesting difference between the substance P effect and that mediated through the other receptors is that the M-current inhibition due to substance P desensitizes rather rapidly (in less than 1 minute) in many cells. Finally, nucleotides such as uridine triphosphate (UTP) inhibit the M-current (Adams et al., 1982b).

The vast majority of the M-current ($\sim$85%) can be inhibited by activation of *any one* of these four receptors. This strongly suggests that the coupling between the receptors and the M-current is not direct and is more consistent with mediation through a common second messenger system. However, most of the plausible candidate second messengers have been ruled out: cyclic AMP, cyclic GMP, and calcium have no effect on the M-current, even when injected directly into the cell (Adams et al., 1982c). Experiments to test the involvement of protein kinase C are in progress.

Other Muscarinic and Peptidergic Effects

It is clear that some of the observed effects of muscarinic agonists (and of LH-RH and substance P) cannot be explained by inhibition of the M-current. In particular, muscarinic agonists and the peptides rather often will depolarize B cells even when the cell is held at very negative potentials, at which inhibition of M-current would have no effect. This effect can also be observed under voltage clamp (Figure 9.6). At hyperpolarized potentials, where the effect is not obscured by the M-current, it is clear that conductance *increases*, that is, channels are *opening*. Furthermore, the effect is (operationally) an increase in the leakage conductance, as no voltage-dependent relaxations are seen. This effect has not been studied in much detail, but several groups have suggested that it is largely due to an increase in conductance to sodium.

In a cell that shows both this response and M-current inhibition, the effect on the steady-state I-V curve is more complex (Figure 9.7). In addition to the net inward current (and reduction in slope) at positive potentials, resulting from M-current inhibition, there is an inward current at hyperpolarized potentials (associated with a slight increase in slope). The difference between the two I-V curves (Figure 9.7B) again gives the agonist-induced current at each voltage. It can be explained entirely by the combination of M-current inhibition and opening of a leakage conductance. Again, this is hardly what would be expected from a traditional neurotransmitter action and was very hard to interpret in the absence of voltage clamp data.

Although we have called the conductance-increase effect a leakage current, it is clear that it is a specific receptor-mediated effect and not an artifact resulting, for example, from nonspecific damage to the cell. The most powerful evidence for this is that the conductance increase, like the M-current inhibition, can be prevented (or reversed) by the appropriate antagonists. The conductance increase effect has some other interesting features. In many cells, its time course is clearly slower than that of the M-current inhibition (see top record in Figure 9.6). It is not seen in all cells—some show pure M-current inhibition—and the relative amounts of M-current inhibition and conductance increase are comparable in a given cell, regardless of which receptor is activated (Figure 9.7B).

The story does not end here—muscarinic and peptidergic agonists have a *third* effect on B cells! The AHP following a directly evoked action potential is reduced in amplitude and duration (Tokimasa, 1984). There are two reasons for this. First,

SUBSTANCE K
90 sec, 300 nM

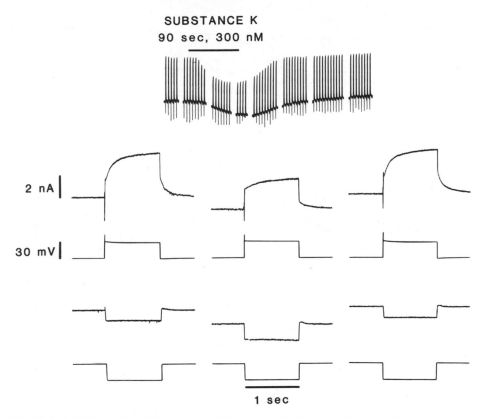

2 nA

30 mV

1 sec

Fig. 9.6. Inhibition of the M-current, and increase in leakage conductance, by substance K. The cell was clamped at -60 mV, with voltage steps to either -40 mV (to activate M-current) or -80 mV (to measure leakage conductance). *(Top)* Records at a slow time scale to show the time course of the effect. Note that inward currents resulted at both -40 and -60 mV and that the time course of the effect was different at the two voltages. *(Below)* Records at a 100 times faster time scale, taken before *(left)*, during *(middle)*, and after *(right)* the substance K response. The depolarizing steps show the decrease in M-current, and the hyperpolarizing steps show a reversible increase in conductance not associated with slow voltage-dependent currents. Substance K is an analog of substance P; the two peptides have similar effects on the bullfrog ganglion.

the conductance increase effect shunts the AHP; that is, the outward potassium current that underlies the AHP is counteracted in part by the transmitter-induced inward leak current. Second, the transmitters also reduce I_{AHP}, the conductance underlying the slow AHP (Figure 9.8). This effect is rather small in the bullfrog ganglion; maximal doses of either muscarinic agonists or peptides reduce I_{AHP} by only 30%, on the average (Pennefather et al., 1985a). It is not firmly established whether these are direct effects on the I_{AHP} channel or are due to changes in the entry or metabolism of calcium (which activates the I_{AHP}).

Once three different modulatory effects have been found, there is little reason

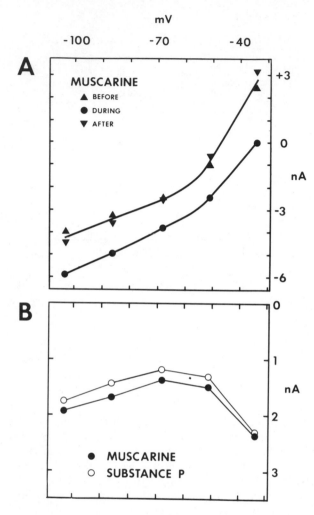

Fig. 9.7. Current-voltage relations for a response to muscarine, showing both M-current inhibition and an increase in leak. (A) The steady-state currents are shown as in Figure 9.5. For comparison, the current induced by substance P in the same cell is also shown (B). Substance P and muscarine (each at 20 μM) were applied by pressure from different barrels of a three-barrel pipette. Note that the effects of muscarine and of substance P are qualitatively similar (from Jones, 1985).

to expect that there will not be others. In fact, several other effects of muscarinic agonists and peptides have been reported on B cells, including inhibition of calcium current, direct effects on action potential shape, and modulation of the nicotinic receptor (Koketsu, 1984). Most of these effects have not been firmly established, however, and they will not be discussed further.

The situation is thus quite complicated—there are four receptors, any one of which can produce three distinct effects (Figure 9.9). This is a very different story from classic receptor mechanisms, in which the receptor and ion channel are more directly coupled. But it is perhaps what would be expected for a second messenger-linked system. Second messengers produce *cascades* of effects. For example, activation of adenylate cyclase leads to phosphorylation of many different proteins in a given cell, and each protein can produce a distinct effect. Furthermore, it is common

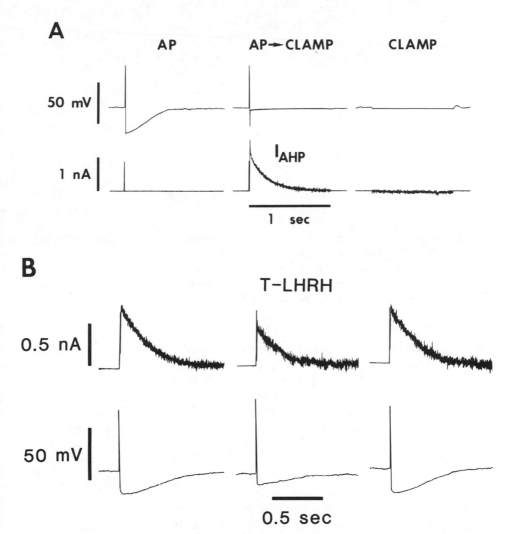

Fig. 9.8. I_{AHP} and the effect of T-LH-RH. (A) The ''hybrid clamp'' protocol used to evoke I_{AHP}. An action potential was evoked by a brief depolarizing current, producing a large AHP lasting for more than half a second *(left)*. When the voltage clamp was turned on just after the action potential, a slowly-decaying outward current resulted *(middle)*. This current (I_{AHP}) is kinetically and pharmacologically distinct from M-current (Pennefather et al., 1985a). When the clamp was turned on without a prior action potential, no current was evoked *(right)*. (B) The effect of teleost LH-RH on I_{AHP} and on the AHP itself. *(Top)* I_{AHP} before, during, and after pressure application of 100-μM T-LH-RH. T-LH-RH caused a 35% reduction of I_{AHP}, in addition to nearly complete abolition of M-current and a large increase in leakage conductance (not shown). *(Bottom)* The effect of T-LH-RH on the AHP. The reduction in amplitude was greater than would be expected from the reduction in I_{AHP} alone and presumably results from shunting of the remaining I_{AHP} by the T-LH-RH-induced leakage conductance. The full amplitude of action potentials is not reproduced by the chart recorder used for this figure (both A and B).

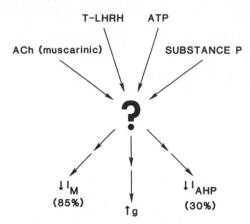

Fig. 9.9. Hypothetical second messenger mechanisms in the bullfrog ganglion. ACh, substance P, LH-RH, and ATP, each acting through a distinct receptor, have the same combination of effects, suggesting that they act on a common pathway (shown by "?"). Since the different effects can differ in time course and involve distinct channels, divergent steps may occur between the common second messenger and the effects on the channels.

for several different receptor types to activate a common second messenger system in a single cell. The complex mixture of effects seen in B cells is therefore not very surprising, and multiple electrophysiological effects resulting from activation of a single receptor type may prove to be the rule rather than the exception for modulatory effects of neurotransmitters. The problem now is to sort the wheat from the chaff—which effects are the important ones, and what are their consequences for cell functioning?

Slow Synaptic Potentials

One obvious question is whether all of the above is simply pharmacology, or whether physiological stimulation can produce inhibition of the M-current (and the other effects). The answer is that the slow (muscarinic) EPSP and the late, slow (peptidergic) EPSP are due to the same mechanisms as are the effects of exogenous muscarinic and peptidergic agonists, as far as has been examined (Adams & Brown, 1982; Kuffler & Sejnowski, 1983; Katayama & Nishi, 1982; Akasu et al., 1984).

Figure 9.10 shows a slow EPSC (i.e., slow EPSP under voltage clamp). When the preganglionic inputs are stimulated, a rapid inward current results (peaking in approximately 2 sec) at the holding potential of −35 mV. Hyperpolarizing voltage steps show that this is due to inhibition of the M-current. The inward current then recovers (along with the M-current) with the same time course as a slow EPSP. In this and some other cells, it is possible to demonstrate a conductance increase effect as well, but that is generally quite small during a slow EPSC. An effect of the slow EPSP on I_{AHP} has not been clearly established.

Figure 9.11 shows a late, slow EPSC. Again, there are two effects: inhibition of the M-current and a conductance increase that is most clear at hyperpolarized

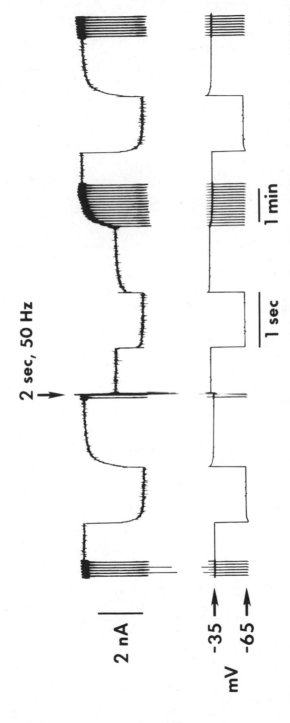

Fig. 9.10. Inhibition of the M-current during the slow EPSC. A protocol similar to that of Figure 9.4 demonstrated a large, rapid inhibition of the M-current following a train of presynaptic stimuli (from Jones, 1985).

173

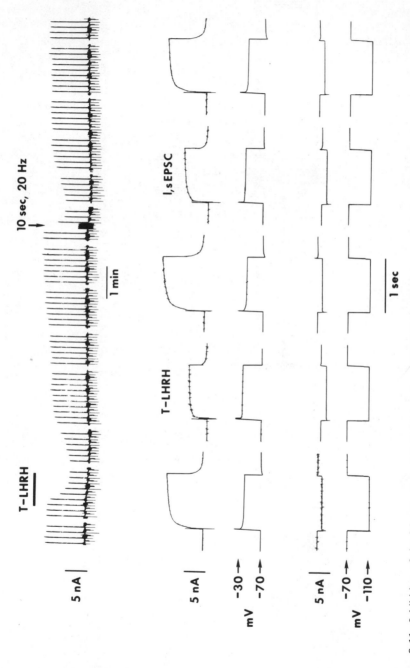

Fig. 9.11. Inhibition of the M-current during the late, slow ESPC. Bath application of T-LH-RH (*left*) and presynaptic stimulation (*right*) produced qualitatively similar inward currents (*top*), inhibition of the M-current (*middle*), and a small increase in leak conductance (*below*). The slow EPSC had been blocked by 1-μ*M* atropine.

174

potentials. Note also that T-LH-RH produces similar effects, with a similar time course, in the same cell. The slow and late, slow EPSCs differ mainly in their time courses: the slow EPSC lasts approximately 1 minute, whereas the late, slow EPSC peaks in about 1 minute and lasts for up to 10 minutes. This difference occurs even though the slow and late, slow EPSPs act on the same underlying currents. The most plausible explanation for the difference is that the transmitters persist for different lengths of time. The rapid time course of the *fast* EPSC in the bullfrog ganglion suggests that ACh is rapidly removed, probably because of hydrolysis by cholinesterase, as at the neuromuscular junction. The time course of the slow EPSC would then reflect not the time course of ACh action but the time course of biochemical processes involved between ACh binding and M-current inhibition. In contrast, the time course of the late, slow EPSC appears to reflect the continued presence of the T-LH-RH-like peptide in the ganglion (Jan & Jan, 1982).

Functional Consequences

The preceding discussion of muscarinic and peptidergic excitatory effects, and of the slow excitatory PSPs, has been entirely in terms of the behavior of the cell under voltage clamp. That was necessary to dissect the complex mixture of effects that can be observed. But what is really important, of course, is the behavior of the cell out of clamp, under physiological conditions. When we say that these effects are excitatory, what do we really mean? Classically, an EPSP is an EPSP because it depolarizes the cell, and the slow and late, slow EPSPs in the bullfrog ganglia under typical circumstances are in fact depolarizations (that is how they were originally discovered). Surprisingly, the excitatory action turns out to have little or nothing to do with the depolarization and can be seen clearly when the depolarization is prevented. In other words, it is somewhat misleading to call the effects EPSPs, as the potential change in the postsynaptic cell is not what is important.

M-Current
We will first consider the effect of the M-current (and of inhibiting it) on the cell. A bullfrog sympathetic neuron with a resting potential of -45 mV will have some steady-state amount of M-current flowing—in fact, most of the resting conductance may result from M-current. Most of the M-current is not activated at -45 mV, however, so anything that would act to depolarize the cell would activate more M-current. The simplest case is a maintained depolarizing current applied through the recording microelectrode (current clamp). If the current is subthreshold for generation of an action potential, the cell will initially depolarize with a more-or-less exponential time course (set by the time constant of the cell). But as the cell depolarizes, M-current is activated with a time constant of ~ 100 msec. Activation of M-current drives the cell back toward E_K, as shown in Figure 9.12. If the depolarizing pulse does reach threshold, the effect of the M-current is similar—activation of M-current tends to hyperpolarize the cell following the action potential. In this way, the M-current acts to inhibit repetitive firing. A depolarization can cause one action potential (and sometimes more) at the beginning, but the slow, voltage-dependent activation of the M-current then hyperpolarizes the cell below threshold. This is the typical

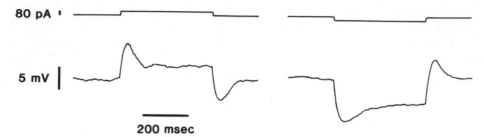

Fig. 9.12. The effect of M-current on subthreshold potentials. Small depolarizing *(left)* and hyperpolarizing *(right)* currents do not produce simple charging curves reflecting the time constant of the membrane. The time constants of the cell and of the M-current interact to produce a highly damped oscillation. The initial positive or negative deflection is followed by a sag in the voltage toward the resting level. The sag results from voltage-dependent activation and deactivation of the M-current (unpublished records of P.R. Adams and D.A. Brown).

Fig. 9.13. The effect of the slow EPSP on excitability. *(Top)* Responses to a depolarizing current of 0.5 nA, applied for 0.3 sec; *(bottom)* the effect of equivalent hyperpolarizing current. Note the changes in the M-current sag; the slow EPSP often causes an increase in the number of anode-break spikes, not seen in this cell.

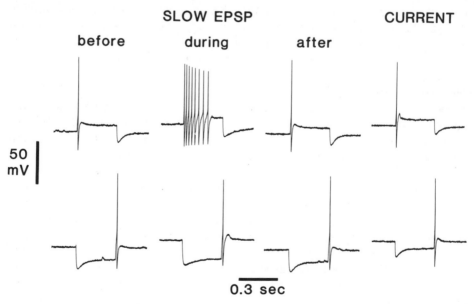

sEPSP

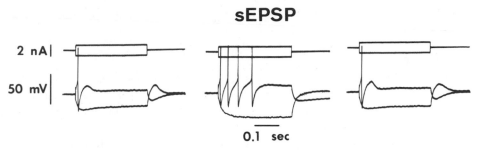

Fig. 9.14. The effect of a manually clamped slow EPSP on excitability. Responses are shown to both depolarizing and hyperpolarizing currents before, during, and after a slow EPSP resulting from a train of nerve stimuli (0.3 sec at 50 Hz) (from Jones, 1985).

behavior of bullfrog sympathetic neurons. It is not a general property of all nerve cells. Other cells may show maintained firing to a maintained depolarization, depending on their mixture of voltage-dependent conductances.

Inhibition of the M-current should increase the excitability of the cell in a specific way, allowing repetitive firing to a maintained depolarizing current. That is actually observed in response to agents that inhibit the M-current in bullfrog sympathetic neurons (Adams et al., 1982b). Figure 9.13 illustrates this for a slow EPSP. A train of presynaptic impulses generated a 10-mV EPSP. During that slow EPSP, the number of spikes generated in response to a 0.5-nA depolarizing current increased from one to eight. That increase in excitability was *not* simply a result of depolarizing the cell; after the slow EPSP, when excitability had returned to normal, a passive depolarization of 10 mV (resulting from steady current passed through the electrode) had no effect on the excitability of the cell. More directly, if the depolarization during the slow EPSP is *prevented* by passing current through the microelectrode to "manually clamp" the cell to its resting potential, the increase in excitability is still seen (Figure 9.14). Figure 9.14 also shows the effect of the slow EPSP on hyperpolarizing potentials: in the control, hyperpolarizing the cell turns off resting M-current, producing a depolarizing "sag." During the slow EPSP, only a simple charging curve is seen in response to hyperpolarizing current; the increased amplitude of the hyperpolarization during the slow EPSP reflects the increased input resistance of the cell (resulting from the M-current blockade).

The primary effect of the slow EPSP, in other words, is not the small depolarization of the cell. When slow EPSPs were first reported, many were skeptical of their physiological importance because small subthreshold depolarizations would seem to have rather little effect on the behavior of a cell, particularly a sympathetic ganglion cell in which the main synaptic input—the fast EPSP—is generally suprathreshold to begin with. The real effect of the slow EPSP is to change the personality of the cell. Rather than being constrained to fire a single action potential to a depolarizing stimulus (a desirable property for a simple relay synapse), the cell can respond with a burst of action potentials. This is a way to change the input-output characteristics of the ganglion for a period of seconds (slow EPSP) or even minutes (late, slow EPSP). Exactly what use the bullfrog makes of this mechanism remains to be investigated.

Increased Conductance

Inhibition of M-current is, however, only one of the observable effects of muscarinic agonists and peptides. What are the consequences of the others? The conductance increase that is often seen should have nowhere near as strong an effect on the cell— unlike the M-current inhibition, the conductance increase would simply act to depolarize the cell, with no effects on repetitive firing (Jones, 1985). It is not even obvious that the conductance increase would be excitatory, as a slow, maintained depolarization could increase the threshold for firing an action potential by causing inactivation of the sodium conductance and by activating potassium conductances (including the M-current). In cells that show both M-current inhibition and the increased conductance effect, it is often possible to show an early increase in excitability (corresponding to the M-current effect) and a late *decrease* in excitability, when the two effects are sufficiently separated in time and when the cell is clamped manually to the resting potential (Jones, 1985).

I_{AHP}

The slow AHP in the bullfrog ganglion plays a role subtly different from that of the M-current. The slow AHP does act to limit repetitive firing by holding the cell below threshold, but as I_{AHP} turns off with time following an action potential, a long depolarizing current pulse still can generate activity, though at a lower frequency. Also, since the AHP current is relatively small, it can be overcome by a sufficiently large depolarizing current. Another (somewhat embarrassing) effect limits the observed influence of I_{AHP}: cells damaged by impalement with the microelectrode do not have slow AHPs, because the AHP is shunted by the leakage current caused by the electrode and because the I_{AHP} tends to run down in damaged cells. The cells in Figures 9.13 and 9.14, for example, had lost most of their slow AHP.

Figure 9.15 shows the effect of inhibiting I_M and I_{AHP} in a cell with a "good" slow AHP. For just suprathreshold currents, blockade of either current produces only a small increase in excitability; blockade of both together gives tonic firing for at

Fig. 9.15. Effects of I_{AHP} and M-current on excitability. 2-nA depolarizing currents were passed for 1 sec in a cell that was manually clamped to −60 mV, under control conditions *(upper left)*, in 10-μM muscarine (musc), 200-μM *d*-tubocurarine (dTC), and in both together. The action potentials were not fully reproduced by the chart recorder (from Pennefather et al., 1985b).

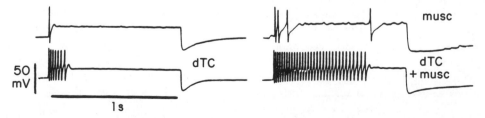

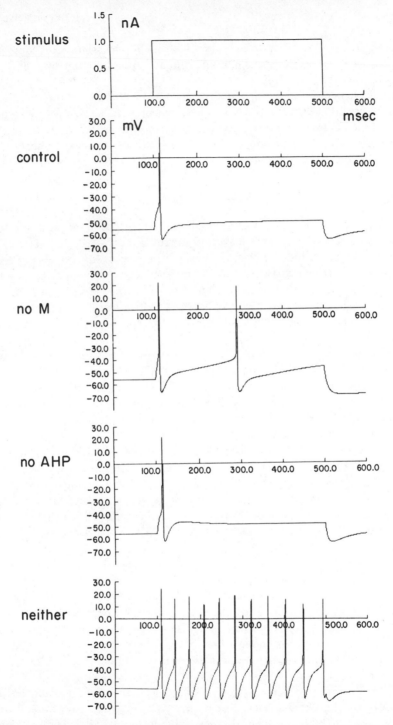

Fig. 9.16. Computer simulation of excitability in the bullfrog ganglion. The simulation included all the known currents in the ganglion, plus the effects of extracellular potassium accumulation and intracellular calcium metabolism. On the model, inhibition of either M-current or I_{AHP} had little effect, but inhibition of both together *(bottom)* led to repetitive firing to a 1-nA depolarizing current (unpublished data of C. Koch and P.R. Adams).

least 1 sec. It is not yet certain whether blockade of I_{AHP} has significant consequences during slow EPSPs, as the transmitters that inhibit the M-current by ~85% inhibit I_{AHP} by only ~30%.

A complementary approach to the issue of control of excitability by these currents is illustrated in Figure 9.16. A computer model of the known voltage-dependent currents of the bullfrog sympathetic neuron can be used to predict the effect of changes in the currents. The effects are remarkably similar to those seen experimentally (compare with Figure 9.15).

C Cells

All of the preceding discussion has centered on one cell type in the bullfrog ganglion, the large B cells. C cells, which may be distinguished on the basis of size or (more reliably) by the conduction velocity of their presynaptic inputs, have somewhat different properties (Dodd & Horn, 1983a). In particular, although C cells generally have clear late, slow EPSPs, they lack a slow muscarinic EPSP. (In fact, C cells have a muscarinic *I*PSP; see Dodd & Horn, 1983b.) This immediately raises the question of whether or not they have an M-current and, if so, why a slow EPSP is not observed.

C cells have a perfectly clear M-current, with properties very similar to those of B cells. In most cells, the M-current is inhibited by LH-RH or T-LH-RH, and a late, slow EPSC can be recorded that is largely due to blockade of M-current (Jones, 1984). However, C cells often show a separate and unexpected effect, a conductance decrease, which is particularly clear hyperpolarized to the M-current range. This effect is rare or absent in B cells.

But even in cells that show clear M-current inhibition to LH-RH agonists, muscarinic agonists have little or no effect. In B cells, 1-μM muscarine inhibits approximately 50% of the M-current. In C cells, 20-μM muscarine inhibits only 20% of the M-current on the average, with most cells showing less than 10% inhibition (Jones, 1984). To a good approximation, the M-current of C cells is not coupled to a muscarinic receptor. (This is somewhat ironic, as the M in M-current stands for muscarinic.)

There is another curious difference between B and C cells. C cells appear to totally lack I_{AHP}. Following a directly evoked action potential, C cells do in fact have an AHP, but even in the best cells the AHP lasts only ~100 msec (compared with more than 500 msec in many B cells). Correspondingly, when C cells are voltage-clamped a few milliseconds after an action potential, the resulting current decays with a time constant of ~40 msec. This residual AHP is not markedly reduced by removal of extracellular calcium, so it does not appear to be an I_{AHP} with a modified time course.

Thus, even within a single ganglion, there are themes and variations. The M-current is present in both B and C cells, but its sensitivity to neurotransmitters is different. In both B and C cells, LH-RH inhibits the M-current and occasionally causes a separate conductance increase. But LH-RH has a small effect on I_{AHP} only in B cells, and occasionally causes a separate conductance *decrease* only in C cells. And B cells have a current, I_{AHP}, which C cells appear to lack totally. Neurons have a repertoire of receptors to choose from and a separate repertoire of currents and a switchboard system of second messengers that can couple receptors to currents in a variety of ways.

SLOW EXCITATION OF HIPPOCAMPAL PYRAMIDAL CELLS

In the bullfrog sympathetic ganglion, the primary effect of the slow EPSPs is to increase the excitability of the cell to other inputs, primarily because of inhibition of a specific potassium current, the M-current. But how general is this mechanism? A large number of synaptic potentials, or effects of putative neurotransmitters, involve a depolarization with associated increase in resistance. Are they all due to blockade of M-current? This question is difficult to answer, as relatively few vertebrate neurons have been studied in detail under voltage clamp. This is largely because of two main technical difficulties. Most vertebrate neurons have cell bodies considerably smaller than those in bullfrog sympathetic ganglia, so they are more difficult to record from, especially with the low-resistance microelectrodes that are necessary for good voltage clamp. A more fundamental limitation is space clamp. A neuron with a large dendritic arbor is not electrically compact—that is, the membrane potential in a distal dendrite can be quite different from that in the cell body. Even if the cell body is well voltage clamped, synaptic potentials in dendrites may not be.

Most studies of slow synaptic potentials of vertebrate neurons have therefore not used voltage clamp. As discussed previously, the effects of a slow EPSP under current clamp can be complex and difficult to interpret. But there are clues: for example, a slow EPSP due to M-current inhibition should not reverse to an IPSP below E_K because of the voltage-dependence of the M-current, the sag in the electronic potential resulting from small hyperpolarizing currents should be reduced (see Figure 9.12), and the action of the transmitter involved should still be seen in the absence of extracellular calcium.

Rather than go through the many examples of slow EPSPs one by one, we will discuss in detail a representative case, the effects of norepinephrine and acetylcholine in the hippocampus.

The effect of norepinephrine on the hippocampus was initially quite mysterious. Iontophoretic application of norepinephrine *in vivo* decreases the spontaneous firing rate of a nearby pyramidal cell, but intracellular recording failed to demonstrate a consistent effect. One extensive study of this problem found that of 119 cells, 21% were depolarized, 44% were hyperpolarized, 19% showed a biphasic effect, and 16% showed no clear effect at all. This is a very common result; except for the classic excitatory and inhibitory transmitters [e.g., glutamate and gamma-aminobutyric acid (GABA)] almost any transmitter, applied to almost any cell in the central nervous system (CNS), will excite about one-third of the cells, inhibit one-third, and do nothing to the rest. To make matters worse, the depolarizations and hyperpolarizations observed in response to norepinephrine were generally tiny (less than 3 mV). The obvious conclusion is that norepinephrine is not doing anything very interesting to the cells; perhaps the *in vivo* effects were due to some complicated presynaptic or polysynaptic action. But this obvious conclusion is wrong. The effect of norepineph-

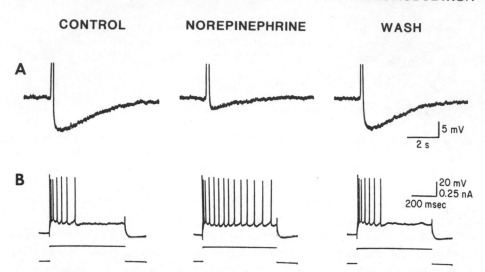

Fig. 9.17. Effects of norepinephrine on hippocampal pyramidal cells. *(Top)* Effects on the slow AHP following a calcium-dependent action potential (in 1-μM TTX and 5-μM TEA); *(Bottom)* the effect of norepinephrine on excitability (in normal medium). (Redrawn from Madison & Nicoll, 1986a.)

rine is on the pyramidal cell itself, but the underlying action is not simply to depolarize or hyperpolarize the cell.

The first problem was that there are two adrenergic receptors on pyramidal cells, hyperpolarizing α-adrenergic receptors and depolarizing β-receptors. But even with specific α and β agonists, the effects on resting potential are still tiny.

The main effect of norepinephrine is to block a slow, calcium-dependent AHP (Madison & Nicoll, 1986a), which is due to a current rather similar to I_{AHP} of the bullfrog ganglion (Lancaster & Adams, 1984). The effect (Figure 9.17) is quite dramatic, and it results in an equally dramatic reduction in spike frequency adaptation (Madison & Nicoll, 1984). By classic criteria, the effect of norepinephrine is through β-receptors and is mediated by an increase in intracellular cyclic AMP (Madison & Nicoll, 1986b). The effect is not secondary to changes in calcium current. The one piece of the puzzle that is still missing is a demonstration that there is a synaptic pathway that blocks the AHP by releasing norepinephrine onto hippocampal pyramidal cells.

Once again, the fundamental effect of a transmitter is nonclassic. Norepinephrine does not open channels. It does not act simply by depolarizing or hyperpolarizing the cell. Even more clearly than for the slow EPSPs in the bullfrog sympathetic ganglion, looking for changes in resting potential was asking the wrong question.

Norepinephrine is not the only neurotransmitter that blocks I_{AHP} in pyramidal cells. ACh, acting through a muscarinic receptor, can block the same current with no effect on I_C. However, the action of ACh is not identical to that of norepinephrine. Muscarinic agonists clearly depolarize the cell, and this action persists in the absence of extracellular calcium, suggesting that it is not due to an action on a resting level of I_{AHP}. Under voltage clamp, muscarinic agonists—but not norepinephrine— inhibit the M-current in hippocampal pyramidal cells (Halliwell & Adams, 1982). In some respects, the muscarinic action on I_M and I_{AHP} in hippocampus is remarkably similar to that in the bullfrog ganglion. But there are some crucial differences. At low concentrations of agonist, I_{AHP} is blocked and I_M is not. In addition, blockade of I_{AHP} can be essentially complete in hippocampus. Another problem is that the muscarinic depolarization cannot easily be explained by the effect on M-current, since blockade of the M-current requires higher concentrations of muscarinic agonists.

A slow muscarinic EPSP can be generated from stimulation of fiber tracts within the hippocampal slice. The fiber tracts contain (among other things) axons of cholinergic neurons originating in the septum. The observed effects are essentially identical to those of exogenous muscarinic agonists: depolarization, blockade of the calcium-dependent AHP, and (only for strong stimulation in the presence of anticholinesterases) blockade of the M-current (Cole & Nicoll, 1984). Similar experiments on explant cultures, in which slices from the septum are allowed to innervate hippocampal slices, also have identified a muscarinic slow EPSP. In the explants, the effect on M-current is more prominent (Gahwiler & Brown, 1985).

Given that the adrenergic effect on I_{AHP} is mediated through cyclic AMP, how can the multiple effects of muscarinic agonists be explained? Clearly, an additional second messenger system is required, instead of or in addition to cyclic AMP. This has not been worked out in detail, but the protein kinase C cascade is a leading candidate. In particular, phorbol esters, which activate protein kinase C directly, depolarize hippocampal pyramidal cells with an decrease in conductance and block the slow AHP (Baraban et al., 1985). Although this explanation must be considered speculative at the moment, it would not be surprising for the effects of two second messenger systems to converge on one endpoint.

CONCLUSIONS

It is clear that slow EPSPs resulting from blockade of potassium currents are widespread phenomena at many levels of vertebrate nervous systems. They selectively enhance the excitability of neurons—in particular, they encourage cells to fire repetitively. These slow EPSPs involve at least two distinct potassium currents, I_M and I_{AHP}. The relative importance of the two currents can differ: in bullfrog sympathetic ganglia, inhibition of I_M is the primary effect, whereas in rat hippocampal pyramidal cells, block of I_{AHP} dominates. In some cells, other effects can be demonstrated (e.g., voltage-independent increases and decreases in conductance), but these generally have minor effects on the behavior of the cell. There are several indications that these slow EPSPs involve second messengers: the slow time courses, the multiple effects, and the multiple receptors that can evoke similar patterns of effects. However, only in the case of norepinephrine in the hippocampus has the second messenger been identified. Future research will undoubtedly concentrate on the biochemical pathways involved in generation of slow EPSPs and on the behavioral functions of these slow, modulatory phenomena.

REFERENCES

Adams, P.R. and Brown, D.A. (1980) Luteinizing hormone-releasing factor and muscarinic agonists act on the same voltage-sensitive K^+-current in bullfrog sympathetic neurones. *Br. J. Pharmacol. 68*, 353–355.

Adams, P.R. and Brown, D.A. (1982) Synaptic inhibition of the M-current: Slow exitatory post-synaptic potential mechanism in bullfrog sympathetic neurones. *J. Physiol. 332*, 263–272.

Adams, P.R., Brown, D.A., and Constanti, A. (1982a) M-currents and other potassium currents in bullfrog sympathetic neurones. *J. Physiol. 330*, 537–572.

Adams, P.R., Brown, D.A., and Constanti, A. (1982b) Pharmacological inhibition of the M-current. *J. Physiol. 332*, 223–262.

Adams, P.R., Brown, D.A., and Jones, S.W. (1983) Substance P inhibits the M-current in bullfrog sympathetic neurones. *Br. J. Pharmacol. 79*, 330–333.

Adams, P.R., Constanti, A., Brown, D.A., and Clark, R.B. (1982c) Intracellular Ca^{2+} activates a fast voltage-sensitive K^+ current in vertebrate sympathetic neurones. *Nature 296*, 746–749.

Adrian, R.H. (1969) Rectification in muscle membrane. *Progr. Biophys. Mol. Biol. 19*, 340–369.

Aghajanian, G.K. (1985) Modulation of a transient outward current in serotonergic neurones by α_1-adrenoceptors. *Nature 315*, 501–503.

Akasu, T., Gallagher, J.P., Koketsu, K., and Shinnick-Gallagher, P. (1984) Slow excitatory post-synaptic currents in bull-frog sympathetic neurones. *J. Physiol. 351*, 583–593.

Baraban, J.M., Snyder, S.H., and Alger, B.E. (1985) Protein kinase C regulates ionic conductance in hippocampal pyramidal neurons: Electrophysiological effects of phorbol esters. *Proc. Natl. Acad. Sci. USA 82*, 2538–2542.

Cole, A.E., and Nicoll R. (1984) Characterization of a slow cholingeric post-synaptic potential recorded *in vitro* from rat hippocampal pyramidal cells. *J. Physiol. 352*, 173–188.

Dodd, J. and Horn, J.P. (1983a) A reclassification of B and C neurones in the 9th and 10th paravertebral sympathetic ganglia of the bullfrog. *J. Physiol. 334*, 225–269.

Dodd, J., and Horn, J.P. (1983b) Muscarinic inhibition of sympathetic C neurones in the bullfrog. *J. Physiol. 334*, 271–291.

Dubinsky, J.M. and Oxford, G.S. (1985) Dual modulation of K channels by thyrotropin-releasing hormone in clonal pituitary cells. *Proc. Natl. Acad. Sci. USA 82*, 4282–4286.

Dufy, B., Dufy-Barbe, L., and Barker, J.L. (1983) Electrophysiological assays of mammalian cells involved in neurohormonal communication. *Meth. Enzymol. 103*, 93–111.

Eiden, L.E. and Eskay, R.L. (1980) Characterization of LRF-like immunoreactivity, in the frog sympathetic ganglia: Non-identity with LRF decapeptide. *Neuropeptides 1*, 29–37.

Gahwiler, B.H. and Brown, D.A. (1985) Functional innervation of cultured hippocampal neurones by cholinergic afferents from co-cultured septal explants. *Nature 313*, 577–579.

Halliwell, J.V. and Adams, P.R. (1982) Voltage-clamp analysis of muscarinic excitation in hippocampal neurons. *Brain Res. 250*, 71–92.

Heuser, J.E., Reese, T.S., Dennis, M.J., Jan, Y., Jan, L., and Evans, L. (1979) Synaptic vesicle exocytosis captured by quick freezing and correlated with quantal transmitter release. *J. Cell Biol. 81*, 275–300.

Hugues, M., Schmid, H., Romey, G., Duval, D., Frelin, C., and Lazdunski, M. (1982) The Ca^{2+}-dependent slow K^+ conductance in cultured rat muscle cells: Characterization with apamin. *EMBO J. 1*, 1039–1042.

Jan, L.Y. and Jan, Y.N. (1982) Peptidergic transmission in sympathetic ganglia of the frog. *J. Physiol. 327,* 219–246.

Jan, Y.N., Jan, L.Y., and Kuffler, S.W. (1979) A peptide as possible transmitter in sympathetic ganglia of the frog. *Proc. Natl. Acad. Sci. USA 76,* 1501–1505.

Jan, Y.N., Jan, L.Y., and Kuffler, S.W. (1980) Further evidence for peptidergic transmission in sympathetic ganglia. *Proc. Natl. Acad. Sci. USA 77,* 5008–5012.

Jones, S.W. (1984) Muscarinic and peptidergic actions on C cells of bullfrog sympathetic ganglia. *Soc. Neurosci. Abstr. 10,* 207.

Jones, S.W. (1985) Muscarinic and peptidergic excitation of bull-frog sympathetic neurones. *J. Physiol. 366,* 63–87.

Kaneko, A. and Tachibana, M. (1985) Effects of L-glutamate on the anomalous rectifier potassium current in horizontal cells of *Carassius auratus* retina. *J. Physiol. 358,* 169–182.

Katayama, Y. and Nishi, S. (1982) Voltage-clamp analysis of peptidergic slow depolarizations in bullfrog sympathetic ganglion cells. *J. Phsyiol. 333,* 305–313.

Klein, M., Camardo, J., and Kandel, E.R. (1982) Serotonin modulates a specific potassium current in the sensory neurons that show presynaptic facilitation in *Aplysia. Proc. Natl. Acad. Sci. USA 79,* 5713–5717.

Koketsu, K. (1984) Modulation of receptor sensitivity and action potentials by transmitters in vertebrate neurons. *Jap. J. Physiol. 34,* 945–960.

Kuba, K. and Koketsu K. (1978) Synaptic events in sympathetic ganglia. *Progr. Neurobiol. 11,* 77–169.

Kuffler, S.W. and Sejnowski, T.J. (1983) Peptidergic and muscarinic excitation at amphibian sympathetic synapses. *J. Physiol. 341,* 257–278.

Lancaster, B. and Adams, P.R. (1984) Single electrode voltage clamp of the slow AHP current in rat hippocampal pyramidal cells. *Soc. Neurosci. Abstr. 10,* 872.

MacDermott, A.B. and Weight, F.F. (1982) Action potential repolarization may involve a transient, Ca^{2+}-sensitive outward current in a vertebrate neurone. *Nature 300,* 185–188.

Madison, D.V. and Nicoll, R.A. (1984) Control of the repetitive discharge of rat CA1 pyramidal neurones *in vitro. J. Physiol. 354,* 319–331.

Madison, D.V. and Nicoll, R.A. (1986a) Actions of noradrenaline recorded intracellularly in rat hippocampal CA1 pyramidal neurones, *in vitro. J. Physiol. 372,* 221–244.

Madison, D.V. and Nicoll,R.A. (1986b) Cyclic adenosine 3′, 5′-monophosphate mediates beta-receptor actions of noradrenaline in rat hippocampal pyramidal cells. *J. Physiol. 372,* 245–259.

Pennefather, P., Jones, S.W., and Adams, P.R. (1985b) Modulation of repetitive firing in bullfrog sympathetic ganglion cells by two distinct K currents, I_{AHP} and I_M. *Soc. Neurosci. Abstr. 11,* 148.

Pennefather, P., Lancaster, B., Adams, P.R., and Nicoll, R.A. (1985a) Two distinct Ca-dependent K currents in bullfrog sympathetic ganglion cells. *Proc. Natl. Acad. Sci. USA 82,* 3040–3044.

Petersen, O.H. (1984) The mechanism by which cholecystokinin peptides excite their target cells. *Biosci. Reports 4,* 275–283.

Romey, G. and Lazdunski, M. (1984) The coexistence in rat muscle cells of two distinct classes of Ca^{2+}-dependent K^+ channels with different pharmacological properties and different physiological functions. *Biochem. Biophys. Res. Commun. 118,* 669–674.

Sherwood, N., Eiden, L., Brownstein, M., Spiess, J., Rivier, J., and Vale, W. (1983) Characterization of a teleost gonadotropin-releasing hormone. *Proc. Natl. Acad. Sci. USA 80,* 2794–2798.

Siegelbaum, S.A., Camardo, J.S., and Kandel, E.R. (1982) Serotonin and cyclic AMP close single K^+ channels in *Aplysia* sensory neurons. *Nature 299*, 413–417.

Stanfield, P.R., Nakajima Y., and Yamaguchi K. (1985) Substance P raises neuronal membrane excitability by reducing inward rectification. *Nature 315*, 498–501.

Tokimasa, T. (1984) Muscarinic agonists depress calcium-dependent g_K in bullfrog sympathetic neurons. *J. Auton. Nerv. Sys. 10*, 107–116.

Trautmann, A. and Marty, A. (1984) Activation of Ca-dependent K channels by carbamoyl choline in rat lacrimal glands. *Proc. Natl. Acad. Sci. USA 81*, 611–615.

10

The S-Current: A Background Potassium Current

STEVEN A. SIEGELBAUM

With the development of single channel recording by Neher and Sakmann and their colleagues (Hamill et al., 1981), it became possible to study transmitter actions at the level of current flow through single ion channels. This technique has greatly advanced our understanding of how conventional transmitter actions, including the effects of ACh at the end-plate (Colquhoun & Sakmann, 1981), and various excitatory (Nowak et al., 1984) and inhibitory (Sakmann et al., 1983) amino acid transmitter effects on central neurons, lead to channel activation. Much less is known, however, about how modulatory transmitter actions regulate the functioning of single ion channels.

This chapter examines a particular example of a modulatory second messenger-dependent transmitter action: the slow excitatory postsynaptic potential (EPSP) produced by serotonin in the abdominal ganglion sensory neurons of *Aplysia* (Kandel & Schwartz, 1982). It reviews experiments that address the general question of how such modulatory synaptic actions alter the behavior of single ion channels. An understanding of the molecular mechanisms in this example is especially interesting because the slow synaptic action is thought to underlie a simple form of learning in *Aplysia*.

SEROTONIN PRODUCES A SLOW EPSP
IN *APLYSIA* NEURONS

The abdominal ganglion in the marine snail *Aplysia californica* contains a cluster of sensory neurons that are involved in the gill withdrawal reflex. A tactile stimulus to the animal's gill or siphon elicits gill withdrawal through a simple reflex arc, illustrated in Figure 10.1. Touching the siphon skin produces an action potential in the periphery of the sensory neuron, which is conducted into the central nervous system. In the abdominal ganglion, the impulse travels to the sensory neuron terminals where it causes release of a transmitter that produces a fast excitatory postsynaptic potential

A

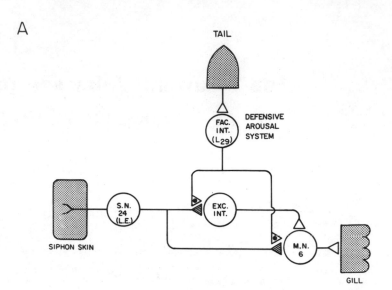

TAIL

FAC. INT. (L₂₉)

DEFENSIVE AROUSAL SYSTEM

SIPHON SKIN

S.N. 24 (L.E.)

EXC. INT.

M.N. 6

GILL

B

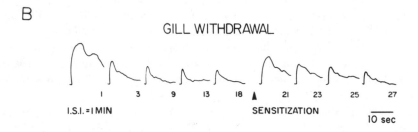

GILL WITHDRAWAL

1   3   9   13   18   21   23   25   27

I.S.I. = 1 MIN   SENSITIZATION

10 sec

C

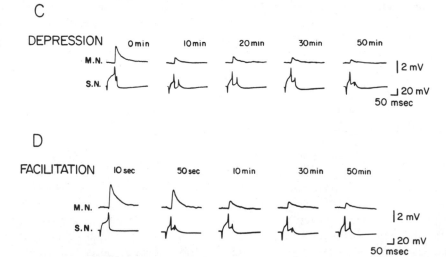

DEPRESSION

0 min   10 min   20 min   30 min   50 min

M.N.

S.N.

| 2 mV

⌐ 20 mV
50 msec

D

FACILITATION

10 sec   50 sec   10 min   30 min   50 min

M.N.

S.N.

| 2 mV

⌐ 20 mV
50 msec

in a cluster of motor neurons that innervate the gill muscle. If the fast EPSP is large enough, it generates an action potential in the follower motor neurons, which produces gill withdrawal.

Several years ago, Kandel and his colleagues showed that this reflex is not fixed but is subject to modification by behavioral experience. Repeated stimulation of the siphon or gill decreases the extent of gill withdrawal—the reflex habituates. If a noxious stimulus is then applied to the animal's tail or head, however, a subsequent stimulus to the siphon or gill will result in a much enhanced gill withdrawal—the reflex becomes sensitized (Figure 10.1B). The mechanism of sensitization is now understood at the cellular level of neuronal function. In response to the sensitizing stimulus, a facilitatory interneuron becomes excited and produces a slow modulatory EPSP in the sensory neurons. Although the identity of the modulatory transmitter remains unknown, serotonin (5-HT) mimics the effects of facilitatory interneuron stimulation and has been used to study the ionic mechanism of the slow EPSP. The slow EPSP in the sensory neuron is accompanied by a decrease in the sensory neuron's resting membrane conductance, a broadening of the action potential duration, and an increase in transmitter release from the sensory neuron terminals. The increase in transmitter release results in a larger fast EPSP in the follower motor neuron, which results in the enhanced gill withdrawal.

What is the ionic mechanism of the slow EPSP and what, if any, relationship does the slow EPSP have with presynaptic facilitation? Using the voltage clamp technique, Klein, Camardo, and Kandel (1982) have shown that the primary effect of serotonin is to decrease a specific outward potassium current (S-current) that is distinct from the previously identified potassium currents in molluscan neurons. Klein and Kandel (1980) originally proposed that presynaptic facilitation could be a consequence of a prolonged action potential at the sensory neuron terminals. The increased action potential duration would allow for a greater total calcium influx into the terminals through the voltage-dependent calcium channels and this increased calcium influx would lead to enhanced transmitter release.

Good evidence now exists that the modulatory effects of serotonin on the S-current are not due to the direct action of serotonin on the S-current channels but are mediated by the second messenger cyclic AMP according to the following general sequence of events (Figure 10.2): (1) The binding of 5-HT to its receptor leads to

---

Fig. 10.1. Habituation and sensitization of the gill-withdrawal reflex are mediated by the same synaptic connection. (A) Simplified wiring diagram of the gill-withdrawal reflex consisting of 24 primary mechanoreceptor sensory neurons *(S.N.)* that receive input from the gill and siphon skin and make excitatory synapses on excitatory interneurons and on six motorneurons *(M.N.)* that innervate the gill muscle. Facilitator interneurons *(Fac. Int.)* receive excitatory input from the tail and facilitate transmitter release from the sensory neuron terminals. (B) Repeated stimulation of the siphon by a water jet results in the habituation of gill withdrawal. Following a sensitizing stimulus, such as tail or head shock, gill withdrawal subsequently increases. (C) Habituation results from depression of transmitter release from the sensory neuron terminals, resulting in a decline in the size of the PSP in the motorneuron. (D) Sensitization is due to facilitation of transmitter release, which restores the PSP to its initial amplitude.

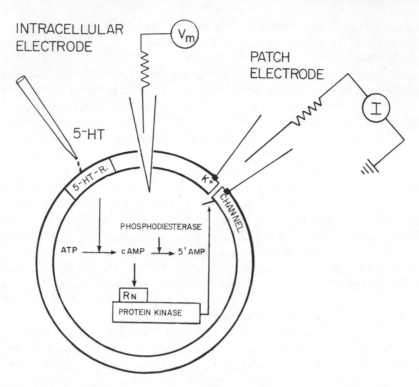

Fig. 10.2. Schematic illustration of experimental protocol and cyclic AMP-dependent model for serotonin action in sensory neurons. A high-resistance gigaohm seal is obtained between the patch electrode and the sensory cell membrane to record single channel currents in the small patch of membrane under the pipette. Normally, both the bath and pipette are filled with artificial seawater containing (in millimolars) 460 NaCl, 10 KCl, 10 CaCl$_2$, 55 MgCl$_2$, and 10 HEPES at pH 7.6. Cell resting potential is recorded with a conventional intracellular microelectrode. Serotonin (10–100 μM) is applied to the cell outside the area of the patch but may still alter the activity of a potassium channel under the pipette by means of the cyclic AMP cascade, illustrated diagramatically.

activation of membrane-bound adenylate cyclase. (2) This leads to a rise in intracellular cyclic AMP. (3) Cyclic AMP then activates cyclic AMP-dependent protein kinase. (4) The catalytic subunit of protein kinase phosphorylates several substrate proteins. (5) This leads to the decrease in S-current by some unknown mechanism. Evidence in support of this scheme includes the finding that intracellular injection of cyclic AMP mimics the electrophysiological effects of serotonin. Serotonin, but not other transmitters, has been shown to produce a specific increase in cyclic AMP levels in signal identified sensory neurons (Bernier et al., 1982). Intracellular injection of the purified catalytic subunit of cyclic AMP-dependent protein kinase also mimics the effects of serotonin (Castellucci et al., 1980), and intracellular injection of the protein kinase inhibitor (PKI) blocks the effects of serotonin (Castellucci et al., 1982).

SINGLE-CHANNEL STUDIES OF SEROTONIN-SENSITIVE POTASSIUM CHANNEL

The techniques of single channel recording have been used to study the slow EPSP produced by serotonin at the molecular level of single channel function (Siegelbaum et al., 1982). Two of the goals of these studies were to identify and characterize the serotonin-sensitive potassium channel and then to investigate the mechanism of S-channel modulation by serotonin and cyclic AMP-dependent protein phosphorylation.

Before discussing the results of these experiments, it will be worthwhile to consider some general mechanisms by which serotonin might produce the observed reduction in the total macroscopic current carried by the S-current channels in the sensory neuron membrane. The magnitude of the macroscopic S-current, I, depends on the number of functional S-channels in the membrane, N_f, the magnitude of the current flow through a single open S-channel, i, and the probability that a given

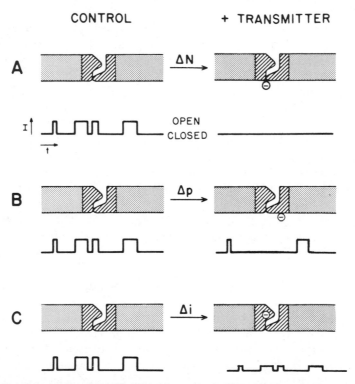

Fig. 10.3. Possible modes of serotonin action on single channel currents. The drawings depict channels as integral membrane proteins with an aqueous pore for ion permeation and a gate for controlling channel opening and closing. Idealized current records show channel openings as an upward current deflection. The transmitter could, in principle, lead to a decrease in the average current carried by a population of such channels by modulating the channel activity at one of several sites, giving rise to different changes in single channel function (modified from Siegelbaum & Tsien, 1983).

channel is open, p, according to the equation, $I = N_f \times i \times p$. In principle, a neurotransmitter could cause a decrease in the magnitude of the net ionic current carried by a population of channels by altering any one of these parameters, as illustrated in Figure 10.3 (see also Chapters 8 and 11). A transmitter could lead to a decrease in overall ionic current by decreasing the magnitude of current flow, i, through a single open channel (Figure 10.3C), by decreasing the probability, p, that a channel is in the open state (Figure 10.3B) or by decreasing the number, N_f, of functional channels in the membrane (Figure 10.3A).

The experimental protocol used to measure single S-channel currents is illustrated in Figure 10.2. Cell membrane potential and resting input resistance were measured with a conventional intracellular microelectrode, allowing sensory neurons to be identified on the basis of their electrophysiological properties and permitting the monitoring of the whole cell's response to serotonin. At the same time, a high-resistance gigaohm seal was obtained between the sensory cell membrane and an extracellular fire-polished glass pipette by pressing the pipette up against the cell membrane and applying gentle suction. Typical seal resistances were greater than 100 gigaohms.

One potential problem that often arises in single channel recording is separating out the contribution of particular ion channel, in this case the S-channel, from the various other single channel currents that contribute to the cell membrane conductance. From the previous voltage clamp studies of Klein, Camardo, and Kandel, it is known that the serotonin-sensitive potassium current is active at the resting potential, does not inactivate with maintained depolarization, and is not dependent on intracellular calcium. Since virtually all other identified ionic currents in molluscan neurons do inactivate to some extent with prolonged depolarizations, the patch potential was generally held at a steady depolarized level (e.g., O mV) to inactivate these other channels. By depolarizing only the small area of membrane under the patch, the total calcium influx into the cell through the voltage-dependent calcium channels is minimized, reducing interference from the calcium-activated potassium current (Marty, 1983). Using such conditions, the patch current records reveal a predominant species of channel that displays many properties expected for the S-channel.

SEROTONIN AND CYCLIC AMP CLOSE THE S-CHANNEL

Figure 10.4 illustrates the action of serotonin on a patch that initially contained four active channels. Figure 10.4B shows a recording of single channel current at an expanded time scale before addition of 5-HT. The current record fluctuates among five discrete levels because of the random openings and closings of the four active channels (0 to 4 channels open). These channels display an identical unit current amplitude when open so they represent a single class of channels. At the holding potential of O mV used here, an open channel carries an outward current of around 3.5 pA in amplitude. Figure 10.4A illustrates the time course of serotonin's action on a slow time scale. Soon after addition of serotonin to the bath, there is a small depolarization of the resting potential, a decrease in cell membrane conductance (data not shown), and a progressive closure of three of the four active channels. The chan-

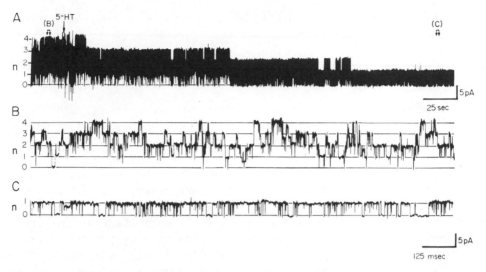

Fig. 10.4. Modulation of single channel currents by serotonin. Patch clamp current records from a sensory neuron membrane patch that initially contained four active channels. (A) Channel current on a slow time base. At the arrow, 100-μM serotonin was added to the bath causing all-or-none closure of three out of four channels. The numbers on the lefthand ordinate indicate current levels corresponding to the number of open channels. Before the addition of serotonin there are a maximum of four open channels. The arrows labeled B and C indicate regions of the trace in A from which the expanded records in the lower two traces (B and C) were obtained. The cell resting potential depolarized from −41 to −37 mV after application of 5-HT, and there was a 33% increase in membrane input resistance. The patch membrane potential was held at 0 mV before 5-HT was applied and +4 mV in the presence of 5-HT (from Siegelbaum & Tsien, 1983).

nels are seen to close in an all-or-none steplike manner: the channels are either completely closed in the presence of serotonin or continue to open and close normally (Figure 10.4B and C). Serotonin does not promote the appearance of channels with reduced conductance or with altered opening probability (see Figure 10.3B and C). Rather, the transmitter appears to cause a decrease in the number of active channels in the membrane by causing prolonged channel closures. The fraction of channels closed by 5-HT varies from patch to patch, but on average around half of all channels are closed.

The experiment of Figure 10.4 also provides indirect support for the idea that the effects of serotonin are mediated by an intracellular messenger. In these experiments, 5-HT is applied to the cell only after the high-resistance gigaohm seal is formed. The contact between the glass pipette and the cell membrane is thought to be so tight that it prevents the diffusion of even small molecules from the bath under the pipette. Since bath application of 5-HT consistently closes channels in the patch under the pipette, it is likely that 5-HT acts to mobilize some intracellular messenger, which can then modulate the channels from inside the membrane. Direct support for this scheme has been obtained in experiments in which injection of cyclic AMP into

sensory neurons from cyclic AMP-filled microelectrodes has been shown to mimic
the effects of serotonin in closing the channels.

SINGLE S-CHANNEL PROPERTIES

The voltage dependence of the serotonin-sensitive channel is shown in Figure 10.5,
where records from a patch that contained only a single active S-channel are shown.
The channel contributes square pulses of outward current over a wide range of membrane potentials. Upon depolarization of the patch, the size of the unit current step
increases because of the increase in outward driving force on ion movement through
the open channel. In this particular patch, however, membrane depolarization has
little effect on the probability that a channel is open, and the channel is open for a
large fraction of time over the entire range of voltages tested. In other patches, channel opening shows a somewhat greater dependence on membrane potential, although
in all cases the channel is open at least part of the time at negative potentials.

The opening of this channel at negative potentials is important because it means
the channel is open at the level of the cell resting potential (around -40 mV). This
means that the channel will contribute to setting the normal level of resting potential
and resting membrane conductance in the sensory neurons. Turning off such a channel by serotonin could thus account for the slow depolarization in the resting potential
and the observed decrease in resting membrane conductance and increase in excitability. As the channel is also open over a wide range of more depolarized potentials,
it will also contribute outward repolarizing current during the entire time course of
the action potential. As a result, turning off such a channel with serotonin can qualitatively explain why serotonin causes action potential broadening.

Fig. 10.5. Voltage-dependence of S-channel. Current records from a patch that contained a
single S-channel at four different patch membrane potentials (indicated at the left of each
trace). The channels are open for a large fraction of time ($p = 0.7$) at all potentials. The
channels show both brief closures lasting around 1 msec and longer closures lasting several
tens of milliseconds. The arrow indicates a closure to a rare subconductance state (from Siegelbaum et al., 1982).

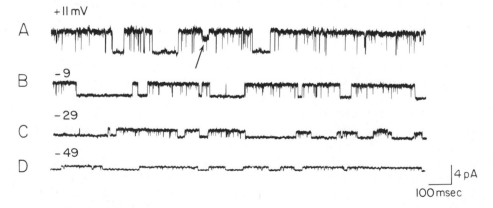

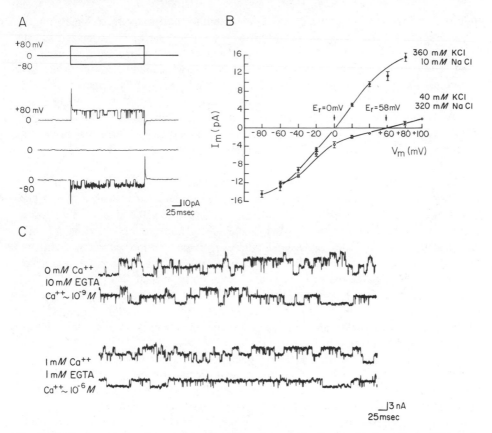

Fig. 10.6. S-channel is voltage independent, potassium selective, and independent of internal calcium. Current records from inside-out membrane patches. (A) The S-channel remains open over a wide voltage range. Recording is done under symmetric ionic conditions with a 360-mM KCl solution in both patch pipette and bath. The patch potential was held at 0 mV (the potassium reversal potential) and stepped up to + 80 mV or down to −80 mV for 200 msec. The channel remains open at both voltages, carrying outward current at +80 mV and inward current at −80 mV. (B) Potassium selectivity of the S-channel measured by substituting sodium for potassium in the bath solution. From the reversal potential shift, the channel is found to be at least tenfold more permeable to potassium than sodium. (C) S-channel gating is shown to be independent of internal calcium by altering the calcium concentration in the bath from around 1 nM up to 1 μM (from Camardo et al., 1983).

S-CHANNELS IN CELL-FREE PATCHES

How do we know that the S-channel is a potassium channel? Will the channel close if the membrane potential is hyperpolarized below -50 mV? Does channel opening require internal calcium, as has been demonstrated for other potassium channels (e.g., see Chapter 8)? To answer these questions, S-channel currents have been recorded from inside-out cell-free patches where the internal surface of the membrane faces the bath (Figure 10.6). Under these conditions, the bath solution contains a high-potassium, low-calcium seawater solution to mimic the intracellular ionic environment. Figure 10.6A shows the results of an experiment designed to investigate the voltage dependence of the channel over a wider potential range from a patch that contained only a single active channel. To record large channel currents at negative potentials, the pipette was filled with the same high-potassium seawater solution as the bath. Under these conditions, no channel current is observed at a holding potential of O mV, since there is no driving force on ionic current flow. Upon stepping the voltage up to +80 mV or down to −80 mV, however, large single channel currents can be seen, confirming the finding that the channel opening is largely voltage independent.

The ionic selectivity of the S-channel is demonstrated in Figure 10.6B in which the single channel current reversal potential has been determined with different concentrations of potassium in the bath (internal surface of the membrane). In symmetrical 360-mM potassium chloride solutions, the channel reversal potential is at O mV, as measured from the single channel current voltage relation. Upon reducing the potassium concentration in the bath to 40 mM, substituting sodium for potassium, the reversal potential shifts in the positive direction to around +55 to +85 mV. If sodium and potassium ions were able to pass through the channel with comparable ease, no shift should have been observed in the reversal potential. Thus, the large shift observed in the reversal potential means that the channel is highly selective for potassium ions over sodium ions.

Recently, it has become clear that many potassium channels are activated primarily by intracellular calcium and not by voltage (Marty, 1983). To examine the question of the calcium dependence of the S-channel, the internal surface of the patch membrane was exposed to various calcium concentrations using the inside-out patch configuration. Under these conditions, the opening of the S-channel persists at very low "intracellular" calcium levels ($<10^{-9}$ M) (Figure 10.6C) and is not altered when the calcium concentration is increased up to 1 mM (data not shown).

Thus, this channel identified in patch clamp recordings has many properties expected for the channel responsible for the S-current based on the previous voltage clamp results. The channel is open at the resting potential and at depolarized voltages, does not inactivate with maintained depolarization, is selective for potassium over sodium, and does not depend on intracellular calcium for its opening. Of course, the most crucial demonstration that this class of channels is responsible for the macroscopic S-current comes from the demonstration that the channel is closed by serotonin.

MECHANISM OF CHANNEL MODULATION BY PROTEIN PHOSPHORYLATION

A major question concerning all cyclic AMP-dependent transmitter actions, including closure of the S-channel, is the nature of the link between protein phosphorylation and channel modulation. Figure 10.7A illustrates that, although the most direct mechanism for S-channel closure involves the direct phosphorylation of the channel by protein kinase, there are several plausible alternatives involving phosphorylation

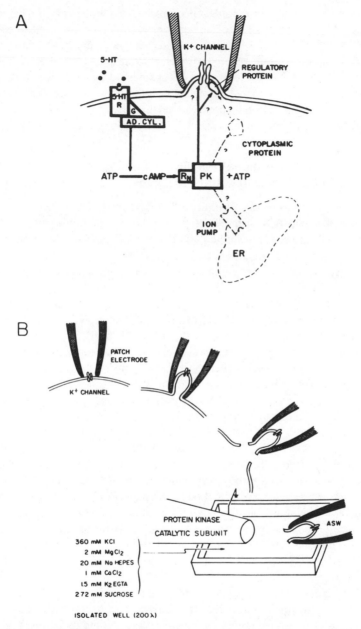

Fig. 10.7. Role of phosphorylation in channel modulation. (A) Illustration of how several different possible substrate proteins—including the channel itself, a membrane-bound regulatory protein, a cytoplasmic protein, or an ion transport protein—for cyclic AMP-dependent protein kinase could participate in channel modulation. (B) Approach to studying the action of catalytic subunit of protein kinase in cell-free patches where cytoplasmic and internal membrane constituents are largely absent. Purified catalytic subunit of cyclic AMP-dependent protein kinase $(0.1-1.0 \ \mu M)$ in the presence of 1 to 2-mM MgATP is directly applied to an inside-out patch in a small 200-μ1 well (from Camardo et al., 1983).

197

of various membrane-bound or cytoplasmic intermediary proteins (see Chapter 1). At present, despite the wide variety of transmitter actions known to be mediated by cyclic AMP-dependent protein phosphorylation, very little is known about the identity or subcellular localization of any of the substrate phosphoproteins that control channel activity. Moreover, while several groups have demonstrated an effect of the catalytic subunit of the cyclic AMP-dependent protein kinase on cellular electrophysiological properties, it is essential to extend such studies to a characterization of the effects of kinase on single channel currents (see also Chapters 8 and 11).

Effects of Cyclic AMP-Dependent Protein Kinase on S-channels in Cell-Free Patches of Membrane

Figure 10.7B shows an approach similar to that described in Chapter 8 to investigating the action of cyclic AMP-dependent protein kinase on single channel function. This involves application of purified catalytic subunit of cyclic AMP-dependent protein kinase (in the presence or absence of MgATP) to cell-free inside-out membrane patches to try to modulate S-channel activity under simplified *in vitro* conditions (Shuster et al., 1985).

An example of the effect of the catalytic subunit on channel currents in an inside-out patch is shown in Figure 10.8. In this patch there were initially four active channels. Upon addition of the catalytic subunit, one channel closes relatively quickly. After a somewhat longer delay, a second channel closes. The channels do not remain closed, even in the maintained presence of kinase, but rather reopen. There is then one more long-lasting channel closure, and this channel does not reopen until after the kinase is washed out of the bath. Such prolonged all-or-none closures are seen in the vast majority (74%) of experiments in which kinase is applied in the presence of ATP, the source of high-energy phosphate. Under these conditions, the catalytic subunit closes 34% of all active S-channels in the patches. These effects of kinase appear to be mediated by a phosphorylation reaction, since the frequency of the kinase-induced closures are reduced three- to fourfold in the absence of ATP.

The prolonged channel closures produced by the kinase in the cell-free patches are qualitatively similar to the all-or-none closures produced by serotonin in cell-attached patches. The effects of catalytic subunit, however are not identical to those of serotonin. The kinase closes a somewhat smaller total fraction of S-channels than does serotonin (34% versus 46% channels closed), and the kinase-induced closures tend to be shorter lasting than those produced with serotonin. With serotonin, channels tend to remain closed for long periods of time, outlasting the duration of transmitter application by about 5 minutes. In contrast, with catalytic subunit, channels tend to close for 1 to 3 minutes and then reopen, even in the maintained presence of the enzyme.

Possible Presence of Phosphoprotein Phosphatase in Cell-Free Patches

One possible explanation for these differences between kinase and serotonin is that the cell-free patches lack some important intracellular component necessary for com-

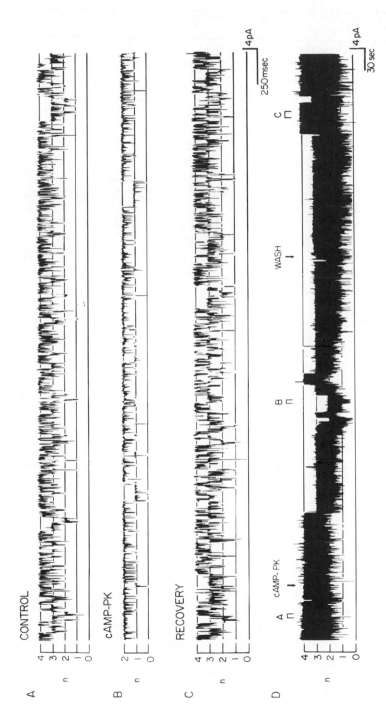

Fig. 10.8. Catalytic subunit of cyclic AMP-dependent protein kinase closes single S-channels in inside-out membrane patches. (A–C) Expanded current records showing S-channel activity taken at times indicated in trace D. (A) Before the addition of kinase four channels are active. (B) In the presence of 0.1-μM kinase, two of the four channels have closed. (C) After washing kinase out of the bath all four channels are active again. (D) The same experiment shown on a slow time scale illustrating the all-or-none step-like channel closures. The trace also shows how channels reopen even in the maintained presence of kinase. The membrane was held at 0 mV. The free calcium concentration in the bath was 0.1 μM (from Shuster et al., 1985).

plete channel modulation. Alternatively, the cell-free patches may contain an endogenous membrane-bound phosphoprotein phosphatase that is capable of cleaving the phosphate from the substrate protein, thus terminating the channel closure. According to this view, the duration of channel closures would reflect the lifetime of the phosphorylated form of the critical substrate protein required for modulation.

Two lines of evidence support a role for phosphatase: (1) Significant phosphoprotein phosphatase activity is associated with the membrane fraction isolated from *Aplysia* nervous tissue by differential centrifugation. The nonspecific phosphatase inhibitor fluoride ion (50 mM) reduces this phosphatase activity to less than half of its control value. (2) Based on this finding, the effects of 50-mM potassium fluoride on the modulation of the S-channel by catalytic subunit have been tested. Fluoride potentiates the action of kinase (Fig. 10.9), increasing both the fraction of successful experiments from 74% (0 potassium fluoride) to 83% (50-mM potassium fluoride), and causing a statistically significant increase in the fraction of channels closed from 34 to 49%. Fluoride also prolongs the periods of channel closure produced by catalytic subunit as much as tenfold. This increase in channel closed time with phosphatase inhibitor is also consistent with the idea that duration of the kinase-induced closures is determined by the rate of protein dephosphorylation.

However, because fluoride ions are nonspecific inhibitors of phosphatase and display many other actions, it is not certain that the effects of fluoride are due to phosphatase inhibition. The action of fluoride nonetheless shows some specificity because it has no effect on channel activity in the absence of kinase. Although fluoride ions are also known to stimulate adenylate cyclase, the possibility that the effects of fluoride on channel modulation are mediated by this action can be ruled out. Direct application of cyclic AMP (0.1–1 mM) to the patch in the presence of ATP neither produces channel closures by itself nor potentiates the effects of the catalytic subunit.

If the cell-free patches do contain phosphatase activity, the obvious question arises as to why the channel closures produced by 5-HT in cell-attached patches last so long. The intact patches should contain at least as much phosphatase activity as the cell-free patches, therefore, the channel closures should be correspondingly brief. One hypothesis is that the sensory neurons contain cytoplasmic inhibitor proteins capable of regulating phosphatase activity in cell-attached patches but lacking in cell-free membrane patches. A number of such inhibitor proteins have been identified that regulate type 1 phosphoprotein phosphatases (Ingebritsen & Cohen, 1983), and preliminary experiments indicate that more than 75% of the membrane-bound phosphatase activity in the *Aplysia* neuronal membranes can be inhibited by such inhibitor proteins purified from mammalian tissue.

One interesting feature of these inhibitor proteins is that they themselves are substrates for cyclic AMP-dependent protein kinase and often are active in inhibiting phosphatases only when they are in the phosphorylated form. This feature provides a means of synergistic regulation of phosphorylation levels in cells, since a rise in cyclic AMP will increase the forward rate of phosphorylation by activating cyclic AMP-dependent protein kinase as well as decrease the rate of dephosphorylation as any phosphatase inhibitor proteins become phosphorylated (Figure 10.10).

According to this model, one would expect the rate of both phosphorylation and dephosphorylation in the sensory neurons to depend on serotonin concentration. And

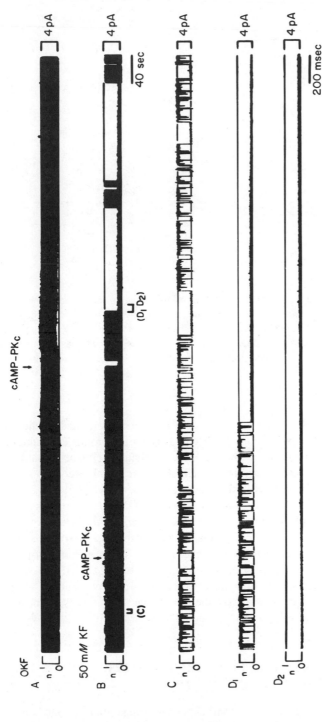

Fig. 10.9. Potassium fluoride potentiates the action of cyclic AMP-dependent protein kinase. The current records are from an inside-out patch containing a single active S-channel. (A) This recording on slow time base shows a lack of effect of cyclic AMP-dependent protein kinase in the absence of potassium fluoride. (B) In the presence of potassium fluoride, the enzyme now produces prolonged channel closures. (C) The record at fast sweep speed shows channel activity in the presence of potassium fluoride but before the addition of kinase. The channel currents appear normal. D and E show continuous recording in the presence of kinase illustrating the all-or-none closure of the channel (from Shuster et al., 1985).

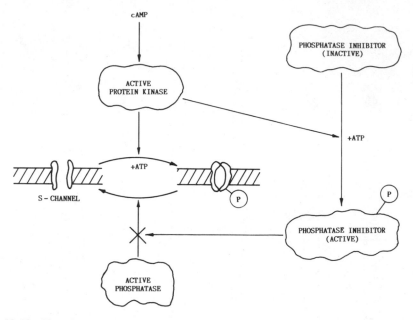

Fig. 10.10. Phosphoprotein phosphatase inhibitors allow for coordinate regulation of phosphorylation reactions. The scheme shows activation of cyclic AMP-dependent protein kinase by cyclic AMP, resulting in phosphorylation of a substrate protein involved in channel modulation (for purposes of illustration shown to be the S-channel) as well as of phosphatase inhibitor proteins. The phosphorylated form of inhibitor protein reduces activity of type I phosphoprotein phosphatase.

if the duration of channel closure is assumed to be inversely related to the rate of protein dephosphorylation, we would predict that as the serotonin concentration is increased a progressive increase in the duration of channel closure should occur. Most experiments with serotonin on the S-channel have used high concentrations of transmitter (100 μM) to maximize effects on channel activity. However, in a few preliminary experiments with lower doses of serotonin (<10 μM), the channel closures are found to be shorter lasting and more closely resemble the effects of catalytic subunit in cell-free patches. Although regulation of phosphatase activity is an intriguing hypothesis to explain aspects of S-channel modulation in *Aplysia,* at present it is only a hypothesis. Future experiments are needed both to test the effects of purified phosphatase inhibitor proteins on channel closures produced by catalytic subunit in the cell-free patches and to demonstrate their presence in the sensory neurons to confirm their physiological role in channel modulation.

CONVERGENT ACTIONS OF MULTIPLE TRANSMITTERS ON A SINGLE ION CHANNEL

One final interesting feature of cyclic AMP-dependent transmitter actions is that they provide a convenient means of allowing convergent actions of different transmitters.

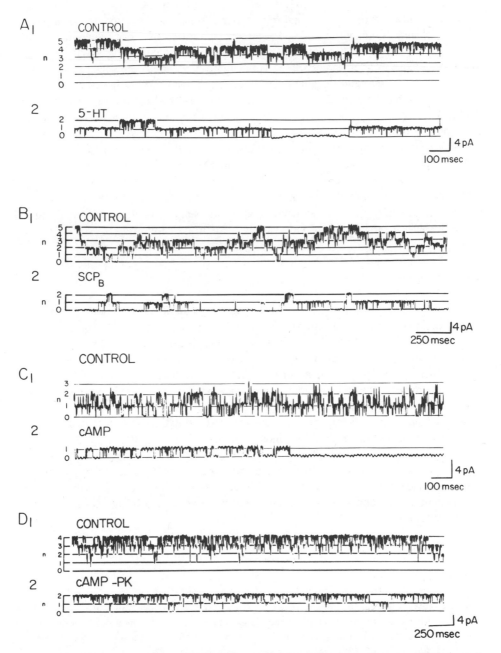

Fig. 10.11. Convergent actions of transmitters, second messengers, and enzymes for channel modulation. (A) Closure of S-channels by serotonin in a patch containing five active channels. Addition of 30-μM serotonin closes three of the active channels in an all-or-none manner. (B) SCP$_B$ (1 μM) also closes three of five active channels from another patch in an all-or-none manner. (C) Intracellular injection of cyclic AMP also closes S-channels. (D) S-channel closure produced by catalytic subunit of cyclic AMP-dependent protein kinase. Similarity of the actions of all the agents results from a final common step of protein phosphorylation mediated by cyclic AMP-dependent protein kinase.

Thus, in contrast with conventional transmitter actions, where activation of a particular ion channel is linked to a single receptor, several modulatory transmitters could influence the activity of the same ion channel (see also Chapter 9) by having multiple receptors linked to adenylate cyclase. This situation occurs in the sensory neurons in which both serotonin and the small cardioactive peptide (SCP) (Abrams et al., 1984) raise cyclic AMP levels and close S-channels. Figure 10.11 summarizes these results and demonstrates the similarity of channel closures produced by application of extracellular transmitter with closures produced by injecting cyclic AMP directly into the sensory neurons or by direct application of cyclic AMP-dependent protein kinase to cell-free patches. It seems likely that in the future other transmitters will be identified that also activate adenylate cyclase in the sensory neurons and close S-channels. As a consequence, S-channel modulation and sensitization of the gill-withdrawal reflex are not limited to a particular synaptic input to the sensory neurons but rather appear to be designed to respond to a wide variety of neuronal stimuli.

CONCLUSIONS

The results reported in this chapter show how the patch clamp technique can be used to explore some of the molecular mechanisms that underlie transmitter modulation of ion channels. The technique has allowed the identification of a class of serotonin-sensitive potassium channels in *Aplysia* sensory neurons and the demonstration that serotonin produces prolonged all-or-none closures of these channels. The channels can be characterized as background conductance potassium channels because they are open at the resting potential, and channel gating is only weakly dependent on membrane potential. In cell-free patches, the purified catalytic subunit of cyclic AMP-dependent protein kinase simulates most, but not all, of the effects of serotonin on cell-attached patches. Although the results do not allow us to distinguish whether the channel itself is phosphorylated or the primary substrate is some other protein that remains attached to the patch, they do suggest that at least some of the important components of the channel modulation reaction are contained in the *in vitro* cell-free patch system.

REFERENCES

Abrams, T.W., Castellucci, V.F., Camardo, J.S., Kandel, E.R., and Lloyd, P.E. (1984) Two endogenous neuropeptides modulate the gill and siphon withdrawal reflex in *Aplysia* by presynaptic facilitation involving cAMP-dependent closure of a serotonin-sensitive potassium channel. *Proc Natl. Acad. Sci. USA 81*, 7956–7960.

Bernier, L., Castellucci, V.F., Kandel, E.R., and Schwartz, J.H. (1982) Facilitatory transmitter causes a selective and prolonged increase in adenosine 3':5'-monophosphate in sensory neurons mediating the gill and siphon withdrawal reflex in *Aplysia*. *J. Neurosci. 2*, 1682–1691.

Camardo, J.S., Shuster, M.J., Siegelbaum, S.A., and Kandel, E.R. (1983) Modulation of a specific potassium channel in sensory neurons of *Aplysia* by serotonin and cAMP-dependent protein phosphoryation. *Cold Spring Harbor Symp. Quant. Biol. 48,* 213–220.

Castellucci, V.F., Kandel, E.R., Schwartz, J.H., Wilson, F.D., Nairn, A.C., and Greengard, P. (1980) Intracellular injection of the catalytic subunit of cyclic AMP-dependent protein kinase stimulates facilitation of transmitter release underlying behavioral sensitization in *Aplysia. Proc. Natl. Acad. Sci. USA 77,* 7492–7496.

Castellucci, V.F., Nairn, A.C., Greengard, P., Schwartz, J.H., and Kandel, E.R. (1982) Inhibitor of adenosine 3′:5′-monophosphate-dependent protein kinase blocks presynaptic facilitation in *Aplysia. J. Neurosci. 2,* 1673–1681.

Colquhoun, D. and Sakmann, B. (1981) Fluctuations in the microsecond time range of the current through single acetylcholine receptor ion channels. *Nature 294,* 464–466.

Hamill, O.P., Marty, A., Neher, E., Sakmann, B., and Sigworth, F.J. (1981) Improved patch-clamp techniques for high resolution current recording from cells and cell-free membrane patches. *Pflugers Arch. 391,* 85–100.

Ingebritsen, T.S. and Cohen, P. (1983) Protein phosphatases: Properties and role in cellular regulation. *Science 221,* 331–338.

Kandel, E.R. and Schwartz, J.H. (1982) Molecular biology of learning: Modulation of transmitter release. *Sci 218,* 433–443.

Klein, M., Camardo, J., and Kandel, E.R. (1982) Serotonin modulates a specific potassium current in the sensory neurons that show presynaptic facilitation in *Aplysia. Proc. Natl. Acad. Sci. USA 79,* 5713–5717.

Klein, M. and Kandel, E.R. (1980) Mechanism of calcium current modulation underlying presynaptic facilitation and behavioral sensitization in *Aplysia. Proc. Natl. Acad. Sci. USA 77,* 6912–6916.

Marty, A. (1983) Ca^{2+}-dependent K^+ channels with large unitary conductance. *Trends in Neurosci. 6,* 262–265.

Nowak, L., Bregestovski, P., Ascher, P., Herbet, A., and Prochiantz, A. (1984) Magnesium gates glutamate-activated channels in mouse central neurones. *Nature 307,* 462–465.

Sakmann, B., Bormann, J., and Hamill, O.P. (1983) Ion transport by single receptor channels. *Cold Spring Harbor Symp. Quant. Biol. 48,* 247–257.

Shuster, M.J., Camardo, J.S., Siegelbaum, S.A., and Kandel, E.R. (1985) Cyclic-AMP-dependent protein kinase closes the serotonin-sensitive K^+ channels of *Aplysia* sensory neurons in cell-free membrane patches. *Nature 313,* 392–395.

Siegelbaum, S.A., Camardo, J.S., and Kandel, E.R. (1982) Serotonin and cyclic AMP close single Kp channels in *Aplysia* sensory neurones. *Nature 299,* 413–417.

Siegelbaum, S.A. and Tsien, R.W. (1983) Modulation of gated ion channels as a mode of transmitter action. *Trends in Neurosci. 6,* 307–313.

11

Calcium Currents
in Heart Cells and Neurons

RICHARD W. TSIEN

It is easy to be chauvinistic about calcium channels. They are found in all known types of neurons and are essential to several aspects of neuronal function. The movement of calcium across cell membranes has special significance beyond that of a transfer of positive charge, important as this may be to the shaping of spikes, pacemaker potentials, or other aspects of neuronal electrical activity. Entry of calcium also represents the flow of a message, to be received by calcium receptor proteins such as calmodulin and decoded with appropriately significant consequences for the cell. Other ions such as sodium, potassium, and chloride are key charge carriers, but probably are not used as messengers per se. The membrane enzymes that make cytoplasmic messengers such as cyclic AMP or inositol trisphosphate are not strikingly voltage dependent. As far as we know, the assignment of transducing electrical signals to chemical messages is unique to calcium ions and calcium channels (see Tsien et al., 1983; Hille, 1984).

Although evolution defies second-guessing, there is logic to this assignment. Consider the following generalizations: (1) The cytoplasmic concentration of calcium ions is universally low, usually of the order of 10 to 100 nM, so rather small ion fluxes can produce large, rapid, localized transients before slower buffering processes take over. (2) This cytoplasmic concentration is typically four orders of magnitude below the extracellular concentration, so there is never a shortage of chemical driving force for calcium influx. (3) Calcium channel pores manage to be highly selective for calcium over other ions while also retaining the capability for supporting high flux rates: relatively large signals can be generated with relatively few channels. (4) Calcium channels open with a probability that depends steeply on membrane potential (like other channels in excitable membranes), so that small voltage changes produce relatively large variations in calcium inflow. All of these factors combine to endow the system of calcium ions and calcium channels with properties of speed, amplification, and reliability. It makes sense that this system lies at the heart of processes such as neurotransmitter release in synaptic terminals, excitation-secretion coupling in gland cells, or contraction coupling in cardiac and smooth muscle.

206

Modulation of Voltage-Dependent Calcium Channels as a Form of Intracellular Calcium Regulation

The main focus of this chapter is on modulation of voltage-gated calcium channels in the surface membrane of excitable cells. We distinguish such modulation from other mechanisms whereby neurochemical substances influence intracellular calcium. These other mechanisms include the following:

1. *Indirect control of calcium entry.* Even if voltage-dependent calcium channels are not directly affected, modulation of other types of channels can change the pattern of cell depolarization and thus alter the flux through voltage-gated calcium channels. Many examples exist of systems of this type, mostly involving modulation of potassium channels (see Chapters 7, 8, and 10).

2. *Chemically gated calcium channels in internal membranes.* There is growing evidence that calcium release from intracellular stores such as endoplasmic reticulum or sarcoplasmic reticulum may be controlled by inositol trisphosphate or other internal transmitters, including intracellular calcium itself.

3. *"Receptor-operated" calcium channels in the surface membrane.* Perhaps the least understood type of calcium channel, these are postulated to be distinct from "voltage-operated" calcium channels (Bolton, 1979, Van Breemen et al., 1979). Receptor-operated calcium channels are thought to be activated by α-adrenergic agents such as norepinephrine in tissues such as liver and smooth muscle. There has been no direct electrophysiological study of their properties, nor any convincing demonstration that they lack voltage dependence.

4. *Control of calcium transport.* This mechanism includes regulation of uptake into intracellular stores or extrusion from the cell. Clear-cut examples are found in the regulation of the sarcoplasmic reticulum calcium pump in heart muscle (see the section on convergence of signals, divergence of effects).

It should be emphasized that these mechanisms are not mutually exclusive and that combinations of these mechanisms have been found to work in parallel in many systems.

Examples of Modulation of Voltage-Dependent Calcium Channels

A wide variety of transmitters and other neurochemicals have been found to modulate voltage-gated calcium channels in neurons and muscle cells. Table 11.1 provides a brief summary of some of the systems in which such modulation has been characterized and, where known, their internal messenger mechanisms.

The following sections deal separately with work in heart cells, vertebrate neurons, and molluscan neurons. The following major questions are considered: What is the biological significance of the modulatory response of calcium channels, and how does it fit in with modulation of other channels? Which type of voltage-dependent calcium channel is modulated? What is the underlying molecular mechanism of the modulatory effect?

Table 11.1. Selected examples of modulation of voltage-gated calcium channels

Tissue	Cell type	Modifier	Messenger mechanism	Response	Functional role	References
Neuron	Chick DRG	Enkephalin, norepinephrine (NE), gamma-aminobutyric acid (GABA), 5-HT, dopamine, somatostatin	Unknown	↓ I	↓ AP duration, ↓ transmitter output	Mudge et al., 1979; Dunlap & Fischbach, 1978
	Rat sympathetic	NE	Unknown	↓ I	↓ AP duration, ↓ transmitter output	McAfee et al., 1981; Galvan & Adams, 1982
	Xenopus, Rohon beard	Met-enkephalin	Unknown	↓ I	↓ AP duration, ↓ transmitter output	Bixby & Spitzer, 1983
	Aplysia, LB,LC	5-HT	cAMP	↑ I	↑ AP duration	Pellmar & Carpenter, 1980
	Aplysia, L10	Histamine	Unknown	↓ I	↓ Transmitter output	Shapiro et al., 1980; Kretz et al., 1984
	Aplysia, bag cell	Unknown	Diacylglycerol (TPA)	↑ I	↑ Afterdischarge	DeRiemer et al., 1985
Heart	All	E,NE (B-adr)	cAMP	↑ I	↑ Rate, ↑ contraction	Reuter, 1967; Tsien et al., 1972
	Atrial, ventricular	Acetylcholine	↓ cAMP	↓ I	↓ Rate, ↓ contraction	Giles & Tsien, 1975; Ikemoto & Goto, 1975; Giles & Noble, 1976
	Purkinje	Angiotensin II	Unknown	↑ I	↑ Contraction	Kass & Blair, 1981

Abbreviations: AP = action potential; B-adr = B-adrenergic receptor; E = epinephrine; 5-HT = 5-hydroxytryptamine; NE = norepinephrine.

MODULATION OF CARDIAC CALCIUM CHANNELS

The biological function and molecular mechanism of calcium channel modulation are better understood in heart cells than in any neuronal preparation. This is not altogether surprising. The cardiac calcium current was the first recognized example of a voltage-gated channel under neurochemical modulation (Reuter, 1967; Vassort et al., 1969) and the first case in which cyclic AMP was shown to be the intracellular messenger for such modulation (Tsien et al., 1972; Tsien, 1973; Watanabe & Besch, 1974). Calcium channels are not only responsive to sympathetic neurotransmitters (norepinephrine, epinephrine) but also to parasympathetic transmitter (acetylcholine). Indeed, extensive studies over the last 15 years have demonstrated responses of cardiac calcium channels to many other agents including histamine, glucagon, adenosine, and angiotensin. The mechanism of β-adrenergic modulation has been particularly well studied at the level of single cells and single calcium channels. In some ways, heart cells have provided a Rosetta stone for neuromodulation comparable to the squid axon for impulse conduction and the frog neuromuscular junction for synaptic transmission.

Convergence of Signals, Divergence of Effects

Figure 11.1 shows the convergence of neuromodulatory signals on cardiac adenylate cyclase activity and the consequent effects on the activity of L-type cardiac calcium channels. The positive responses are mediated, respectively, by beta$_1$ receptors for β-adrenergic agonists such as norepinephrine, epinephrine, and isoproterenol, as well as receptors for histamine and glucagon. The inhibitory responses are produced by acetycholine binding to muscarinic receptors or adenosine interaction with adenosine receptors. All of these agents are thought to act through appropriate guanosine triphosphate (GTP)-binding proteins—N_S or N_i—to stimulate or inhibit adenylate cyclase. The resulting variations in the level of cyclic AMP bring about changes in the activity of L-type calcium channels as a result of cyclic AMP-dependent phosphorylation of the calcium channel or a closely associated protein.

  Changes in the magnitude of the calcium current affect several aspects of cardiac function, including (1) rhythmic firing of the sinoatrial node, the heart's natural pacemaker, (2) impulse conduction through the atrioventricular node, and (3) the strength of contraction of working heart muscle (for general reviews, see Tsien, 1977; Katz,

Fig. 11.1. Convergence of neurohormonal signals on cardiac calcium channels.

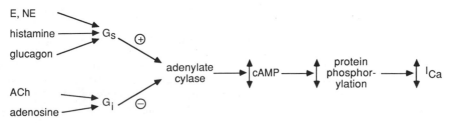

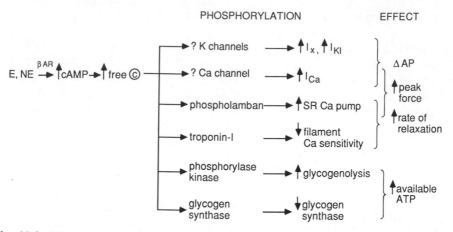

Fig. 11.2. Divergence of cyclic AMP-mediated effects of sympathetic stimulation of β-adrenergic receptors, combining to give multifaceted effect on heartbeat.

1983; Reuter, 1983). A prime example of the multifaceted nature of the cardiac response is seen during sympathetic stimulation. Enhanced calcium channel activity helps to accelerate sinus pacemaker activity, to quicken impulse spread through the atrioventricular (A-V) node, and to increase the strength of contraction in working heart muscle.

Modulation of calcium channels does not occur in isolation. The rise in intracellular cyclic AMP not only modulates calcium channel activity but also helps control other cellular processes (Figure 11.2). Enhancement of potassium channel currents keeps the action potential from becoming greatly prolonged as a result of increased I_{Ca}. Stimulation of the calcium pump in the sarcoplasmic reticulum membrane increases stores of releasable calcium, but also helps keep the intracellular calcium transient from becoming inappropriately long. Decreased calcium sensitivity of contractile proteins also favors rapid relaxation and allows the heart enough time to fill with blood despite the increased heart rate associated with sympathetic activity. Increased glycogenolysis helps supply ATP to meet increased energy demands. All of these changes combine with calcium channel modulation to produce an appropriately coordinated response; some of them are balanced against the effect of calcium channel modulation in a series of checks and balances. As a neuromodulatory system, the cardiac response to sympathetic stimulation provides a leading example of how a single second messenger can rapidly orchestrate divergent but harmonious cellular effects.

Hypotheses for the Mechanism of Calcium Channel Modulation

Proposals that cyclic AMP-dependent protein phosphorylation might mediate β-adrenergic modulation of cardiac ionic channels were made as early as 1973 (Tsien, 1973), soon after the initial evidence for the involvement of cyclic AMP. The next few years saw further support for the cyclic AMP hypothesis (reviewed by Spere-

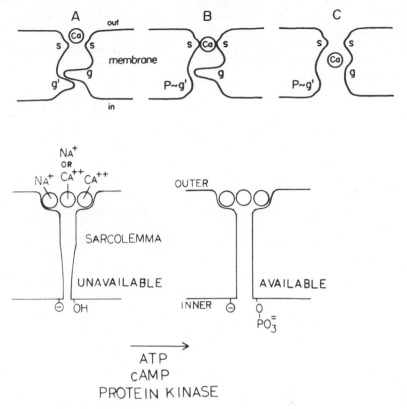

Fig. 11.3. Specific proposals that cyclic AMP-dependent protein phosphorylation increases the availability of functional calcium channels (RSSS hypothesis) [(A) from Reuter, 1979. (B) from Sperelakis & Schneider, 1976.]

lakis, 1985) and improved descriptions of the changes in calcium current during β-adrenergic stimulation (e.g., Reuter & Scholz, 1977). Several groups (e.g., Niedergerke & Page, 1977) put forward proposals of mechanisms for regulation of calcium channels by phosphorylation.

The specific mechanisms proposed by Reuter and Scholz (1977; Reuter, 1979) and Sperelakis and Schneider (1976) are shown in Figure 11.3. These schemes are so similar that we will refer to them collectively as the RSSS hypothesis. The basic idea is that voltage-dependent gating and phosphorylation-dependent gating occur independently (e.g., through opening and closing of the chemically controlled gates labeled g and g' in Figure 11.3). Phosphorylation by cyclic AMP-dependent protein kinase has a permissive effect in making a given channel available for opening in response to membrane depolarization. Since phosphorylation by protein kinase can be reversed by dephosphorylation through a protein phosphatase, individual channels may undergo transitions between the unavailable pool and the available pool. β-adrenergic stimulation would alter the steady-state balance between pools, producing what Reuter and Scholz called "an increase in the number of functional conductance channels."

It is important to define at this point what we mean by the number of functional channels and to indicate what other factors determine the overall calcium channel current in a cell (I). One way of stating this is as follows:

$$I = N_f.p_0.i \qquad (1)$$

where

N_f = the number of channels in the available pool.
p_0 = the probability that the channel will be open, given that it is available.
i = the unitary current or flux through the open pore.
   Another way of expressing this subdivides N_f into two factors:

$$N_f = N_T.p_f \qquad (2)$$

   where

N_T = the total number of channels (available or unavailable) in the sarcolemmal membrane.
p_f = the probability that a given channel is available, giving

$$I = N_T.p_f.p_0.i \qquad (3)$$

In the single channel experiments, the factors p_f and p_0 are sometimes lumped together and simply called p. As we shall discuss later, p_f and p_0 are easily distinguished because they reflect processes operating on very different time scales.

The increase in N_f (or p_f) proposed by Reuter and Scholz and Sperelakis and Schneider is one of a number of possible modulatory mechanisms, represented schematically in Figure 11.4 in a manner similar to that of Figure 10.3. Each of the panels depicts a change in one of the factors Equation in 2. Panel A shows an increase in the ion flux through the open calcium channel, seen as an increase in the amplitude of the unitary current pulses (i) in single channel recordings. Such an effect could conceivably arise from phosphorylation of a site involved in ion permeation (Siegelbaum & Tsien, 1983). Figure 11.4B depicts the possibility of a change in p_0, the fraction of time an available channel spends open. Increased openness could arise from alterations in the millisecond kinetics of channel opening and closing, such as prolonged opening times (t_0) or abbreviated closed periods (t_c), or both. Figure 11.4C describes the possibility of increased availability of functional channels. During repeated depolarizations in a control run (left), sweeps containing openings (the channel available) are shown interspersed with blank sweeps (the unavailable channel). The righthand panel shows an increase in the proportion of nonblank sweeps with β-adrenergic stimulation and cyclic AMP-dependent protein phosphorylation, following the RSSS hypothesis. Another possibility is an increase in N_T (Panel D). In the extreme, this might occur if channels were recruited by fusion of channel-containing intracellular vesicles with the sarcolemmal membrane. Such a mechanism has been proposed for antidiuretic hormone (ADH)-stimulated water transport in the toad bladder (Wade et al., 1981). The main point here is that any of

CONTROL   + TRANSMITTER

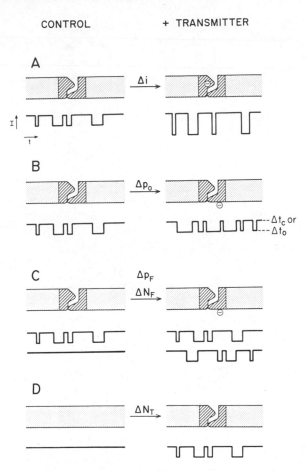

Fig. 11.4. Various hypothetical mechanisms for calcium channel modulation. (A) Increased open channel flux *(i)* through modification of a site along the path of ion permeation; (B) increased probability of channel openness (p_0) through altered millisecond kinetics of channel opening or closing; (C) increased availability of functional channels (p_f or N_f), seen as a decrease in the proportion of blank sweeps, (D) increase in total number of channels (N_T) (after Siegelbaum & Tsien, 1983).

these mechanisms could plausibly be linked to cyclic AMP-dependent protein phosphorylation, and all of them might be at least roughly consistent with information from voltage clamp experiments in multicellular preparations.

    Experimental tests of these hypotheses became possible with the advent of patch clamp methods for studying unitary properties of calcium channels. Investigators have relied largely on two particular variations of the patch clamp method: recordings from cell-attached patches, aimed at studying the properties of individual channels, and whole cell recordings, designed to analyze properties of the entire pool of functional calcium channels. These approaches are inherently complementary and lead to a mutually consistent set of conclusions about the mechanism of β-adrenergic modulation.

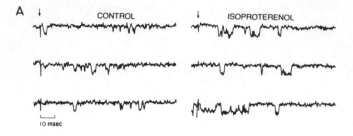

A   ↓   CONTROL   ↓   ISOPROTERENOL

10 msec

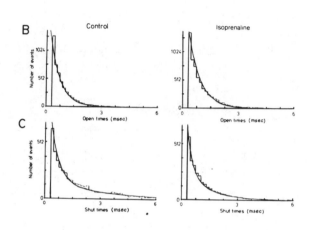

B   Control   Isoprenaline

C

D   Brum et al. (1984)

$(p_o)_{max}$

control   C1 ⇌ C2 ⇌ O   0.308
          1178   1606
          1696   1482

                                         1.58

B-stim   C1 ⇌ C2 ⇌ O   0.488
          1994   2125
          1187   1143

E   Cachelin et al. (1983)

$(p_o)_{max}$

control   C1 ⇌ C2 ⇌ O   0.0376
          162   334
          656   1695

                                         1.82

8-Br-cAMP   C1 ⇌ C2 ⇌ O   0.068
          211   444
          631   1515

Changes in Rapid Kinetics Studied with Unitary Current Recordings

Figure 11.5 illustrates the results obtained with unitary current recordings in cell-attached patches. Panels A and B show single channel records from a neonatal rat ventricular cell. Following depolarization steps of appropriate strength imposed across the membrane patch, openings of calcium channels appear as downward pulses of current, typically lasting 1 msec. The unitary amplitude of fully resolved current pulses is ≈ 1 pA, with isotonic barium as the extracellular charge carrier in the patch pipette, large enough to be easily distinguished from the background noise. The unitary current amplitude corresponds to a flux of about 3 million divalent ions per second. Records taken in a control run (A) may be compared with sweeps taken after calcium channel activity was stimulated following exposure of the cell to isoproterenol (B). The main point of this illustration is that the unitary current size remains unchanged with β-adrenergic stimulation. This has been a general finding in studies with β-agonists or exogenous derivatives of cyclic AMP, and it rules out the mechanism of channel modulation illustrated in Figure 11.4A.

There is also general agreement that increased calcium channel activity arises at least in part through elevation of p_0, the opening probability of available calcium channels, and that this comes about through changes in the milisecond kinetics of channel opening and closing. Figure 11.5B and C show histograms of open and closed times obtained in a cell-attached patch recording from guinea pig ventricular cell (Brum et al., 1984). In this particular illustration, the open time distribution is fitted with single exponentials, with time constants of 0.54 msec in the absence of drug and 0.63 msec after administration of isoproterenol (B). The closed time distributions (D) are fitted by the sum of two expotentials, with time constants that de-

---

Fig. 11.5. (A) Effect of isoproterenol on current through a single calcium channel, recorded from a cell-attached membrane patch on a cultured cell from neonatal rat heart. Patch pipette contained 96-mM Ba^{2+} as the charge-carrying species and 20-μM tetrodotoxin to block sodium channels. Calcium channel openings were evoked by depolarizations from Vm -90 mV to Vm $+10$ mV; step change occurred at the time marked by the arrow and was associated with a downward spike of imperfectly subtracted capacitative current. Traces show selected records from a control run *(left)* and after exposure of the cell to 10-μM isoproterenol *(right)* (experiment of H. Reuter, C.F. Stevens. R.W. Tsien, and G. Yellen). (B and C) Altered millisecond kinetics of calcium channel activation. Analysis of isoproterenol effect in a single channel recording from a guinea pig ventricular cell. Open and closed time histograms in the absence *(left)* and presence *(right)* of isoproterenol. In B, open time distributions are fitted with single exponentials, with $\tau_0 = 0.54$ msec (control) and $\tau_0 = 0.63$ msec (isoproterenol). In C, closed time distributions are fitted with the sum of two exponentials, with $\tau_s = 0.42$ msec and $\tau_{ag} = 2.7$ msec in control, and $\tau_s = 0.28$ msec and $\tau_{ag} = 1.27$ msec after exposure to isoproterenol. (D and E) Averaged kinetic parameters describing changes in millisecond opening kinetics with β-stimulation or cyclic AMP administration (from Brum et al., 1984). (D) Effect of β-adrenergic stimulation in ventricular myocytes of bovine, cat, and guinea pig hearts with depolarizations to $+15$ mV at 36°C (from Brum et al., 1984). (E) Effect of exposure to 8-bromocyclic AMP in neonatal rat ventricular cells at 24 to 26°C (Cachelin et al., 1983).

crease with β-stimulation. The overall result is an increase in the probability of openness.

This type of histogram analysis has been presented within the framework of a closed-closed-open scheme for channel gating. Figure 11.5 D and E summarizes the collected results from experiments using β-agonists in various mammalian myocytes by Trautwein's group (D) and experiments using 8-bromo cyclic AMP by Reuter and colleagues (E). The prolongation of openings corresponds to a decrease in the rate constant k_{-2}, and the abbreviation of closings is represented by an increase in k_1 and k_2. Although quantitative discrepancies exist in the details of how the kinetics are altered, resulting perhaps from differences in experimental preparation and temperature, the results match fairly well in supporting the type of mechanism in Figure 11.4B.

Changes in Rapid Kinetics—Sufficient to Explain the Overall Enhancement?

An obvious question is whether changes in p_0 associated with rapid kinetic changes account completely for the overall effect of β-adrenergic stimulation. Figure 11.6A and B shows changes in the time course and amplitude of the calcium channel current predicted from the kinetic data summarized in Figure 11.5E and F. The predicted increases in p_0 are 1.8-fold in neonatal rat ventricular cells (A) and 1.6-fold in adult guinea pig ventricular myocytes (B). For comparison, Figure 11.6C shows whole cell recordings from frog ventricular heart cells. In this case, the enhancement of peak calcium channel current was six-fold in collected results from 25 cells (Bean et

Fig. 11.6. (A and B) Average changes in calcium channel current predicted from the kinetic parameters reported for the C↔C↔O model by Cachelin et al. (A) or Brum et al. (B), as indicated in Figure 11.5D and E. The vertical scale has been normalized to make the control current amplitude roughly equal in all panels. (C) Experimentally observed enhancement of whole-cell calcium channel current in frog ventricular cells. The five-fold increase in this particular example is close to the six-fold increase seen in 25 cells (from Bean et al., 1984).

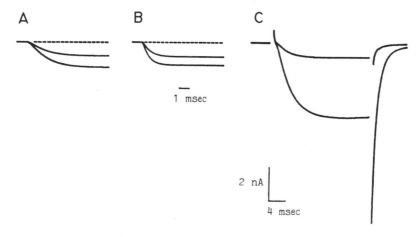

al., 1984), far larger than the 1.5- to 2.0-fold enhancement seen in other preparations. This comparison raises the question of whether or not β-adrenergic modulation of calcium channels might, under certain circumstances, involve changes other than increased p.

Evidence of Increased Availability of Channels from Fluctuation Analysis

Bean et al. (1984) looked specifically for an increase in the availability of functional channels as proposed in the RSSS hypothesis. Taking advantage of the large and consistent β-adrenergic response in frog ventricular cells, they studied single channel properties with the technique of fluctuation analysis of whole cell recordings (Sigworth, 1980a, b). Figure 11.7 illustrates this method. Repeated depolarizations (a) evoke whole cell current records (b–d) that contain fluctuations reflecting opening and closing of individual channels. Subtracting one current record from the next gives the pairwise difference currents in traces e through g. The fluctuations may be seen more clearly because the smooth onset of inward current common to adjacent records (h) is eliminated by the pairwise subtraction. The fluctuations express the collective behavior of the population of calcium channels that are opening and closing during one or both of the sweeps. For analysis of single channel properties, individual difference records are squared, divided by 2, and averaged to give the variance (j), and the relationship between the variance and the mean current is plotted (k) and then fitted by a theoretical curve. The curve is part of a parabola with parameters reflecting properties of single channels,

$$\text{variance} = \frac{iI - I^2}{N_f}$$

where $I = N_f \cdot p_0 \cdot i$.

The portion of the parabola that is plotted extends from $p = 0$ to $p = p_{\max}$. This is the behavior expected theoretically for a homogeneous pool of available channels that respond independently to membrane depolarization and show one level of nonzero conductance (Sigworth, 1980). N_f refers to the number of channels that are readily available. If an individual channel remain dormant for several consecutive sweeps, it does not contribute to pairwise difference currents and is therefore not counted toward N_f.

The parabola can be given an intuitive explanation. The theoretical curve must start at the origin: just after the depolarization, when all channels are still closed and p_0 and inward current are zero, the variance must also be zero, since it is certain that there is no current. At the other extreme, the theoretical curve must come back toward the abscissa, toward an intercept corresponding to complete certainty of opening ($p_0 = 1$). At this intercept (not reached by the actual data), the total inward current is $N_f \cdot i$. Between the intercepts the variance undergoes a maximum for $p_0 = \frac{1}{2}$, when closed and open states are equally likely. Variance piles up quickly when $p_0 = \frac{1}{2}$ because individual channels are either closed or open but never half open. The

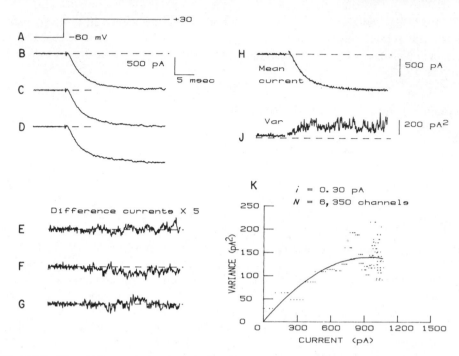

Fig. 11.7. Fluctuation analysis of a whole-cell recording of barium current through calcium channels. Cultured neonatal rat heart cell (day 2): (A) voltage protocol; (B–D) current traces accompanying three consecutive voltage steps; (E–G) difference signals, obtained by subtracting each trace from the trace immediately following, after a small (1%) correction for drift; (H) mean current obtained by averaging individual sweeps as in b through d; (J) variance calculated as the average of squared difference currents (the dashed line is zero baseline), (K) plot of variance against mean current. Background variance is subtracted. The horizontal streaks were obtained by averaging the variance over successive time bins. Smooth parabolic curve with parameters indicated was obtained by least squares fit (from Tsien et al., 1983).

parabolic relationship fits the data well enough to give some confidence in the assumptions of the theory.

Figure 11.8 compares the mean current and variance record before and after β-adrenergic stimulation in a frog ventricular cell. Isoproterenol-induced enhancement of mean current is associated with a large increase in variance in pairwise analysis of successive sweeps. Variance versus mean current plots (B and C) indicate that the large increase in current in frog cells is accompanied by (1) no significant change in i, (2) an appreciable increase in peak p_0, from 0.40 to 0.58, and (3) a roughly threefold increase in N_f, from 11,000 to 37,000. These results are representative of collected data from a large number of frog ventricular cells. On the average, peak p_0 increased from 0.34 to 0.49, and N_f increased from 11,000 to 31,000 (Bean et al., 1984).

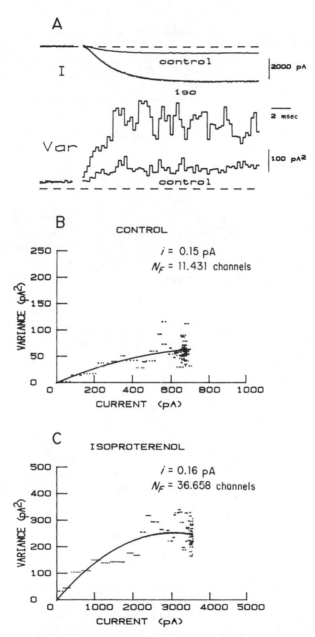

Fig. 11.8. Effect of isoproterenol (0.5 μM), studied with fluctuation analysis of whole cell recordings from a bullfrog ventricular cell. (A) Mean current and variance recorded during a control run and after the cell was exposed to isoproterenol; (B and C) plots of variance versus the mean current. Smooth curves obey Equation 3 with the parameters indicated and are least squares fits to the data (from Bean et al., 1984). Note that the assumption of a single homogenous population of calcium channels has been supported by whole-cell experiments in frog ventricular cells (from Bean, 1985).

Evidence for Increased Channel Availability
from Unitary Recordings

The basis for the increase in N_f observed with fluctuation analysis can be studied further with unitary current recordings. As Figure 11.9 illustrates, changes in the availability of calcium channels can be seen in guinea pig ventricular cells, as well as in frog myocytes. When studied at the level of individual channels, the increase in availability is expressed as a decrease in the percentage of null sweeps (see also Cachelin et al., 1983; Brum et al., 1984).

In the experiment shown in Figure 11.9, channel availability in a cell-attached patch was assayed with depolarizations at 3-sec intervals. Representative groups of consecutive current records show unitary calcium channel activity during runs taken in the absence of drug *(left)* and after bath application of isoproterenol *(right)*. Averaged current records from these runs are shown below the individual sweeps. The β-agonist more than doubles the peak inward current and slows its time course of decay. The maximal number of conductance levels remains constant, indicating that N_T is unchanged, as previously reported (Brum et al., 1984). As the individual records indicate, nulls sweeps are relatively common in the control run and rare after β-stimulation.

The importance of changes in channel availability is further illustrated in Figure 11.10, which presents results from a patch where the peak of the averaged inward current record increased about fivefold (A and B). To show temporal variations in channel availability, we plot the open state probability for individual sweeps as a function of time during 10-minute runs (C and D). The probability values for individual sweeps also contribute to the histograms in panels E and F. There is a dramatic difference between the behavior in the absence of drug (C and E) and in the presence of β-adrenergic agonist (D and F). Isoproterenol largely eliminates nulls, raising the proportion of nonblank sweeps from $41/176 = 24\%$ to $204/215 = 95\%$. After exposure to the drug, the nonblank sweeps tend to have a slightly higher value of p_0. However, changes in the channel availability are clearly the dominant factor in the overall increase in activity.

Experiments like those shown in Figures 11.9 and 11.10 explain the results obtained with fluctuation analysis. The cell-attached patch recordings indicate that individual channels tend to remain unavailable for several consecutive sweeps. During a prolonged dormant period, there is no difference between consecutive single channel traces other than background noise; the channel would therefore be counted as nonfunctional in fluctuation analysis of pairwise difference currents (see Figures 11.7 and 11.8). As Bean et al. (1984) point out, their choice of pairwise analysis is important in the distinction between changes in N_f and in p_0, the key being the length of the analysis period in relation to the average period that the channel is unavailable. Sigworth (1980b) made the same point when he described tetrodotoxin and saxitoxin block of sodium currents at the node of Ranvier in terms of a decrease in the number of available channels. In the case of fluctuation analysis of β-adrenergic modulation, the operational definition of N_f is consistent with the definition used by Reuter and Scholz (1977) and the RSSS hypothesis of a slow exchange between functional and nonfunctional channels (see also Niedergerke & Page, 1977).

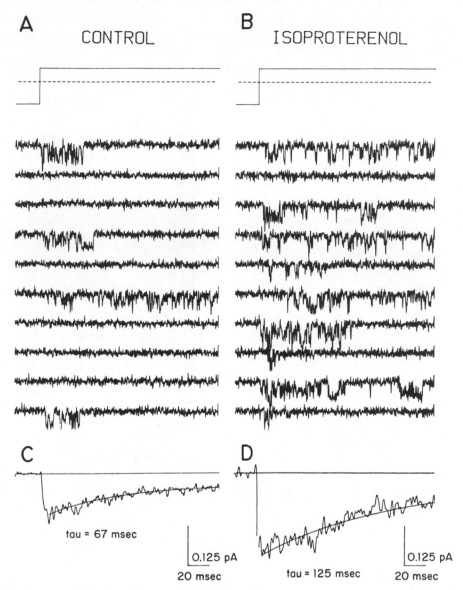

Fig. 11.9. Effect of β-adrenergic stimulation on unitary calcium channel activity. Cell-attached patch containing two calcium channels as judged from the appearance of two nonzero conductance levels. (A and B) Representative groups of consecutive current records in the absence of drug (A) and in the presence of 14-μM isoproterenol (B). The voltage clamp protocol is shown above the current records. (C and D) Averaged current records from corresponding runs (cell B08E).

221

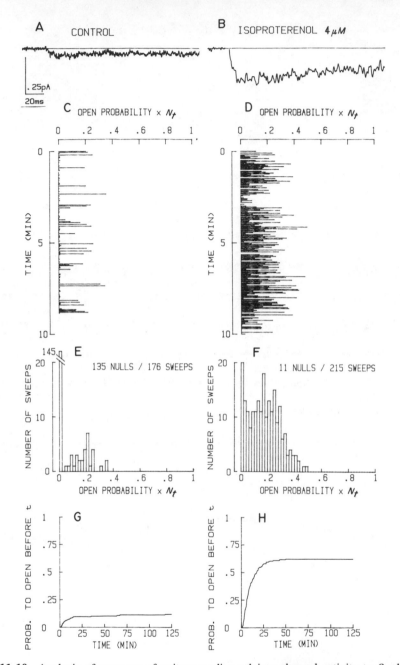

Fig. 11.10. Analysis of response of unitary cardiac calcium channel activity to β-adrenergic stimulation. The cell-attached patch contains two channels. (A and B) Averaged current records without drug (A) and after the cell was exposed to 4-μM isoproterenol (B); voltage clamp pulse (not shown) from -60 mV to $+20$ mV. (C and D) The p values for individual sweeps plotted against time, in the absence and presence of isoproterenol. (E and F) Histograms of p values. (G and H) Cumulative distributions of the latency to first opening. The distribution saturates at levels corresponding to the chances of the channel being available (i.e., not being in mode 0). Correction has been made for the presence of two channels in the patch. As a result, the saturating probability of opening is $1\sqrt{(135/176)} = 0.124$ in G, and $1\sqrt{(11/215)} = 0.774$ in H (cell B14E).

MODULATION OF CALCIUM CHANNELS IN INVERTEBRATE NEURONS

The large size of certain molluscan neurons and the relatively extensive knowledge about their synaptic interactions has led many investigators to look for possible neuromodulation of calcium channels in these cells. In this section, we review specific cases in which calcium channel currents may be under direct modulatory control. One theme that runs through both this section and the next is the idea that modulation of calcium channels may be important in controlling transmitter release from synaptic terminals.

Presynaptic Inhibition in the *Aplysia* Abdominal Ganglion

Figure 11.11 shows presynaptic interactions in a system of neurons in the *Aplysia* abdominal ganglion that has been investigated by Shapiro, Kandel, and associates (Shapiro et al., 1980; Kretz et al., 1984). This system has the great advantage that the L32 interneurons that cause the presynaptic inhibition have been identified and are large enough to allow intracellular recording (Byrne, 1980). As Figure 11.11 illustrates, the monosynaptic excitatory connection between the presynaptic cell (L10) and the follower cell (RB) is depressed by stimulation of the L32 cells or the pleuroabdominal connective that drives the L32 cells. The presynaptic inhibitory effect of L32 activity occurs without any conductance change in the postsynaptic follower cells. The presynaptic effect on L10 has two components: (1) a hyperpolarization of L10, seen as an increase in outward current when L10 is voltage-clamped at the resting potential and attributed to activation of potassium channels; (2) a decrease in the inward current activated by depolarization, attributed to a down-modulation of calcium channel activity. (This change in calcium current is somewhat attenuated in Figure 11.11B because of the presence of calcium-activated potassium current.) The second factor is important because eliminating the hyperpolarization with the voltage clamp fails to abolish the presynaptic inhibition.

Histamine is the putative presynaptic inhibitory transmitter. Effects of L32 stimulation are mimicked by bath application of histamine (but not other candidate transmitters); the histamine antagonist cimetidine blocks effects of L32 on L10, just as it blocks the response to histamine (Kretz et al., 1984). Bath application of histamine reduces voltage-dependent barium influx through calcium channels without shifting the apparent voltage-dependence of calcium channel activation (Figure 11.11D).

Up-Modulation of Calcium Currents by Serotonin

Increases in calcium current in *Aplysia* neurons have been described by Pellmar and Carpenter (1980; see Pellmar, 1981, for review). In LB and LC cells of the abdominal ganglion, iontophoretic application of serotonin evokes a slowly developing and decaying inward current with striking voltage dependence (Figure 11.12). In subsequent work, Pellmar (1981) showed that similar voltage-dependent responses could also be evoked by iontophoretic application of dopamine and octapamine. The evidence suggests that calcium channels are involved. In all cases, the transmitter-induced inward current component is not seen at potentials negative to -30 or 40 mV;

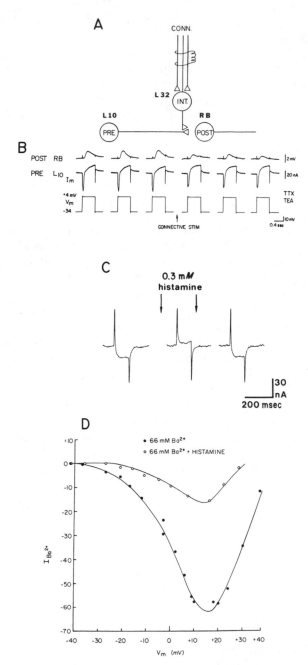

Fig. 11.11. Presynaptic inhibition in *Aplysia*. (A) Neural elements; (B) connective stimulation decreases inward calcium current in cell L10 and the postsynaptic potential in cell RB. Currents recorded with calcium as the charge carrier and TTX and TEA to reduce sodium and potassium currents (from Shapiro et al., (1980). (C) Inward barium currents in cell L10, before, during, and after exposure of the cell to 0.3-m*M* histamine; (D) voltage dependence of barium current in the absence and presence of histamine (from Kretz et al., 1984)

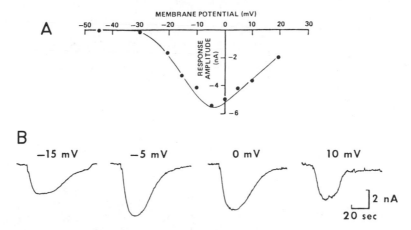

Fig. 11.12. Enhancement of calcium current in LB neurons of *Aplysia* produced by ionto-phoretic application of serotonin. (A) Current changes measured with steady holding potentials as indicated; (B) magnitude of current changes plotted against holding potential (from Pellmar 1981).

its amplitude reaches a maximum near 0 mV and becomes progressively smaller with further depolarization. The inward current is largely insensitive to manipulations of most external ions, including chloride replacement by acetate, elevated potassium, and sodium substitution by glucosamine. The response is strongly diminished in amplitude by conventional calcium channel blockers such as cobalt, cadmium, or manganese ions; it is not appreciably reduced by application of calcium-poor solutions, but Pellmar and Carpenter (1980) argued that this may reflect imperfect exchange of extracellular solutions or the channel's intrinsic affinity for calcium ions. Thus, their overall conclusion was that the serotonin-induced, regeneratively voltage-dependent current was carried by calcium ions.

Superficially similar responses to serotonin and dopamine appear in *Helix* neurons and have been attributed to a decrease in a calcium- and voltage-dependent potassium current rather than an induction of a voltage-dependent calcium current (Paupardin-Tritsch et al., 1981; Deterre et al., 1981). Measurements of intracellular calcium transients in voltage-clamped neurons of *Aplysia* and *Helix* suggest genuine differences between species (Boyle, 1983; Boyle et al., 1984).

Up-Modulation of Bag Cell Neuron Calcium Currents by Phorbol Ester

Another example of a direct enhancement of neuronal calcium channel activity comes from studies of *Aplysia* bag cell neurons (see Chapter 7). When stimulated by brief electrical stimulation or exposure to peptides from the reproductive tract, this group of neurons undergoes a stereotyped sequence of changes in electrical properties, starting with the generation of a half-hour afterdischarge. The associated release of egg-laying hormone and other neuroactive peptides leads to a complicated set of behav-

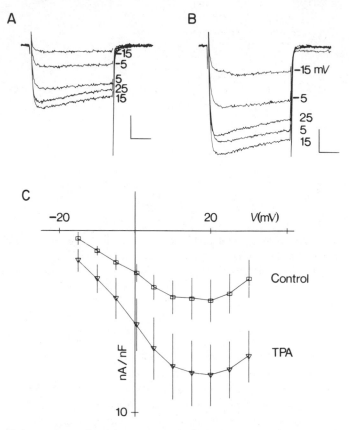

Fig. 11.13. Enhancement of calcium current in *Aplysia* bag cell neurons by stimulation of kinase C. (A) Inward currents evoked by depolarizing pulses to levels indicated in a cell pretreated with the inactive phorbol ester 4-α-phorbol; (B) inward currents in a cell pretreated with the active phorbol ester, TPA; (C) voltage dependence of calcium current in collected results from seven cells as in A, and seven paired cells as in B (from DeRiemer et al., 1985).

iors culminating in the laying of eggs. Because many lines of evidence suggest that calcium ions and cyclic AMP play important roles in shaping the bag cell activity, attention has been focused on the possible involvement of the enzyme targets of these messengers. The known effects of cyclic AMP-dependent protein kinase involve various types of potassium channels rather than calcium channels per se (Chapter 7). On the other hand, calcium channel activity is modulated by protein kinase C.

Evidence for the involvement of protein kinase C comes from experiments of DeRiemer et al. (1985). Bag cell action potentials are increased in height by exposure to the phorbol ester 12-0-tetradecanoyl-phorbol-13-acetate (TPA), a known stimulated of C kinase, but not by 4-α-phorbol, an inactive analog. Direct intracellular injection of protein kinase C increases action potential height in much the same way. The ionic basis for these effects was studied with voltage clamp experiments comparing TPA-pretreated cells with control cells, under ionic conditions where potas-

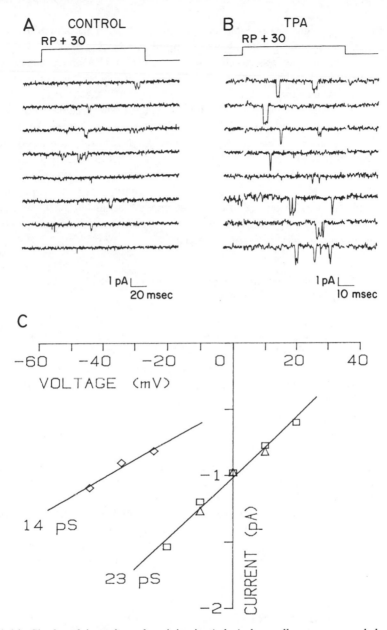

Fig. 11.14. Single calcium channel activity in *Aplysia* bag cell neurons recorded with cell-attained patch pipettes containing 330-m*M* barium. (A) Small-amplitude openings (14-pS slope conductance) in a 4-α-phorbol pretreated cell; (B) small-amplitude and large-amplitude openings (23-pS) in a TPA-pretreated cell; (C) unitary current-voltage relations for small and large conductance channels (from Strong et al., 1986).

227

sium channel or calcium channel currents could be studied in isolation. Outward currents through potassium channels were essentially unaffected by TPA. In contrast, the calcium channel current was roughly twice as large in TPA-pretreated cells as in controls (Figure 11.13). There was no obvious change in the voltage or time dependence of the inward calcium current.

An obvious question is whether the enhancement of I_{Ca} results from increased activity of the normal population of calcium channels or recruitment of additional channels. This was investigated with cell-attached patch recordings from control and TPA-pretreated cells (Strong et al., 1986). Figure 11.14 illustrates recordings made with 330-mM barium as the charge carrier. In control cells, the predominant form of calcium channel activity appears as relatively small unitary currents (open channel conductance 14 pS). In TPA-pretreated cells, openings of the small conductance channel are seen in combination with activity of a larger conductance calcium channel (23 pS) that was essentially absent in control cells.

Stimulation of Calcium Current in *Helix* Neurons by Extracellular ATP

The calcium current in certain *Helix* neurons can be increased by about 30% with extracellular application of ATP or its nonhydrolyzable analog AMP-PNP (Yatani et al., 1982). The $K_{0.5}$ for ATP is 1 μM; the $K_{0.5}$ for AMP-PNP is 3 nM. Neither compound is effective when applied intracellularly at comparable concentrations. Putative antagonists for purinergic receptors such as apamin, quinidine, or propranolol failed to interfere with the response to external ATP. Thus, the receptor mechanism of the nucleotide effect is unknown.

MODULATION OF CALCIUM CHANNELS IN VERTEBRATE NEURONS

Calcium channels in vertebrate neurons can be modulated by a wide variety of neurotransmitter substances, including enkephalin, norepinephrine (NE), GABA, serotonin (5-HT), dopamine, and somatostatin (see Table 11.1). There is much interest in the possibility that neuromodulation of presynaptic calcium channels is a mechanism for presynaptic inhibition (see Dunlap, 1981).

Presynaptic Inhibition: Control of Pain Transmission?

Melzack and Wall (1965) proposed that presynaptic inhibition is a major factor in the flow of information in pain pathways in the spinal cord. In their "gate control theory" (Figure 11.15A) they tried to explain how transmission of nociceptive signals from C-fiber afferent terminals to output neurons might be modulated by descending inputs and incoming information from pathways for touch. They postulated that substantia gelatinosa interneurons produced presynaptic inhibition of primary afferent terminals.

Experimental approaches to the mechanism of pain transmission have increased

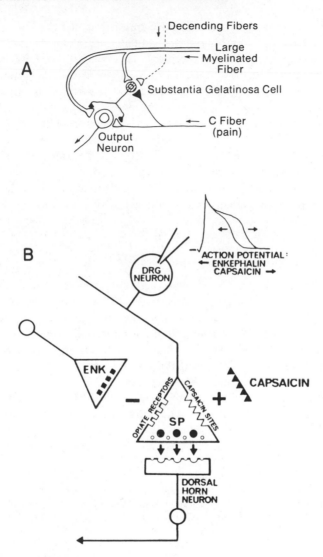

Fig. 11.15. (A) Simplified diagram illustrating the gate-control theory of Melzack and Wall (1965) (from Shepherd, 1983). The postulated excitatory terminals are shown as open profiles and inhibitory as shaded profiles. (B) Diagrammatic representation of the possible interactions of enkephalin and other opiates with substance P-containing terminals of primary sensory neurons in the dorsal horn of the spinal cord (from Jessell, 1982).

with growing interest in substance P as a putative pain transmitter, and the development of antibody methods for assaying substance P release. The release of substance P in spinal cord or trigeminal nucleus can be inhibited by opiate analgesics such as morphine or enkephalinlike peptides (Jessell & Iversen, 1977; Yaksh et al., 1980). These results led Jessell and Iversen (1977) to propose a specific neuronal basis for the general gating mechanism of Melzack and Wall. This scheme (see Figure 11.15B) postulates that substance P is the excitatory transmitter at the synapse between C-fiber primary afferent and dorsal horn cells and that release of substance P is inhibited by enkephalin acting on presynaptic receptors. This type of hypothesis is easily modified to take account of descending inputs from the locus coeruleus (norepinephrine) and nucleus raphe magnus (5-HT), which are also capable of modifying the transmission of sensory information in the spinal cord (Basbaum et al., 1976; Segal & Sandberg, 1977), possibly at a presynaptic site of action (Headley et al., 1978). The serotonergic input from the raphe may have a detectable anatomical substrate in the form of presynaptic axo-axonic contacts (LaMotte & de Lanerolle, 1980). On the other hand, there is no good evidence for enkephalin-containing terminals presynaptic to other synaptic terminals (Hunt et al., 1979; LaMotte & de Lanerolle, 1980). This leaves room for the idea that enkephalin may act at sites somewhat distant from the point of release.

Opiate-Induced Depression of Synaptic Transmission

Clear-cut effects of opiates have been observed on transmitter release at a number of synapses. Figure 11.16 illustrates recordings in cell culture from a synapse between a dorsal root ganglion (DRG) cell and a spinal cord cell (Macdonald & Nelson, 1978). Stimulation of the DRG neuron with an intracellular current pulse evoked an action potential (A-DRG) that was followed with appropriate latency by a 10 to 12-mV excitatory postsynaptic potential (EPSP) in the spinal cord cell. Application of the opiate etorphine produced clear attenuation of the EPSP amplitude (A–E and B–E). The etorphine effect was almost completely reversed by the presence of the opiate antagonist naloxone (panel B, E + N). The individual traces in B–E show an important feature of the etorphine effect: relatively large variations in the size of the epsp. This is as expected if the number of transmitter quanta is decreased. Indeed, quanti-

Fig. 11.16. Etorphine antagonizes synaptic transmission from DRG neuron to spinal cord neuroin in cell culture by reducing the quantal content (from Macdonald & Nelson, 1978).

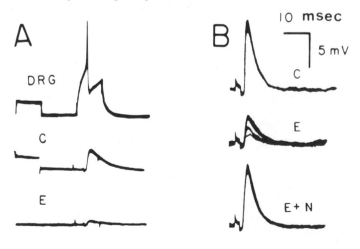

tative analysis of such experiments showed a substantial reduction in the average number of quanta without any significant change in the amplitude of the quantal event. From these results, Macdonald and Nelson concluded that the primary action of the opiate was presynaptic.

In related experiments, naloxone-blocked presynaptic inhibitory effects have been observed in cholinergic synapses in sympathetic ganglia (Konishi et al., 1981) and at the frog neuromuscular junction (Bixby & Spitzer, 1983). The inhibition was produced by application of an enkephalin analog at the neuromuscular junction and by repetitive stimulation of preganglionic nerves to the sympathetic ganglia. In both cases, quantal content was strongly reduced. Additional support for a presynaptic site of opiate action was provided by ruling out changes in postjunctional sensitivity by direct iontophoresis of the transmitter acetylcholine.

Enkephalin Depresses Substance P Release and Calcium Action Potentials

What is the basis for the presynaptic inhibition? An important step forward was provided by experiments by Mudge, Leeman, and Fischbach (1979) in cell cultures containing sensory neurons from chick DRG, free of other cell types. They demonstrated a potassium-evoked, cobalt-blocked release of substance P, consistent with a release of transmitter mediated by activation of voltage-sensitive calcium channels. The evoked release was largely inhibited by exposure to the enkephalin analog D-ala2-enkephalin amide (DAEA), and this inhibition was reversed by naloxone. Mudge et al. went on to study the electrophysiological effects of DAEA and enkephalin on calcium-dependent action potentials recorded from DRG cell bodies (Figure 11.17). They found a reversible reduction in the duration of the calcium spike with enkephalin (A) as well as with DAEA; both responses were blocked by naloxone (B). The opiate effect was heightened in the presence of barium ions, an experimental condition in which repolarizing potassium currents are largely inhibited; it remained clear when fast sodium currents were blocked by tetrodotoxin. Mudge et al. also found similar effects with somatostatin, but not with bradykinin, neurotensin, thyrotropin-releasing factor, or substance P itself.

Working in the same laboratory as Mudge et al., Dunlap and Fischbach (1978) had previously reported effects of other agents in the same system: serotonin, GABA, and norepinephrine abbreviate the action potential in DRG soma in much the same way as is found for the opiates (Figure 11.17C–F). In all of these cases, the agents altered calcium spikes without significantly altering the resting membrane potential and membrane resistance.

The most obvious interpretation of these results is that neurotransmitters decrease transmitter release and calcium spikes by a direct action on calcium channels. The main reservations about this conclusion are the following:

1. Changes in calcium spikes could come about through modulation of outward currents through potassium channels, electrically in parallel with calcium channels. This mechanism is known to operate in *Aplysia* bag cell neurons (see Chapter 7) and sensory neurons (see Chapter 10). Similar phenomena

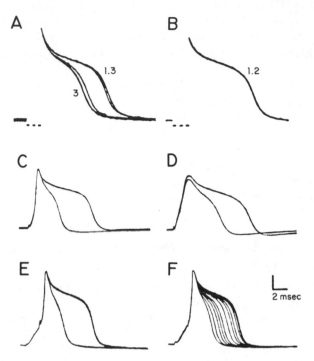

Fig. 11.17. Abbreviation of calcium-dependent action potentials in chick DRG neurons by various neurochemicals. (A) Records taken before (1), during (2), and after (3) puffer application of $0.1\text{-}\mu M$ enkephalin; (B) sweeps recorded before and during enkephalin application in the presence of $1\text{-}\mu M$ naloxone (from Mudge et al., 1979); (C–E) similar action potential shortening with application of $10\text{-}\mu M$ 5-HT, $100\text{-}\mu M$ GABA, or $100\text{-}\mu M$ norepinephrine; (F) slow recovery from norepinephrine-induced action potential shortening shown with records taken every 10 sec (C–F from Dunlap & Fischbach, 1978).

are to be expected in vertebrate neurons since neurochemical modulation of potassium channels is commonplace (see Chapters 6, 7, 8, and 9).

2. The interpretation of the electrical recordings depends on the assumption that electrophysiological responses in the cell body are representative of those at the nerve terminal. This assumption is plausible and widely precedented (see Chapter 10) but unproven.

Evidence for Direct Modulation of Neuronal Calcium Channels

In any given instance, several approaches can be taken to test whether or not enhanced potassium channel activity accounts for the inhibition of calcium spikes. To begin with, most investigators try to minimize the confounding effect of other types of ion channel with pharmacological blockers such as TEA and TTX. Possible changes in the activity of calcium-activated potassium current ($I_{K(Ca)}$) may be assessed by

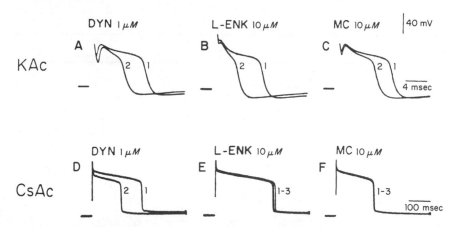

Fig. 11.18. Action potentials in a mouse DRG neuron recorded before (1) and during (2) application of various opioid peptides with different selectivities. The columns show responses to dynorphin (kappa-receptors), leu-enkephalin (delta-receptors), and morphiceptin (mu-receptors). In this particular cell, all three agents shorten the calcium-dependent plateau when recordings are made with a potassium-containing pipette. Cesium injection abolishes abbreviation of calcium plateau by leu-enkephalin and morphiceptin but not by dynorphin (from Werz & Macdonald, 1984).

monitoring the amplitude of afterhyperpolarizations indicative of $I_{K(Ca)}$. This approach is exemplified in a study by McAfee et al. (1981) of norepinephrine inhibition of calcium spikes in sympathetic ganglion cells.

Werz and Macdonald (1984) have used intracellular cesium injection as a means of minimizing potassium channel currents and dissecting possible contributions of calcium channel modulation. Figure 11.18A–C shows recordings from a neuron that exhibited clear-cut abbreviation of calcium-dependent action potentials with exposure to dynorphin, leucine-enkephalin (L-ENK) and morphiceptin (MC). Following reimpalement of the same neuron with a cesium-filled recording electrode and intracellular iontophoresis of cesium ions, the dynorphin effect remains, but the response to leucine-enkephalin and morphiceptin are completely abolished. The most reasonable interpretation is that dynorphin directly modulates calcium channels, while L-ENK and MC act indirectly, through enhancement of potassium channels.

Voltage clamp studies represent a third approach. The most extensive analysis has been aimed at analyzing modulation by norepinephrine (chick DRG neurons: Dunlap & Fischbach, 1981; rat sympathetic neurons: Galvan & Adams, 1982). Calcium currents were recorded in the presence of TTX to block sodium channels and TEA to inhibit potassium currents (Figure 11.19). The voltage clamp provides two arguments in favor of a direct modulation of calcium channels. First, the effects of norepinephrine on peak current shows similar voltage dependence to that expected and found for the putative calcium current (B). Second, as illustrated in Figure 11.19C, norepinephrine strongly reduces inward tail currents measured with step hyperpolarization to E_K (where currents through potassium channels should be minimal).

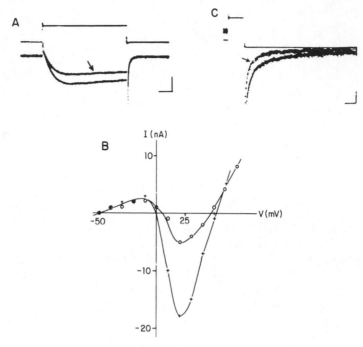

Fig. 11.19 Voltage clamp analysis of norepinephine of calcium current in chick DRG neurons. (A) Membrane current recorded from a cell bathed in 10-mM calcium solution with TTX plus TEA. The arrow marks the trace taken after application of 100-μM norepinephrine (B) I-V relations under similar ionic conditions, in control (+) and after norepinephine administration (o) (from Dunlap, 1981). (C) The calcium current "tail" evoked by repolarization to -70 mV (E_K) is reduced by norepinephrine (from Dunlap & Fischbach, 1981).

Assignment of Modulatory Responses to Different Calcium Channel Types

Most of the experimental information about calcium channel modulation in vertebrate neurons was obtained before investigators were fully aware of the coexistence of multiple types of calcium channels. The first indications that this might be the case came from studies of cerebellar and olivary neurons (Llinas & Sugimori, 1980; Llinas & Yarom, 1981) and neuroblastoma cells (Fishman & Spector, 1980); the existence of multiple components of calcium currents has been a general finding in a number of preparations. The most extensive studies have been carried out with conventional dorsal root ganglion cells (e.g., Carbone & Lux, 1984; Fedulova et al., 1985; Bossu et al., 1985; Nowycky et al., 1985b). Single channel recordings from the cell body of chick DRG neurons distinguish between three types of calcium channel with different single channel conductance, kinetics, and pharmacology (Nowycky et al., 1985b). Some key properties of the three channel types are summarized in Table 11.2. The main distinguishing features are (1) voltage dependence of activation, (2) voltage and time-dependence of inactivation, (3) sensitivity to inorganic

Table 11.2. Properties of three types of calcium channels in chick DRG neurons

Properties	T	N	L
Activation range (10 calcium)	Positive to -70 mV	Positive to -10 mV(?)	Positive to -10 mV
Inactivation range	-100 to -60 mV	> -100 to -40 mV	-60 to -10 mV
Relaxation rate (0 mV, 10 calcium or 10 barium)	Moderate (tau $\sim$20–50 msec)	Moderate (tau $\sim$20–50 msec)	Very slow (tau $>$ 500 msec)
Single channel conductance	8–10 pS	11–15 pS	23–27 pS
Single channel kinetics	Late opening, brief burst, inactivation	Long burst, inactivation	Hardly any inactivation
Cadmium block	Resistant	Sensitive	Sensitive
Cobalt block	Sensitive	Less sensitive	Less sensitive
w-CGTX block	Weak, reversible	Persistent	Persistent
Dihydropyridine sensitivity	No	No	Yes

Source: Fox et al., 1986.

calcium channel blockers (e.g., cadmium ions), (4) responsiveness to organic agents, particularly dihydropyridine (DHP) compounds, and (5) sensitivity to peptide toxins.

Knowledge of the coexistence of three types of calcium channels is only recent, so it is not surprising that little systematic study of how the three types of channels respond to various modulators has been done. For example, in their important study of norepinephrine action in DRG neurons, Dunlap and Fischbach (1981) used a holding potential of -50 mV, a voltage protocol that would be expected to evoke L currents but not N or T currents. In more recent studies of modulatory effects on I_{Ca} in neuroblastoma cells, Tsunoo et al. (1984, 1985) have used voltage protocols that distinguish between long-lasting (L-type) calcium currents and transient calcium currents (type I in their classification, probably T-type). They have found that the long-lasting calcium current is increased by exogenous cyclic AMP and decreased by leucine-enkephalin or somatostatin at doses that leave the transient current unchanged. The peptide effects are generally consistent with the idea that L-type calcium channels help trigger transmitter release and are targets for presynaptic effects of opioid peptides. The effects of cyclic AMP run parallel to effects seen with L-type calcium channels in heart.

Studies of the Mechanism of Norepinephrine or Dopamine Modulation

Recent experiments have focused on the several related questions about the mechanisms of calcium channel regulation by amines: (1) the nature of the amine receptor(s), (2) the possible involvement of intracellular or intramembrane messengers, and (3) the basis for the modulation at the level of single calcium channels.

Nature of Amine Receptor

There is general agreement that norepinephrine inhibition of neuronal calcium channels is mediated by α-adrenergic receptors, not by β-receptors. Whether the receptor
is either the classically defined alpha$_1$ or alpha$_2$ receptor or neither is presently under
investigation (see McAfee et al., 1981; Canfield & Dunlap, 1984).

Mediation by Diacylglycerol Stimulation of Protein Kinase C

Recent work has explored the possible involvement of putative second messengers
such as calcium ions, cyclic AMP, cyclic GMP, and metabolites of phosphatidyl
inositol. Inhibition of calcium current in DRG neurons is not affected by strongly
buffering internal calcium or by introducing millimolar concentrations of cyclic AMP
or cyclic GMP by means of the internal solution in a suction pipette (Forscher &
Oxford, 1985). On the other hand, Rane and Dunlap (1985) find that the norepinephrine response is mimicked by exposing DRG neurons to 1,2-oleoyl acetyl glycerol
(OAG), a membrane-permeant analog of diacylglycerol, the natural stimulator of
protein kinase C; the effects of norepinephrine and OAG on calcium current are
mutually occlusive. Since the response of calcium spikes to norepinephrine, dopamine, and serotonin are also nonadditive (Canfield & Dunlap, 1984), it appears likely
that the final pathway for all of these amines is stimulation of protein kinase C.

Modulation by Dihydropyridine Agonists and Antagonists

Calcium channels in a wide variety of excitable cells can be inhibited by dihydropyridine (DHP) calcium antagonists such as nifedipine or enhanced by closely related
DHP calcium agonists such as Bay K 8644 (Figure 11.20 A and B). These drugs
may be thought of as honorary neuromodulators, presumed mimics of as yet undis-
covered endogenous substances that regulate calcium channels (see Schramm et al.,
1983). Their action on calcium channels involves shifts between different modes of
gating and is of general interest as a mechanism of channel modulation (see Hess et
al., 1984; Fox et al., 1986).

   Figure 11.20 illustrates cell-attached patch recordings of unitary calcium channel
current from a chick DRG neuron (Nowycky et al., 1985). Depolarizing pulses are
applied every 4 sec to evoke calcium channel activity. With 110-mM barium in the
patch pipette, open events are seen as downward pulses of current, ~1 pA in amplitude. In control recordings (A), the sweeps are dominated by two patterns of activity:
(1) sweeps with no detectable openings, in which the channel appears to be unavailable; (2) sweeps with brief openings, of the order of 1 msec in duration. Every so
often, as in the first sweep in panel A, a channel shows a series of much longer
openings. These three patterns of activity have been referred to as mode 0 (null
mode), mode 1, and mode 2 (Hess et al., 1984). They have been studied in patches
containing only one calcium channel in heart cells and smooth muscle cells (Fox et
al., 1986), although in neurons it is much more common to find several channels in
the same patch, as illustrated here. A given channel will often stay in a particular
mode of gating for a period extending over several stimulus intervals, during which
time the channel may open hundreds or thousands of times. It is as if a set of dice
were occasionally loaded and unloaded during a long series of throws.

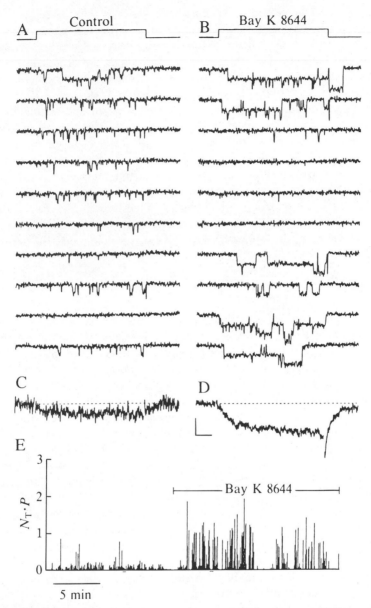

Fig. 11.20. Effect of Bay K 8644 on L-type Ca channel activity. Cell-attached patch recording from a chick DRG neuron with 110 mM Ba as the external charge carrier in the recording pipette. Patch contains three functional Ca channels. (A and B) Sets of consecutive sweeps before and after application of 5 μM Bay K 8644 to the external solution bathing the cell. Small horizontal bars in E indicate when sweeps were taken. "Mode 2" activity is apparent in first current record in A and in sweeps 1, 2, 7, 8, 9 & 10 in B. C, D, averaged currents obtained from sweeps in control run and sweeps taken after drug application. Horizontal scale bar indicates 20 ms; vertical scale bar indicates 2 pA in A & B and 0.2 pA in C and D. E, plot of channel openness on a sweep by sweep basis. From Nowycky et al. (1985a).

Panel B shows the pattern of calcium channel gating after the cell is exposed to the calcium agonist Bay K 8644. This compound acts quickly, within seconds, presumably because it reaches calcium channels under the patch pipette by rapid diffusion within the plane of the lipid bilayer. A large increase occurs in the average calcium channel current (compare C and D); this comes about because individual channels spend an increased proportion of their time in mode 2.

It remains to be seen whether or not investigators will find naturally occurring compounds whose action resembles that of Bay K 8644. The main point here is that the gating properties of calcium channels are intrinsically complex and contain the potential for multiple mechanisms of up- or down-modulation. In this context, it is important to emphasize that the mechanism of calcium channel modulation by Bay K 8644 and other DHP calcium agonists is significantly different from the action of cyclic AMP-dependent protein phosphorylation in the heart, which can be described primarily as a shift of cardiac calcium channels from mode 0 to mode 1, and secondarily as an alteration of the rapid millisecond kinetics within mode 1.

CONCLUSIONS

In surveying systems in which calcium channel modulation has been studied, the most obvious characteristic is diversity. Many neurochemicals, and a multiplicity of messengers, influence calcium channel activity. The direction of the modulatory effect varies from one cell type to another. For example, in heart, epinephrine and norepinephrine act in large part through β-receptors and cyclic AMP, while in sensory neurons these catecholamines act through α-receptors and, possibly, diacylglycerol. Cyclic AMP increases I_{Ca} in heart but produces no clear modulatory effect on I_{Ca} in most neurons other than prolonged survival in whole cell recordings. Protein kinase C stimulation increases I_{Ca} in *Aplysia* bag cell neurons but decreases I_{Ca} in DRG cells. One can almost imagine a kind of menu for evolutionary mixing and matching, with transmitters in column A, messengers in column B, and modulatory mechanisms in column C.

Future studies of calcium channel modulation have the rather obvious agenda of working out the relationships between natural transmitters, messengers, and channel mechanisms in individual cases. In a system like the bag cell neurons of *Aplysia,* it seems very likely that calcium channel modulation involves diacylglycerol as an internal messenger, but the identity of the natural transmitter that stimulates diacylglycerol production is not known. On the other hand, there are many cases in which the transmitter *is* known but the messenger system and single channel mechanisms remain uncharacterized. This is the case for opioid peptides acting in vertebrate neurons; the same may be said about the actions of angiotensin II and α-agonists in heart. One very productive area of research may be the study of final common pathways for actions of multiple transmitter substances. A prime example of such convergence comes from studies of cardiac calcium channel modulation by β-agonists and muscarinic agents, which up- or down-modulate I_{Ca} by raising or lowering intracellular cyclic AMP (Kameyama et al., 1986).

The existence of multiple calcium channel types makes analysis of calcium channel modulation more difficult but more interesting. Much of the earlier evidence will need to be reevaluated or extended. Inferences about modulation of calcium channels at nerve terminals based on extrapolations from recordings at cell bodies must be viewed with increased caution, given the possibility that the soma and nerve terminals express different calcium channels (e.g., Llinas & Sugimori, 1980). On the other hand, the existence of different calcium channel types greatly increases the functional capabilities of the cell and the potential richness of modulatory phenomena.

REFERENCES

Basbaum A.I., Clanton, D.H., and Fields, H.L. (1976) Opiate and stimulus-produced analgesia: functional anatomy of a medullo-spinal pathway. *Proc. Natl. Acad. Sci. USA 73*, 4685–4688.

Bean, B.P. (1985) Two types of calcium channel in canine atrial cells. Differences in kinetics, selectivity and pharmacology. *J. Gen. Physiol. 86*, 1–30.

Bean, B.P., Nowycky, M.C., and Tsien, R.W. (1984) β-Adrenergic modulation of calcium channels in frog ventricular heart cells. *Nature 307*, 371–375.

Bixby, J.L. and Spitzer, N.C. (1983) Enkephalin reduces calcium action potentials in Rohon-Beard neurons in vivo. *J. Neurosci. 3*, 1014–1018.

Bolton, T.B. (1979) Mechanisms of action of transmitters and other substances on smooth muscle. *Physiol. Revs. 59*, 606–718.

Bossu, J.L., Feltz, A., and Thomann, J.M. (1985) Depolarization elicits two distinct calcium currents in vertebrate sensory neurones. *Pflugers Arch., 403*, 360–368.

Boyle, M.B. (1983) Long-lasting changes induced by serotonin in intracellular free calcium and calcium-activated outward current in molluscan neurons. Doctoral Thesis, Yale University, New Haven, CT.

Boyle, M.B., Klein, M., Smith, S.J., and Kandel, E.R. (1984) Serotonin increases intracellular Ca^{2+} transients in voltage-clamped sensory neurons of *Aplysia californica*. *Proc. Natl. Acad. Sci. USA 81*, 7642–7646.

Brum, G., Osterrieder, W., and Trautwein, W. (1984) β-adrenergic increase in the calcium conductance of cardiac myocytes studied with the patch clamp. *Pflugers Arch. 401*, 111–118.

Byrne, J. (1980) Identification of neurons contributing to presynaptic inhibition in *Aplysia californica*. *Brain Res. 199*, 235–239.

Cachelin, A.B., dePeyer, J.E., Kokubun, S., and Reuter, H. (1983) Ca^{2+} channel modulation by 8-bromocyclic AMP in cultured heart cells. *Nature 304*, 462–464.

Canfield, D.R. and Dunlap, K. (1984) Pharmacological characterization of amine receptors on embryonic chick sensory neurones. *Br. J. Pharmacol. 82*, 557–563.

Carbone, E. and Lux, H.D. (1984) A low voltage-activated fully inactivating Ca channel in vertebrate sensory neurones. *Nature 310*, 501–502.

DeRiemer, S.A., Strong, J.A., Albert, K.A., Greengard, P., and Kaczmarek, L.K. (1985) Enhancement of calcium current in *Aplysia* neurones by phorbol ester and protein kinase C. *Nature 313*, 313–316.

Deterre, P., Paupardin-Tritsch, D., Boackaert, J., and Gerschenfeld, H.M. (1981) Role of cyclic AMP in a serotonin-evoked slow inward current in snail neurons. *Nature 290*, 783–785.

Dunlap, K. (1981) Neurotransmitter modulation of voltage-dependent channels: Possible mechanism for presynaptic inhibition? In *The Mechanism of Gated Calcium Transport Across Biological Membranes* (eds. S.T. Ohnishi and M. Endo), pp. 87–97. Academic Press, New York.

Dunlap, K. and Fischbach, G.D. (1978) Neurotransmitters decrease the Ca component of sensory neurone action potentials. *Nature 276*, 837–838.

Dunlap, K. and Fischbach, G.D. (1981) Neurotransmitters decrease the Ca conductance activated by depolarization of embryonic chick sensory neurones. *J. Physiol. 267*, 281–298.

Fedulova, S.A., Kostyuk, P.K., and Veselovsky, N.S. (1985) Two types of calcium channels in the somatic membrane of new-born rat dorsal root ganglion neurones. *J. Physiol. 359*, 431–446.

Fishman, M.C. and Spector, I. (1981) Potassium current suppression by quinidine reveals additional calcium currents in neuroblastoma cells. *Proc. Natl. Acad. Sci. USA 78*, 5245–5249.

Forscher, P. and Oxford, G.S. (1985) Modulation of calcium channels by norepinephrine in internally dialyzed avian sensory neurons. *J. Gen. Physiol. 85*, 743–763.

Fox, A.P., Nowycky, M.C., and Tsien, R. W. (1986). Single channel properties of three types of Ca channel in chick sensory neurons, in preparation.

Galvan, M. and Adams, P.R. (1982) Control of calcium current in rat sympathetic neurones by noradrenaline. *Brain Res. 244*, 135–144.

Giles, W. and Tsien, R. W. (1975). Effects of acetylcholine on membrane currents in frog atrial muscle. *J. Physiol. 246*, 64–66.

Headley, P.M., Duggan, A.W., and Griersmith, B.T. (1978) Selective reduction by noradrenaline and 5-hydroxytryptamine of nociceptive responses of cat dorsal horn neurones. *Brain Res. 145*, 185–189.

Hess, P., Lansman, J.B., and Tsien, R.W. (1984) Different modes of Ca channel gating behavior favored by dihydropyridine Ca agonists and antagonists. *Nature 311*, 538–544.

Hille, B. (1984) *Ionic Channels of Excitable Membranes*. Sinauer Assoc., Sunderland, MA.

Holz, G.G., Kream, R.M., and Dunlap, K. (1985) Norepinephrine inhibits field stimulation-evoked release of substance P from chick dorsal root ganglion cells in culture. *Soc. Neurosci. Abstr. 11*, 126.

Hunt, S.P., Emson, P.C., and Kelly, J.S. (1979) The immunohistochemical localization of met-enkephalin within the rat spinal cord: light and electronmicroscopic observations. *Neurosci. Letts. Suppl. 3*, 200.

Jessell, T.M. and Iversen, L.L. (1977) Opiate analgesics inhibit substance P release from rat trigeminal nucleus. *Nature 268*, 549–551.

Kass, R.S. and Blair, M.L. (1981) Effects of angiotensin II on membrane current in cardiac Purkinje fibers. *J. Mol. Cell. Cardiol. 13*, 797–809.

Katz, A. (1983) Cyclic adenosine monophosphate effects on the myocardium: A man who blows hot and cold with one breath. *J. Am. Coll. Cardiol. 2*, 143–149.

Konishi, S., Tsunoo, A., and Otsuka, M. (1981) Enkephalin as a transmitter for presynaptic inhibition in sympathetic ganglia. *Nature 294*, 80–82.

Kretz, R., Shapiro, E., Connor, J. and Kandel, E.R. (1984) Posttetanic potentiation, presynaptic inhibition and the modulation of the free Ca^{2+} level in the presynaptic terminals. *Exp. Br. Res. Suppl. 9*, 240–283.

LaMotte, C. and de Lanerolle, N. (1981) Substance P, enkephalin and serotonin: ultrastructural basis of pain transmission in primate spinal cord. *Pain Suppl I*, S19.

Llinas, R. and Sugimori, M. (1980) Electrophysiological properties of *in vitro* Purkinje cell somata in mammalian cerebellar slices. *J. Physiol. 305*, 171–195.

Llinas, R. and Yarom, Y. (1981) Electrophysiology of mammalian inferior olivary neurones *in vitro*. Different types of voltage dependent ionic conductances. *J. Physiol. 315*, 549–567.

Macdonald, R.L. and Nelson, P.G. (1978) Specific-opiate-induced depression of transmitter release from dorsal root ganglion cells in culture. *Science 199*, 1449–1451.

Marchetti, C., Carbone, E., and Lux, H.D. (1986) Effects of dopamine and noradrenaline on Ca channels of cultured seonsory and sympathetic neurons of chick. *Pflugers Arch.*, in press.

McAfee, D.A., Henon, B.K., Horn, J.P., and Yarowsky, P. (1981) Calcium currents modulated by adrenergic receptors in sympathetic neurons. *Fed. Proc. 40*, 2246–2249.

Melzack, R. and Wall, P.D. (1965) Pain mechanisms: A new theory. *Science 150*, 971–979.

Mudge, A., Leeman, S., and Fischbach (1979) Enkephalin inhibits release of substance P from sensory neurons in culture and decreases action potential duration. *Proc. Natl. Acad. Sci. USA 76*, 526–530.

Niedergerke, R. and Page, S. (1977) Analysis of catecholamine effects in single atrial trabeculae of the frog heart. *Proc. R. Soc. London B 197*, 333–367.

Nowycky, M.C., Fox, A.P., and Tsien, R.W. (1985a) Long-opening mode of gating of neuronal calcium channels and its promotion by the dihydropyridine calcium agonist Bay K 8644. *Proc. Natl. Acad. Sci. USA 82*, 2178–2182.

Nowycky, M.C., Fox, A.P., and Tsien, R.W. (1985b) Three types of neuronal calcium channel with different calcium agonist sensitivity. *Nature 316*, 440–443.

Paupardin-Tritsch, D., Deterre, P., and Gerschenfeld, H.M. (1981) Relationship between two voltage-dependent serotonin responses of molluscan neurons. *Brain Res. 217*, 210–206.

Pellmar, T.C. (1981) Transmitter-induced calcium current. *Fed. Proc. 40*, 2631–2636.

Pellmar, T.C. and Carpenter, D.O. (1980) Serotonin enduces a voltage-sensitive calcium current in neurons of *Aplysia californica*. *J. Neurophysiol. 44*, 423–439.

Rane, S.G. and Dunlap, K. (1985) The kinase C activator 1,2-oleoyl acetyl glycerol mimicks norepinephrine's effect on the voltage dependent calcium current of embryonic chick dorsal root ganglion neurons. *Soc. Neurosci. Abstr. 11*, 748.

Reuter, H. (1967) The dependence of the slow inward current on external calcium concentration in Purkinje fibres. *J. Physiol. 192*, 497–492.

Reuter, H. (1979) Properties of two inward membrane currents in the heart. *Annu. Rev. Physiol. 41*, 413–424.

Reuter, H. (1983) Calcium channel modulation by neurotransmitters, enzymes and drugs. *Nature 301*, 569–574.

Reuter, H. (1985) A variety of calcium channels. *Nature 316*, 391.

Reuter, H. and Scholz, H. (1977) The regulation of the Ca conductance of cardiac muscle by adrenaline. *J. Physiol. 264*, 49–62.

Segal, M. and Sandberg, D. (1977) Analgesia produced by electrical stimulation of catecholamine nuclei in the rat brain. *Brain Res. 123*, 369–372.

Shapiro, E., Castellucci, V.F., and Kandel, E.R. (1980) Presynaptic inhibition in *Aplysia* involves a decrease in the Ca^{2+} current of the presynaptic neuron. *Proc. Natl. Acad. Sci. USA 77*, 1185–1189.

Siegelbaum, S.A. and Tsien, R.W. (1983) Modulation of gated ion channels as a mode of transmitter action. *Trends in Neurosci. 6*, 307–313.

Sigworth, F.J. (1980a) The variance of sodium current fluctuations at the node of Ranvier. *J. Physiol. 307*, 97–129.

Sigworth, F.J. (1980b) The conductance of sodium channels under conditions of reduced current at the node of Ranvier. *J. Physiol. 307*, 131–142.

Sperelakis, N. (1985) Phosphorylation hypothesis of the myocardial slow channels and control of Ca^{2+} influx. In *Cardiac Electrophysiology and Arrhythmias, A Symposium in Honor of Gordon K. Moe* (ed. D. Zipes and J. Jalife), pp. 123–135. Grune & Stratton, Orlando, FL.

Sperelakis, N. and Schneider, J. (1976) A metabolic control mechanism for calcium ion influx that may protect the ventricular myocardial cell. *Am. J. Cardiol. 37,* 1079–1085.

Strong, J.A., Fox, A.P., Tsien, R.W., and Kaczmarek, L.K. (1986) Phorbol ester promotes a large conductance Ca channel in *Aplysia* bag cell neurons. *Biophys. Soc., 49,* 430a.

Tsien, R.W. (1973) Adrenaline-like effects of intracellular iontophoresis of cyclic AMP in cardiac Purkinje fibres. *Nature New Biol. 245,* 120–122.

Tsien, R.W. (1977) Cyclic AMP and contractile activity in heart. *Adv. Cyclic Nucl. Res. 8,* 363–420.

Tsien, R.W. (1983) Calcium channels in excitable cell membranes. *Annu. Rev. Physiol. 45,* 341–358.

Tsien, R.W., Bean, B.P., Hess, P., and Nowycky, M. (1983) Calcium channels: Mechanisms of β-adrenergic modulation and ion permeation. *Cold Spring Harbor Symp. Quant. Biol. 48,* 201–212.

Tsien, R.W., Giles, W., and Greengard, P. (1972) Cyclic AMP mediates the action of adrenaline on the action potential plateau of cardiac Purkinje fibres. *Nature New Biol. 240,* 181–183.

Tsunoo, A., Yoshii, M., and Narahashi, T. (1984) Different properties of two types of calcium channels in neuroblastoma cells. *Biophys. J. 47,* 433a.

Tsunoo, A., Yoshii, M., and Narahashi, T. (1985) Enkephalin and somatostatin block of calcium channel in neuroblastoma cells. *Soc. Neurosci. Abstr. 11,* 517.

van Breemen, C., Aaronson, P., and Loutzenhiser, R. (1979) Na-Ca interactions in mammalian smooth muscle. *Pharmacol. Rev. 30,* 167–208.

Vassort, G., Rougier, O., Garnier, D., Sauviat, M.P., Coraboeuf, E., and Gargouil, Y.M. (1969) Effects of adrenaline on membrane inward currents during the cardiac action potential. *Pflugers Arch. 309,* 70–81.

Wade, J.B., Stetson, D.L., and Lewis, S.A. (1981) ADH action: Evidence for a membrane shuttle mechanism. *Ann. N.Y. Acad. Sci. 372,* 106–117.

Watanabe, A.M. and Besch, H.R., Jr. (1974) Cyclic adenosine monophosphate modulation of slow calcium influx channels in guinea pig hearts. *Circ. Res. 35,* 316–324.

Werz, M.A. and Macdonald, R.L. (1984) Dynorphin reduces calcium-dependent action potential duration by decreasing voltage-dependent calcium conductance. *Neurosci. LETT 46,* 185–190.

Werz, M.A. and Macdonald, R.L. (1985) Phorbol esters: Opposing effects on calcium-dependent action potentials of dorsal root ganglion neurons. *Soc. Neurosci. Abstr. 11,* 747.

Yaksh, T.L., Jessell, T.M., Gamse, R., Mudge, A.W., and Leeman, S.E. (1980) Intrathecal morphine inhibits substance P release from mammalian spinal cord *in vivo*. *Nature 286,* 155–157.

Yatani, A., Tsuda, Y., Akaike, N., and Brown, A.M. (1982) Nanomolar concentrations of extracellular ATP active membrane Ca channels in snail neurones. *Nature 296,* 169–171.

12

Neurotransmitter Release
and Its Modulation

ROBERT S. ZUCKER

The nature of synaptic interactions between cells is either excitatory or inhibitory. Activity in one cell either enhances or reduces activity in the target neuron. The strength of this influence and its duration are quite variable among synapses, and the mechanisms responsible for the postsynaptic effect are also variable. The classic synaptic action is to open ion channels, causing excitatory current to flow inward or inhibitory current to flow outward. Inhibitory synapses can also operate by increasing the postsynaptic conductance, shunting other synaptic responses. More recently, as documented in Chapter 9 and elsewhere in this volume, synaptic interactions have been observed in which ion channels are closed rather than opened, or in which voltage-dependent ion channels are modulated so as to change their voltage sensitivity. In all cases, the effect is to alter the postsynaptic neuron's electrical activity and its responsiveness to other inputs, thus changing the relationship between the cell and its environment.

Synaptic messages are transmitted by the presynaptic release of a transmitter substance that acts on postsynaptic receptors. The neurotransmitter is packaged presynaptically in vesicles, variable numbers of which fuse with the presynaptic membrane immediately following an action potential and release their contents into the synaptic cleft by exocytosis (Heuser et al., 1979; Zimmermann, 1979; Ceccarelli & Hurlbut, 1980). The evidence for this vesicle hypothesis of transmitter release is not completely compelling, and alternatives have been proposed (Tauc, 1982; Dunant & Israël, 1985). It is clear, however, that spike-evoked transmission involves the release of multiple packages of about 5,000 to 10,000 molecules of transmitter (Kuffler & Yoshikami, 1975), called quanta, within a millisecond or so after invasion of the presynaptic terminals by an action potential or other more slowly changing electrical signal.

In the absence of presynaptic activity, quanta are released spontaneously at a very low rate (typically about 1 per second at a neuromuscular synapse). These quanta evoke tiny postsynaptic responses, called miniature excitatory postsynaptic potentials (MEPSPs). Presynaptic depolarization increases the frequency of MEPSPs exponentially (Liley, 1956); thus, an action potential leads to an intense phasic acceleration of MEPSP frequency. These quanta, released nearly simultaneously after an action potential, summate to form the full spike-evoked EPSP.

Synapses do not transmit information statically. Rather, their effectiveness depends in a sensitive and complex manner on the pattern of prior presynaptic activity. This plastic or modulatable property of synaptic efficacy has been appreciated since the earliest electrophysiological studies of synaptic transmission (Feng & Li, 1941) and has been termed *homosynaptic plasticity*. In addition, transmitter release can be regulated by the activity of another neuron, and the molecular mechanisms underlying such *heterosynaptic plasticity* are discussed in Chapter 10. This chapter discusses basic mechanisms of transmitter release and modulation by means of homosynaptic plasticity.

HOMOSYNAPTIC PLASTICITY

The effects of prior activity are quite varied at different synapses. Sometimes, a brief train of action potentials evokes rapidly increasing transmitter release to successive spikes. This effect dissipates equally rapidly, lasting between tens and hundreds of milliseconds (Magleby, 1973). The process is called synaptic facilitation. A minor component of facilitation, lasting several seconds, is sometimes distinguished and

Fig. 12.1. Sequence of events in homosynaptic plasticity at a "typical" synapse. Changes in the number of quanta released per impulse are shown for the successive spikes in a tetanus and for single test spikes at intervals following the end of the tetanus. During the tetanus, facilitation develops faster than depression, but depression is a larger effect and soon exceeds facilitation. A slowly developing potentiation appears as a reduction in tetanus depression. After the tetanus, the rapidly decaying facilitation can be seen at brief intervals after the last spike. Subsequently, depression decays, revealing posttetanic potentiation. The relative magnitudes and actual durations of facilitation, depression, and potentiation are quite variable among synapses and depend on the frequency and number of spikes in the tetanus (Hubbard, 1963).

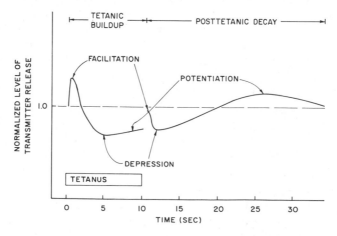

called augmentation (Magleby & Zengel, 1976). At other synapses, successive spikes release less and less transmitter, until presynaptic spikes are almost ineffective on target neurons (Liley & North, 1953). This process, which is also reversible although somewhat more slowly than facilitation, is called synaptic depression. At some synapses, another process is evident in which spike-evoked release grows only very gradually during repeated presynaptic activity, and this slowly growing potentiation also lasts a long time, for minutes or even hours (Magleby & Zengel, 1975). Finally, at some synapses, long-term potentiation can last for hours or days (see Chapter 13), although in this case it is not clear whether the changes are in the presynaptic release of transmitter or in the response of the postsynaptic cell.

Many synapses display a mixture of these processes. Some neuromuscular junctions, for example, show superimposed facilitation, depression, and potentiation (Figure 12.1). The three processes accumulate during a train of spikes and afterward decay at different rates. Because potentiation requires a tetanus (train of many spikes) and can be observed in isolation only after the tetanus, when recovery from facilitation and depression have occurred, it is often referred to as posttetanic potentiation.

Depression

These signs of homosynaptic plasticity, or variation in strength of synaptic transmission dependent on prior activity in the same synapse, are interesting for two reasons: (1) they determine the information-transmitting characteristics of the synapse, and (2) they shed light on the physiological mechanisms underlying synaptic transmission. Synaptic depression, for example, is most pronounced when synaptic transmission is operating at high levels. Procedures that depress the amount of transmitter release by spikes also reduce the depression occurring to successive spikes (Thies, 1965). This suggests that depression is due to a depletion of transmitter stores available for release, with a slow recovery between impulses. A simple model of synaptic depression due to depletion (Figure 12.2) makes a number of testable predictions: (1) the magnitude of depression depends on the fraction of a transmitter store released by each impulse; (2) reducing this fraction, for example, by lowering external calcium concentration, reduces depression; (3) recovery from depression is exponential with a characteristic rate constant independent of the magnitude of depression; (4) tetanic depression accumulates exponentially at a predictable rate and to a predictable steady-state level, both of which are dependent on frequency of impulses, faction of release, and the recovery rate. This model of depression provides an adequate description of the process at some synapses but not at others (Zucker & Bruner, 1977; Klein et al., 1980).

Facilitation

The mechanism of synaptic facilitation has also been the subject of intensive study. This is largely because it seems to be intimately tied to the process of transmitter release. To understand facilitation, we first need to review current ideas about the mechanism of release. When an action potential invades a nerve terminal, the depolarization of the terminal opens voltage-dependent calcium channels, which admit

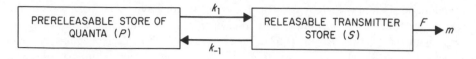

k_1 = RATE OF REFILLING RELEASABLE STORE (S)
k_{-1} = LEAKAGE RATE OUT OF S
F = FRACTION OF S RELEASED BY EACH IMPULSE
$m(t)$ = NUMBER OF QUANTA RELEASED BY AN IMPULSE AT TIME t
f = FREQUENCY OF STIMULATION

DURING A TRAIN:

$dS/dt = k_1 P - k_{-1} S - fFS, \quad m = FS$

$m(t) = FS_s - F(S_r - S_s)e - (fF + k_{-1})t$

S_r = RESTING LEVEL OF S = $k_1 P/k_{-1}$

S_s = STEADY-STATE LEVEL OF S = $k_1 P/(fF + k_{-1})$

AFTER A TRAIN OF DURATION T:

$m(t) = FS_r + F(S_i - S_r)e - k_{-1}t$

S_i = LEVEL OF S AT END OF TRAIN

$= S_s - (S_r - S_s)e - (fF + k_{-1})T$

Fig. 12.2. Mathematical outline of depression due to depletion of a releasable store of transmitter (Zucker & Bruner, 1977).

calcium into the terminal (Llinás et al., 1981a), where resting calcium concentration is very low—about 100 nM. Transmitter release is closely correlated to the calcium entry (Katz & Miledi, 1967a,b; Llinás et al., 1981b). Release by action potentials is very nonlinearly sensitive to the calcium concentration in the external medium, suggesting a cooperative action of several calcium ions in releasing transmitter once they have crossed the membrane (Dodge & Rahamimoff, 1967). Raising intracellular calcium by any means, such as microinjection, exposure to calcium-transporting ionophores, or fusion with calcium-loaded liposomes, elicits transmitter release whereas reducing calcium by opening calcium channels in a calcium-free medium reduces MEPSP frequency. The idea that calcium is a necessary and sufficient agent in causing neurosecretion is called the calcium hypothesis of synaptic transmission (Figure 12.3).

The phasic release of transmitter after a spike is thought to be terminated by the rapid diffusion of calcium away from presynaptic sites of transmitter release. However, some of the calcium entering during action potentials will linger near release

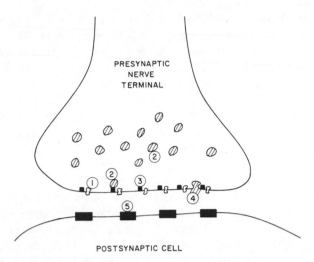

Fig. 12.3. Sequence of events involved in synaptic transmission. Presynaptic depolarization→calcium channels (1) open→calcium enters→active calcium rises→vesicles (2) fuse with release sites (3)→transmitter is liberated (4)→diffuses across synaptic cleft→binds to postsynaptic receptors (5)→postsynaptic ion channels open→postsynaptic current flows→postsynaptic potential generated.

Fig. 12.4. Nonlinear relationship between transmitter release and free calcium. Calcium entering during a spike (Ca_E) triggers more release in the presence of residual calcium (Ca_R) from prior activity.

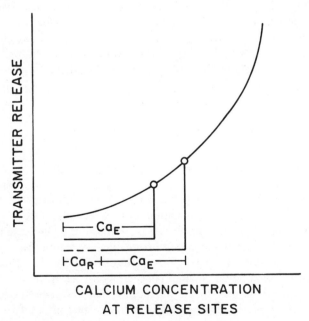

sites, as the late phases of diffusional equilibrium are established or as the terminal begins to fill up with calcium (Zucker & Stockbridge, 1983). This "residual calcium" may be too little to elicit more than an acceleration of the frequency of spontaneously released MEPSPs (Miledi & Thies, 1971; Zucker & Lara-Estrella, 1983). The influx of calcium accompanying a test action potential, however, will add to this residual calcium, and the peak calcium concentration at release sites will be higher than for isolated action potentials. Because of the nonlinearity of the relation between calcium and release, even a small augmentation in the peak calcium will release significantly more transmitter, leading to synaptic facilitation (Figure 12.4). This is the residual calcium hypothesis of synaptic facilitation.

Evidence for this hypothesis of synaptic facilitation comes from several experiments. Katz and Miledi (1968) showed that facilitation by an action potential requires calcium entry during the action potential. Furthermore, injecting calcium into the presynaptic terminal of the squid giant synapse facilitates release evoked by spikes without changing the spike waveform (Charlton et al., 1982). Charlton and Bittner (1978b) had earlier shown that facilitation is not due to a change in spike waveform or presynaptic afterpotentials. In addition, facilitation to a test pulse can be obtained even though the amount of calcium entering the cell during the pulse is not changed (Charlton et al., 1982).

Potentiation

The third form of homosynaptic plasticity, potentiation, has recently also come under experimental scrutiny. The magnitude of the effect depends on the presence of external sodium, suggesting that internal sodium accumulation causes potentiation (Lev-Tov & Rahamimoff, 1980). This idea is supported by findings that microinjection of sodium ions, exposure to sodium ionophores, fusion with sodium-loaded liposomes, or treatments that encourage sodium accumulation, such as blockade of the sodium pump, all enhance potentiation (Charlton & Atwood, 1977; Meiri et al., 1981; Rahamimoff et al., 1978; Birks & Cohen, 1968; Atwood et al., 1975). The long duration of potentiation is believed to reflect the slow kinetics of sodium accumulation and removal. How internal sodium influences transmitter release is unknown, although it is often assumed that it operates by increasing intracellular calcium and is really a sodium-activated form of synaptic facilitation (Figure 12.5).

RECENT CHALLENGES TO THE CALCIUM HYPOTHESIS

The field of presynaptic physiology has always been exciting and full of ferment. The last 10 years have been no exception, as new techniques have been developed and applied to the study of transmitter release. Only in the last decade has a presynaptic terminal been voltage clamped, with consequent experimental control over ionic fluxes, especially calcium, intimately involved in synaptic transmission. Only in the last decade has the presynaptic calcium concentration been measured during synaptic transmission. And it is largely in the last decade that evidence has accumulated for the hypotheses of the processes involved in homosynaptic plasticity.

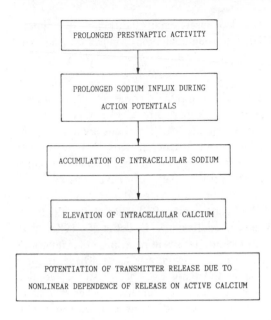

Fig. 12.5. Hypothetical scheme of events underlying synaptic potentiation.

As data have accumulated, however, their interpretation has been neither unambiguous nor unanimous. In fact, even the basic calcium hypothesis of transmitter release has come under attack. Recent experiments at the squid giant synapse (a huge junction in the stellate ganglion where the presynaptic terminal is up to 1 mm long and 50 μm wide) and at frog and crayfish neuromuscular junctions have suggested that, under certain circumstances, changes in presynaptic membrane potential can elicit transmitter release even in the absence of calcium influx or a change in calcium concentration at release sites. This can be called the voltage hypothesis of transmitter release. This issue is fundamental to our understanding of synaptic function, and an exploration of these recent challenges to the calcium hypothesis will occupy the remainder of this chapter.

The Squid Synapse

One indication of a direct role of membrane voltage in triggering neurosecretion came from observations at the squid giant synapse. Rodolfo Llinás and his colleagues (Llinás et al., 1981b) found that the same calcium influx can occur during pulses to low or high membrane potentials. Small depolarizations open few calcium channels with a large current per channel. Large depolarizations open all calcium channels, but as the calcium equilibrium potential is approached, the current per channel drops. According to the calcium hypothesis, a given calcium influx should elicit a given transmitter release, whatever the size of the pulse. On the contrary, Llinás and his associates found that a calcium current caused by a large depolarization elicits more release than the same calcium current caused by a small depolarization. This suggested a direct effect of membrane potential on the release process. However, as will be shown later, this phenomenon is a simple consequence of diffusion of calcium ions in three dimensions following their entry through calcium channels (see below).

Neuromuscular Junctions

The other indications of a direct effect of potential on release come from experiments on neuromuscular junctions. An early observation, reported by Cooke, Okamoto, and Quastel (1973), was that depolarization can accelerate MEPSP frequency at frog neuromuscular junctions in the absence of added external calcium ions. This result was initially interpreted as an indication of a direct voltage effect, but later results indicated that the omission of a calcium chelator from the bath may have allowed external calcium to reach significant levels and that ions other than calcium might contribute to release in the absence of calcium (Hubbard et al., 1968; Kita et al., 1981).

More recently, Dudel (1983, 1984) and his colleagues (Dudel et al., 1983) have observed some surprising responses to depolarizing pulses at neuromuscular junctions that appear to contradict the calcium hypothesis of transmitter release. These findings can be readily explained, however, by the spatial inhomogeneity of stimuli applied through the large extracellular electrodes used in these experiments (Zucker & Landò, 1986). Furthermore, several other experiments described below provide direct evidence that transmitter release cannot be evoked by depolarization without calcium entry.

TRANSMITTER RELEASE REQUIRES CALCIUM INFLUX

Since the voltage hypothesis suggests that presynaptic depolarization can evoke release if intracellular calcium at release sites is already high, several methods have been used to elevate free calcium, and then depolarize terminals while blocking calcium influx. Hypertonic media accelerate MEPSP frequency, apparently by raising internal calcium in terminals uniformly throughout cytoplasm (Shimoni et al., 1977). This effect depends on the internal elevation of sodium ions (Muchnik & Venosa, 1969), suggesting a similarity to potentiation. The voltage hypothesis predicts that depolarization will elicit phasic release without calcium influx in hypertonic media. On the contrary, it was found (Zucker & Landò, 1986), in agreement with Shimoni et al. (1977), that depolarization reduces MEPSP frequency under such conditions, probably because of the efflux of calcium from terminals when calcium channels open in the presence of a reversed calcium gradient. Action potentials also fail to evoke release under such conditions.

In another series of experiments (Zucker & Landò, 1986), mitochondrial uncouplers were used to raise intracellular calcium. Such agents deplete terminals of ATP and cause mitochondria to release bound calcium. Uncouplers such as carbonyl cyanide m-chlorophenylhydrazone (CCCP) cause a dramatic rise in MEPSP frequency (Glacoleva et al., 1970), but electrical depolarization of the terminals still fails to increase transmitter release. Cobalt ions are commonly used as a calcium channel antagonist. When calcium influx is blocked by substituting cobalt for calcium ions and raising internal calcium with CCCP, still no release is evoked by action potentials (Figure 12.6).

EPSP   MEPSPs

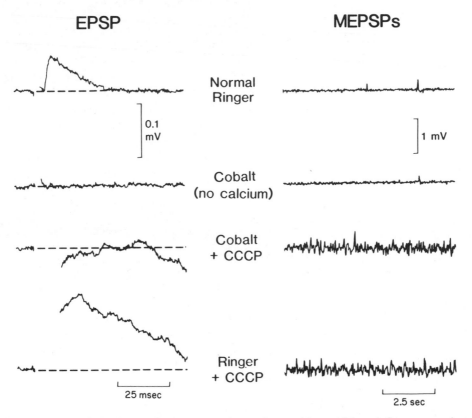

Fig. 12.6. Depolarization evokes no transmitter release without calcium influx, even when intracellular calcium at release sites is high. All traces are intracellular recordings from a muscle fiber in the leg opener muscle of crayfish. Replacing calcium in normal Ringer with cobalt blocks calcium influx and spike-evoked transmitter release. In CCCP, elevated free calcium increases MEPSP frequency from 1 per 8 sec to about 3 per second. CCCP also raises the threshold of the nerve, but when a larger stimulus is used to excite the nerve (causing a larger stimulus artifact), there is still no transmitter release and no EPSP. Restoring the normal calcium-containing Ringer restores transmission, which is facilitated by the elevated presynaptic calcium. Extracellular recordings from nerve terminals (not shown) indicated that the terminals were invaded by action potentials in all the solutions (unpublished results provided by L. Landò).

MODELS OF DYNAMIC BEHAVIOR OF ACTIVE CALCIUM AND TRANSMITTER RELEASE

The argument remains that the apparent voltage dependence of release in squid is inconsistent with calcium hypothesis of transmitter release. We shall now consider whether a mathematical formulation of the calcium hypothesis can account for this apparent discrepancy.

One-Dimensional Calcium Diffusion

The problem can be approached by considering the behavior of calcium entering a cylindrical terminal at the surface and diffusing radially inward following action potentials (Zucker & Stockbridge, 1983). This situation may be simulated by solving the diffusion equation in cylindrical coordinates with a brief pulsatile calcium influx at the surface corresponding to each spike. Intracellular calcium ions are known to be bound rapidly by cytoplasmic proteins, with two effects: (1) most of the calcium entering the terminal does not remain free, but is adsorbed to binding sites, and (2) diffusion is slowed substantially in relation to aequeous solutions. It is also known that calcium is extruded from cytoplasm by surface pumps and by uptake into intra-

Fig. 12.7. Simulations using a one-dimensional calcium diffusion model. Equation 4 from Zucker and Stockbridge (1983) was modified by dividing pump and influx terms by the ratio of bound to free calcium (correcting an error), and a term was included in Equations 2 to 4 to represent calcium uptake into endoplasmic reticulum. (A) Diagram of the system of equations; (B) total free cytoplasmic calcium during and after a 2-sec, 33-Hz tetanus. Calcium measurements by microspectrophotometric absorbance changes in a calcium-sensitive dye are compared to simulations. (C) The postsynaptic response (EPSC) to a presynaptic spike is compared to the time course of submembrane calcium raised to the second power. Events other than the rise and fall of submembrane calcium determine the time course of the postsynaptic response. (D) Simulations and experimental observations of facilitation (the fractional increase of the second response relative to the first) measured by the responses to two spikes separated by a variable interval.

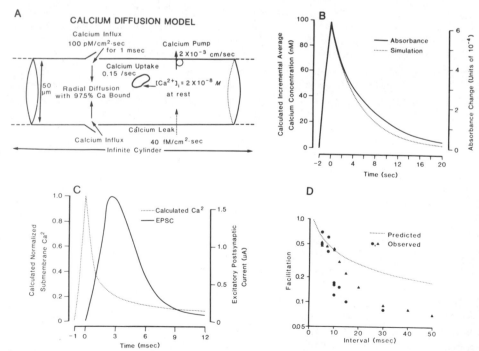

cellular oganelles. Finally, a square-law relationship between transmitter release and active calcium was assumed, based on measurements of the relationship between transmitter release and calcium current under voltage clamp (Charlton et al., 1982). Provisions for all of these processes were included in the simulation.

The initial results with this one-dimensional model were quite successful (Figure 12.7). The model predicts that the total free calcium in the terminal rises during a tetanus or single spike and declines afterwards with a half-time of several seconds. This corresponds to the kinetics of the change in presynaptic calcium measured using arsenazo microspectrophotometry (Charlton et al., 1982). The model predicts that phasic transmitter release would last only a few milliseconds or less, even if transmitter release is dependent only on the square of submembrane calcium. Higher stoichiometries lead to even more rapid release, but other processes subsequent to calcium action may be rate limiting. Finally, the model predicts that facilitation following one spike would peak at about 100% and decline with two time constants, about 6 and 60 msec, similar to experimental observation (Charlton & Bittner, 1978a). The success of these simulations was particularly significant because there were no free parameters. The calcium influx, geometrical dimensions, cytoplasmic binding efficiency, and extrusion and uptake rates were set according to independent measurements reported in the literature.

Simulation of Tetanic Responses

The effects of long tetani (100 spikes in 5 sec) were also simulated. The model succeeds in predicting an accumulating facilitation with several time constants, including one lasting seconds and corresponding to augmentation (Figure 12.8). This is caused by the filling of the terminal with calcium, so that a component of submembrane residual calcium is removed by extrusion processes. The faster phases of facilitation correspond to diffusion away from the membrane. Facilitation after a tetanus shows these same components, which correspond to similar time constants of decay following one spike. These characteristics are similar to those seen experimentally (Magelby & Zengel, 1982).

Simulations with this model, however, produce a major discrepancy with experimental data. After the last spike in the tetanus, the model predicts that submembrane calcium will remain higher than the peak active calcium reached in the first spike for an extended period. This would correspond to a posttetanic phasic transmitter release lasting well over 50 msec, which is never observed experimentally. Clearly, something is wrong with either the formulation of this model or the underlying assumptions (the calcium hypothesis of transmitter release).

Calcium Domains Near Calcium Channels

Simon and Llinás (1985) pointed out that calcium does not enter uniformly across the membrane, but rather through discrete calcium channels. Each calcium channel is surrounded by a little independent "calcium domain" (Figure 12.9A). Shortly after a spike, these calcium domains will collapse as calcium diffuses rapidly in three dimensions away from each channel. Within a few milliseconds, equilibration in the

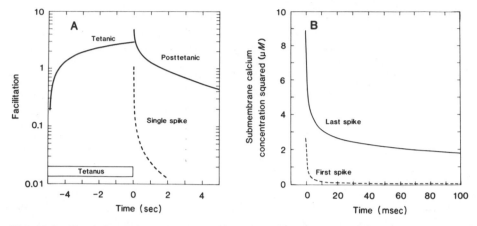

Fig. 12.8. Simulations of tetanic responses using a one-dimensional calcium diffusion model (adapted from Fogelson & Zucker, 1985). (A) The solid curve predicts facilitation of transmitter release to successive stimuli in a 5-sec, 20-Hz tetanus (rising phase) and to single test stimulus delivered at various times after the tetanus (falling phase). The dashed curve represents the decay of facilitation after a single spike. (B) Assuming transmitter release is proportional to the square of submembrane or active calcium, the time course of transmitter release is plotted for the first and last spikes in the tetanus. Release by the last spike is fallaciously predicted to continue for 50 msec at a level higher than the peak rate of release by the first spike. This problem is independent of the assumed cooperativity of calcium ions in releasing transmitter.

plane of the membrane will be established, and thereafter calcium will diffuse radially in one dimension, as in the model described previously. In this case, the peak calcium concentration near channel mouths at the end of a spike will be much greater than in the model with uniform calcium entry, although residual calcium will be the same. Thus, residual calcium will never approach the level of the peak calcium near release sites in a spike, and the major problem with the one-dimensional diffusion model disappears (Figure 12.9B). With a reduced ratio of residual to peak calcium, however, a higher calcium stoichiometry of release will be needed to account for facilitation. The mathematical formulation of these ideas requires the solution of the diffusion equation in three dimensions for an array of hundreds of thousands of calcium channels, with cytoplasmic binding and extrusion (Fogelson & Zucker, 1985).

Where Are Calcium Channels?

Before simulations with the three-dimensional model can be performed, some parameter choices must be made. The number of calcium channels can be determined by dividing the total calcium current (measured in squid synapses; Llinás et al., 1982) by the single channel calcium current (measured in snail neurons; Lux & Brown, 1984). The disposition of these channels is not very obvious. In early simulations

A

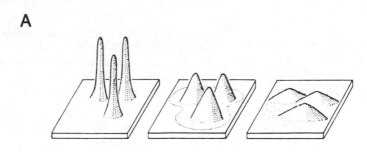

B

I. 1-D diffusion away from membrane

Peak calcium at
release sites

Residual calcium

II. Initial rapid 3-D diffusion, followed by

1-D radial diffusion after surface equilibration

Peak calcium at
release sites

Residual calcium

Fig. 12.9. Implications of calcium domains surrounding single calcium channels. (A) Sketch of hypothetical calcium concentrations near calcium channels at various times after the end of an action potential (adapted from Hartzell et al., 1975). Initially, calcium is confined to the regions surrounding channel mouths and diffuses away from them in three dimensions. Later, equilibration in the plane of the membrane is nearly complete, and subsequent diffusion is essentially one-dimensional (radial). (B) Comparison of models in which calcium influx is uniform (B-I) or is confined to discrete calcium channels (B-II). In the former case, residual calcium *(dotted line)* reaches a higher fraction of the peak active calcium than in the latter case.

255

calcium channels were distributed uniformly in the presynaptic membrane face in contact with the postsynaptic cells. Ultrastructural observations, however (Pumplin et al., 1981), indicate that synaptic vesicles and intramembranous particles thought to represent calcium channels are actually clustered into about 10,000 "active zones," each about 0.65 μm^2 in area. Such an array of calcium channels has been used for more realistic simulations.

How far from calcium channels does exocytosis occur? The synaptic delay of 0.2 msec between calcium channel opening and exocytosis (Llinás et al., 1981b) allows calcium ions to diffuse only about 50 nm from channel mouths. Freeze fracture observations of exocytosis at frog neuromuscular junctions (Heuser et al., 1979) also show vesicle fusion occurring about 50 nm from putative calcium channels. If fusion occurred much closer than this, it would obliterate calcium channels in the process. Thus, transmitter release can be taken to be proportional to some power of calcium concentration 50 nm from calcium channel mouths. Since transmitter release depends on up to the fourth power of external calcium (Dodge & Rahamimoff, 1967; Katz & Miledi, 1970), and this dependence probably underestimates the stoichiometry or cooperativity of calcium action in releasing transmitter (Barton et al., 1983), a fifth-power relation between active calcium and transmitter release has been assumed for simulations.

Three-Dimensional Calcium Diffusion Simulations

Simulations with these parameter choices and other parameters (binding and extrusion) chosen as in the one-dimensional simulations provide gratifying fits to experimental results (Figure 12.10). The model simulates well the removal of total calcium from cytoplasm and facilitation during trains and after trains and single spikes. Most important, the chief problem with the one-dimensional model no longer exists. Transmitter release, as determined by the fifth power of calcium 50 nm from calcium channels, remains almost as short-lived after 100 spikes as after a single spike. Release decays in both situations with a half-time of less than 1 msec.

An unexpected result arises from simulations with a uniform distribution of channels. When calcium channels are not clustered in active zones, calcium does not diffuse rapidly away from each active zone in three dimensions; instead, equilibration in the plane of the membrane and the situation of the one-dimensional model are attained more rapidly. In these simulations, phasic transmitter release is prolonged to several milliseconds after the one-hundredth spike in a tetanus. The problem is similar to but not as exaggerated as the problem with the purely one-dimensional model. Only by boosting the rate of calcium extrusion by pumps to unphysiological levels can the model be made to account adequately for the removal of excess calcium from release sites. Apparently, the clustering of channels into active zones is necessary, to ensure the rapid diffusion of calcium away from regions containing release sites after long tetani. This may explain why the release machinery, consisting of calcium channels and synaptic vesicles, is clustered into separate active zones in all the chemical synapses studied so far.

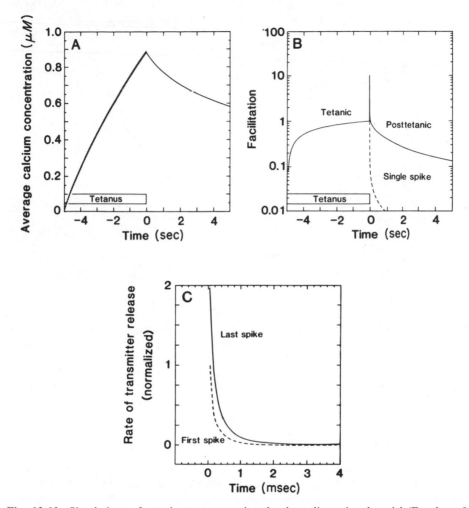

Fig. 12.10. Simulations of tetanic responses using the three-dimensional model (Fogelson & Zucker, 1985). (A) Prediction of average free cytoplasmic calcium concentration during and after a 5-sec, 20-Hz tetanus; (B) tetanic accumulation of synaptic facilitation and its posttetanic decay *(solid curve)* and facilitation following a single spike *(dashed curve);* (C) time course of decay of submembrane active calcium, 50 nm from calcium channel mouths in the center of active zones, for the first and last spike in the tetanus.

Relationship between Transmitter Release and Calcium Current

The three-dimensional model can also account for the finding that large depolarizations evoke more transmitter release than small ones, even when both depolarizations elicit the same calcium current (Llinás et al, 1981b; Smith et al., 1985). A third-order relation appears to exist between transmitter release and calcium current (Smith

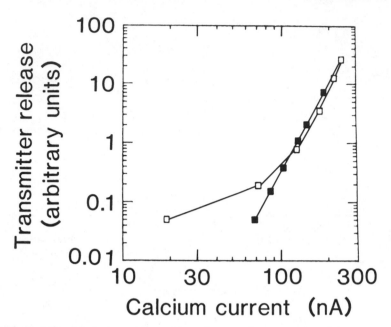

Fig. 12.11. Relationship between transmitter release and presynaptic calcium current at the end of a pulse, using different size depolarizations. The simulations are using the three-dimensional calcium diffusion model (Zucker & Fogelson, 1986). The open symbols indicate 2.5 msec pulses to 0 mV or less; the filled symbols indicate pulses to 10 mV or greater. Simulations of longer pulses are not possible, because they require calcium channels to reopen randomly in time and space during the pulse.

et al., 1985), somewhat lower than the calcium stoichiometry necessary to account for facilitation. It is also lower than the degree of calcium cooperativity suggested by the dependence of release on external calcium. Consideration of the effect of calcium domains, however, helps us to understand this result. If calcium domains during depolarizing pulses are entirely independent and nonoverlapping, then as more calcium channels are opened, more domains will be recruited, each releasing the same average number of transmitter quanta. A linear relationship between transmitter release and total calcium current would then result. (Actually, since larger depolarizations approach the calcium equilibrium potential, the single channel influx declines, and a less-than-linear relation results; Simon and Llinás, 1985.) This situation is analogous to the postsynaptic situation, in which the postsynaptic actions of individual quanta sum linearly, because of nonoverlapping quantal release sites, despite a nonlinear relation between transmitter concentration and postsynaptic current (see Hartzell et al., 1975).

   If all calcium domains overlapped completely, then doubling the calcium current would double the number of channels opening and the submembrane calcium concentration. The relation between transmitter release and calcium current would then reflect faithfully the degree of calcium cooperativity in activating neurosecretion. In reality, when a few calcium channels are opened, their calcium domains remain entirely distinct. As more channels open, their domains approach each other and begin to overlap. Thus, over much of the range of the relation between transmitter release and calcium current, a situation intermediate between complete independence and complete overlap should prevail.

It is impossible to intuit what the power of this relationship would be. The three-dimensional model, with calcium channels clustered in active zones, can predict this relationship for different size depolarizations (Figure 12.11). Assuming a fifth-order calcium cooperativity in releasing transmitter, the predicted power, 3.3, in the mid-range of depolarizations is strikingly close to that observed experimentally, from 2.4 to 3.5 (Smith et al., 1985).

Apparent Voltage Dependence of Transmitter Release

The model can also be used to predict the behavior of this relationship for very large depolarizations. The effects of brief pulses are simulated as opening calcium channels once during the pulse. Large pulses with a given calcium current at the end of the pulse differ from small pulses in two ways: (1) they open more calcium channels, with greater overlap of calcium domains, and (2) they admit less calcium through each channel during the pulse because of the lower driving force for calcium entry. These effects combine to make large depolarizations that elicit a given calcium current more effective than small depolarizations (Figure 12.11), as is seen in the experimental observations (Smith et al., 1985). Thus, the apparent voltage dependence of release is a natural consequence of the effect of variable overlap of calcium domains at different voltages and is not a sign of direct regulation of synaptic transmission by membrane potential.

CONCLUSIONS

These experiments and simulations leave us with restored confidence in the utility of the calcium hypothesis of transmitter release and its corollary, the residual calcium hypothesis of synaptic facilitation. Several challenges to the calcium hypothesis have withstood careful experimental and theoretical scrutiny. At present, no evidence exists that membrane potential can elicit transmitter release in the absence of calcium influx. The calcium hypothesis therefore remains the most useful model on which to base further experiments.

Although presynaptic voltage may not *elicit* transmitter release directly, recent experiments by Dudel (1984b) suggest that voltage may *modulate* release caused by calcium influx. These workers reported that small depolarizing (or hyperpolarizing) pulses, either immediately preceding or following a major depolarizing test pulse, enhance (or diminish) release by this major test pulse. However, they do not affect release evoked by a subsequent identical test pulse. Because the two major test pulses are identical, they should activate the same synaptic terminals under the electrode. The absence of an effect on synaptic facilitation suggests that the small pulses do not alter calcium influx evoked by the major test pulse or the resulting residual calcium.

Thus, presynaptic potential may modulate synaptic transmission without affecting calcium entry. More work on this interesting idea is needed.

It should be emphasized that, besides the possibility of a modulatory role of voltage, the calcium hypothesis does not account perfectly for all experimental observations. Certainly its formulation, even in the three-dimensional diffusion model, is not completely accurate. It is unlikely that exactly five or any other single number of calcium ions always cause a synaptic vesicle to fuse with the plasma membrane and release its contents. Neither calcium channels nor vesicle fusion sites occur in regular arrays, and calcium channels do not open synchronously, even in action potentials. In longer depolarizations, especially, the stochastic nature of different channels opening and closing repeatedly in random spatial and temporal patterns, as well as the local exhaustion of release sites and replenishment with releasable vesicles, is likely to affect significantly the properties of transmitter release. These imperfections may well be partly responsible for the imperfect fit of simulations to observations when fine details are considered. Nevertheless, the experimental results and simulations suggest that we are probably still on the right track, although nowhere near the final station.

REFERENCES

Atwood, H.L., Swenarchuk, L.E., and Gruenwald, C.R. (1975) Long-term synaptic facilitation during sodium accumulation in nerve terminals. *Brain Res. 100*, 198–204.

Barton, S.B., Cohen, I.S., and van der Kloot, W. (1983) The calcium dependence of spontaneous and evoked quantal release at the frog neuromuscular junction. *J. Physiol. 337*, 735–751.

Birks, R.I. and Cohen, M.W. (1968) The influence of internal sodium on the behaviour of motor nerve endings. *Proc. Royal Soc. London B 170*, 401–421.

Bliss, T.V.P. and Lomo, T. (1973) Long-lasting potentiation of synaptic transmission in the dentate area of the anaesthetized rabbit following stimulation of the perforant path. *J. Physiol. 232*, 331–356.

Brown, T.H. and McAfee, D.A. (1982) Long-lasting synaptic potentiation in the superior cervical ganglion. *Science 215*, 1411–1413.

Ceccarelli, B. and Hurlbut, W.P. (1980) Vesicle hypothesis of the release of quanta of acetylcholine. *Physiol. Rev. 60*, 396–441.

Charlton, M.P. and Atwood, H.L. (1977) Modulation of transmitter release by intracellular sodium in squid giant synapse. *Brain Res. 134*, 367–371.

Charlton, M.P. and Bittner, G.D. (1978a) Facilitation of transmitter release at squid synapses. *J. Gen. Physiol. 72*, 471–486.

Charlton, M.P. and Bittner, G.D. (1978b) Presynaptic potentials and facilitation of transmitter release in the squid giant synapse. *J. Gen. Physiol. 72*, 487–511.

Charlton, M.P., Smith, S.J., and Zucker, R.S. (1982) Role of presynaptic calcium ions and channels in synaptic facilitation and depression at the squid giant synapse. *J. Physiol. 323*, 173–193.

Cooke, J.D., Okamoto, K., and Quastel, D.M.J. (1973) The role of calcium in depolarization-secretion coupling at the motor nerve terminal. *J. Physiol. 228*, 459–497.

Dodge, F.A., Jr. and Rahamimoff, R. (1967) Co-operative action of calcium ions in transmitter release at the neuromuscular junction. *J. Physiol. 193*, 419–432.

Dudel, J. (1983) Transmitter release triggered by a local depolarization in motor nerve terminals of the frog: Role of calcium entry and of depolarization. *Neurosci. Letts. 41*, 133–138.

Dudel, J. (1984) Control of quantal transmitter release at frog's motor nerve terminals. II. Modulation by de- or hyperpolarizing pulses. *Pflugers Arch. 402*, 235–243.

Dudel, J., Parnas, I., and Parnas, H. (1983) Neurotransmitter release and its facilitation in crayfish muscle. VI. Release determined by both intracellular calcium concentration and depolarization of the nerve terminal. *Pflugers Arch. 399*, 1–10.

Dunant, Y. and Israël, M. (1985) The release of acetylcholine. *Scientific Amer. 252*, 58–66.

Erulkar, S.D., Rahamimoff, R., and Rotshenker, S. (1978) Quelling of spontaneous transmitter release by nerve impulses in low extracellular calcium solutions. *J. Physiol. 278*, 491–500.

Feng, T.P. and Li, T.H. (1941) Studies of the neuromuscular junction. XXIII. A new aspect of the phenomena of eserine potentiation and post-tetanic facilitation in mammalian muscles. *Chin. J. Physiol. 16*, 37–50.

Fogelson, A.L. and Zucker, R.S. (1985) Presynaptic calcium diffusion from an array of single channels: Implications for transmitter release and synaptic facilitation. *Biophys. J. 48*, 1003–1017.

Glacoleva, I.M., Liberman, Y.A., and Khashayev, A.Kh.M. (1970) Effect of uncoupling agents of oxidative phosphorylation on the release of acetylcholine from nerve endings. *Biophysics 15*, 74–82.

Hartzell, H.C., Kuffler, S.W., and Yoshikami, D. (1975) Post-synaptic potentiation: Interaction between quanta of acetylcholine at the skeletal neuromuscular synapse. *J. Physiol. 251*, 427–463.

Heuser, J.E., Reese, T.S., Dennis, M.J., Jan, Y., Jan, L., and Evans, L. (1979) Synaptic vesicle exocytosis captured by quick freezing and correlated with quantal transmitter release. *J. Cell Biol. 81*, 275–300.

Hubbard, J.I. (1963) Repetitive stimulation at the mammalian neuromuscular junction, and the mobilization of transmitter. *J. Physiol. 169*, 541–662.

Hubbard, J.I., Jones, S.F., and Landau, E.M. (1968) On the mechanism by which calcium and magnesium affect the spontaneous release of transmitter from mammalian motor nerve terminals. *J. Physiol. 194*, 355–380.

Huxley, A.F. and Taylor, R.E. (1958) Local activation of striated muscle fibres. *J. Physiol. 144*, 426–441.

Katz, B. and Miledi, R. (1967a) The release of acetylcholine from nerve endings by graded electric pulses. *Proc. Royal Soc. London B 167*, 23–38.

Katz, B. and Miledi, R. (1967b) A study of synaptic transmission in the absence of nerve impulses. *J. Physiol. 192*, 407–436.

Katz, B. and Miledi, R. (1968) The role of calcium in neuromuscular facilitation. *J. Physiol. 195*, 481–492.

Katz, B. and Miledi, R. (1970) Further study of the role of calcium in synaptic transmission. *J. Physiol. 207*, 789–801.

Kita, H., Narita, K., and van der Kloot. W. (1981) Tetanic stimulation increases the frequency of miniature end-plate potentials at the frog neuromuscular junction in Mn^{2+}, Co^{2+}, and Ni^{2+}-saline solutions. *Brain Res. 205*, 111–121.

Kita, H. and van der Kloot, W. (1976) Effects of the ionophore X-537A on acetylcholine release at the frog neuromuscular junction. *J. Physiol. 259*, 177–198.

Klein, M., Shapiro, E., and Kandel, E.R. (1980) Synaptic plasticity and the modulation of the Ca^{2+} current. *J. Exp. Biol. 89*, 117–157.

Kuffler, S.W. and Yoshikami, D. (1975) The number of transmitter molecules in a quantum:

An estimate from iontophoretic application of acetylcholine at the neuromuscular synapse. *J. Physiol. 251*, 465–482.

Lev-Tov, A. and Rahamimoff, R. (1980) A study of tetanic and post-tetanic potentiation of miniature end-plate potentials at the frog neuromuscular junction. *J. Physiol. 309*, 247–273.

Liley, A.W. (1956), The effects of presynaptic polarization on the spontaneous activity at the mammalian neuromuscular junction. *J. Physiol. 134*, 427–443.

Liley, A.W. and North, K.A.K. (1953) An electrical investigation of effects of repetitive stimulation on mammalian neuromuscular junction. *J. Neurophysiol. 16*, 509–527.

Llinás, R., Steinberg, I.Z., and Walton, K. (1981a) Presynaptic calcium currents in squid giant synapse. *Biophys. J. 33*, 289–322.

Llinás, R., Steinberg, I.Z., and Walton, K. (1981b) Relationship between presynaptic calcium current and postsynaptic potential in squid giant synapse. *Biophys. J. 33*, 323–352.

Llinás, R., Sugimori, M., and Simon, S.M. (1982) Transmission by spike-like depolarization in the squid giant synapse. *Proc. Natl. Acad. Sci. USA 79*, 2415–2419.

Lux, H.D. and Brown, A.M. (1984) Patch and whole cell calcium currents recorded simultaneously in snail neurons. *J. Gen. Physiol. 83*, 727–750.

Magleby, K.L. (1973) The effect of repetitive stimulation on facilitation of transmitter release at the frog neuromuscular junction. *J. Physiol. 234*, 327–352.

Magleby, K.L. and Zengel. J.E. (1975) A quantitative description of tetanic and post-tetanic potentiation of transmitter release at the frog neuromuscular junction. *J. Physiol. 245*, 183–208.

Magleby, K.L. and Zengel, J.E. (1976) Augmentation: A process that acts to increase transmitter release at the frog neuromuscular junction. *J. Physiol. 257*, 449–470.

Magleby, K.L. and Zengel, J.E. (1982) A quantitative description of stimulation-induced changes in transmitter release at the frog neuromuscular junction. *J. Gen. Physiol. 80*, 613–638.

Meiri, H., Erulkar. S.D., Lerman, T., and Rahamimoff, R. (1981) The action of the sodium ionophore, monensin, on transmitter release at the frog neuromuscular junction. *Brain Res. 204*, 204–208.

Miledi, R. (1973) Transmitter release induced by injection of calcium ions into nerve terminals. *Proc. Royal Soc. London B 183*, 421–425.

Miledi, R. and Thies, R. (1971) Tetanic and post-tetanic rise in frequency of miniature end-plate potentials in low-calcium solutions. *J. Physiol. 212*, 245–257.

Muchnik, S. and Venosa, R.A. (1969) Role of sodium ions in the response of the frequency of miniature end-plate potentials to osmotic changes in the neuromuscular junction. *Nature 222*, 169–171.

Parnas, I., Dudel. J. and Parnas, H. (1984) Depolarization dependence of the kinetics of phasic transmitter release at the crayfish neuromuscular junction. *Neurosci. Letts. 50*, 157–162.

Pumplin, D.W., Reese, T.S., and Llinás, R. (1981) Are the presynaptic membrane particles the calcium channels? *Proc. Natl. Acad. Sci. USA 78*, 7210–7213.

Rahamimoff, R., Meiri, H., Erulkar, S.D., and Barenholz, Y. (1978) Changes in transmitter release induced by ion-containing liposomes. *Proc. Natl. Acad. Sci. USA 75*, 5214–5216.

Shimoni, Y., Alnaes, E., and Rahamimoff, R. (1977) Is hyperosmotic neurosecretion from motor nerve endings a calcium-dependent process? *Nature 267*, 170–172.

Simon, S.M. and Llinás, R.R. (1985) Compartmentalization of the submembrane calcium activity during calcium influx and its significance in transmitter release. *Biophys. J. 48*, 485–498.

Simon, S., Sugimori, M., and Llinas, R. (1984) Modelling of submembranous calcium-concentration changes and their relation to rate of presynaptic transmitter release in the squid giant synapse. *Biophys. J. 45,* 264a.

Smith, S.J., Augustine, G.J., and Charlton, M.P. (1985) Transmission at voltage-clamped giant synapse of the squid: Evidence for cooperativity of presynaptic calcium action. *Proc. Natl. Acad. Sci. USA 82,* 622–625.

Statham, H.E. and Duncan, C.J. (1975) The action of ionophores at the frog neuromuscular junction. *Life Sci. 17,* 1401–1406.

Stockbridge, N. and Moore, J.W. (1984) Dynamics of intracellular calcium and its possible relationship to phasic transmitter release and facilitation at the frog neuromuscular junction. *J. Neurosci. 4,* 803–811.

Tauc, L. (1982) Nonvesicular release of neurotransmitter. *Physiol. Rev. 62,* 857–893.

Thies, R.E. (1965) Neuromuscular depression and the apparent depletion of transmitter in mammalian muscle. *J. Neurophysiol. 28,* 427–442.

Zimmermann, H. (1979) Vesicle recycling and transmitter release. *Neuroscience 4,* 1773–1804.

Zucker, R.S. (1974) Excitability changes in crayfish motor neurone terminals. *J. Physiol. 241,* 111–126.

Zucker, R.S. and Bruner, J. (1977) Long-lasting depression and the depletion hypothesis at crayfish neuromuscular junctions. *J. Comp. Physiol. 121,* 223–240.

Zucker, R.S. and Fogelson, A.L. (1986) Relationship between transmitter release and presynaptic calcium influx when calcium enters through discrete channels. *Proc. Natl. Acad. USA 83,* 3032–3036.

Zucker, R.S. and Landò, L. (1986) Mechanism of transmitter release: Voltage hypothesis and calcium hypothesis. *Science 231,* 574–579.

Zucker, R.S. and Lara-Estrella, L.O. (1983) Post-tetanic decay of evoked and spontaneous transmitter release and a residual-calcium model of synaptic facilitation at crayfish neuromuscular junctions. *J. Gen. Physiol. 81,* 355–372.

Zucker, R.S. and Stockbridge, N. (1983) Presynaptic calcium diffusion and the time courses of transmitter release and synaptic facilitation at the squid giant synapse. *J. Neurosci. 3,* 1263–1269.

13

Some Examples of Neuromodulation in Mammalian Brain

VALENTIN K. GRIBKOFF
F. EDWARD DUDEK

The concept of neuromodulation, in the most general sense, relates to virtually every action on a mature neuron that results in a change of cell properties. The previous chapters have dealt with neuromodulation at the level of the single channel and membrane currents; these studies have exploited model systems particularly suitable for biophysical analyses of neuromodulatory mechanisms. This chapter is concerned with complex neuromodulatory actions in mammalian brain that have been studied with electrophysiological techniques. The goal is to describe examples of modulation of electrical activity, and to discuss the need for further studies aimed at determining whether the mechanisms known to occur in model systems, such as invertebrates, also apply to the mammalian brain.

This chapter provides a brief and selective overview of the large body of literature in this exciting and diverse field. We will discuss only phenomena associated with the "normal" function of the neuron, although epileptiform bursting will be used for studying modulation of neuronal discharge properties at the population level. Representative examples of phenomena will be chosen from a few systems, without an exhaustive listing of pertinent studies. It is hoped that the reader will gain a theoretical and practical appreciation of some of the electrophysiological phenomena in mammalian brain encompassed by the term neuromodulation. By presenting examples from model systems in mammals, the enormous complexity of neuromodulatory interactions that must exist in the human brain will ideally be recognized. Each example of neuromodulation in this chapter is associated with numerous unanswered questions, and we will emphasize some areas where further research is needed to determine fundamental mechanisms in the complex systems of the mammalian brain.

SYNAPTIC PLASTICITY

Short-term Effects

Under certain conditions, repetitive stimulation of a presynaptic pathway results in significant enhancement of subsequent postsynaptic potentials. This effect has been observed for end-plate potentials at the neuromuscular junction (see Chapter 12), and for excitatory postsynaptic potentials (EPSPs) in the spinal cord and at many central synapses. This enhancement, usually termed post-tetanic potentiation, is relatively short lasting (seconds to minutes). In most cases, post-tetanic potentiation appears to involve a mechanism, possibly mediated by calcium ions, that leads to increased transmitter release by subsequent stimuli. The physiological significance of post-tetanic potentiation, particularly in mammalian brain, is unknown and deserves more attention.

Long-term Potentiation (LTP)

LTP in Hippocampus

Brief, high-frequency stimulation of afferent fibers in the hippocampus causes a long-lasting enhancement of subsequent postsynaptic responses, a robust phenomenon that can be differentiated from post-tetanic potentiation by its much slower decay kinetics. Hippocampal LTP, first observed following repetitive stimulation of afferents to granule cells of the dentate gyrus (Bliss & Gardner-Medwin, 1973), is extremely durable; the enhanced synaptic efficacy that follows conditioning stimuli has been reported to last for weeks *in vivo* (Bliss & Gardner-Medwin, 1973; Douglas & Goddard, 1975). Figure 13.1A shows an example of LTP recorded from hippocampal neurons *in vivo*. Enhanced population and single-cell EPSPs, plus greatly increased synchronous cell discharges (population "spikes"), can be elicited from neurons in all regions of the *in vitro* hippocampal slice preparation. In this isolated system a brief, high-frequency

Fig. 13.1. Long-term potentiation in the hippocampus. (A) Examples of extracellularly recorded population responses obtained *in vivo* from the dentate gyrus in response to electrical stimulation of an afferent pathway before and after a series of high-frequency stimulus trains. The initial transients are stimulus artifacts, and the slow positive-going waves are synaptic responses of the population. The sharp, negative deflection is the population spike, which represents the synchronous discharge of hippocampal neurons. (B) Increased response amplitude after stimulus trains. The mean relative increase in response amplitude is plotted as a function of time during a series of high-frequency stimulus trains. The control data show the enduring nature of LTP. Pretreatment with 6-hydroxydopamine or reserpine was used to reduce norepinephrine (NA), which decreased LTP (from Bliss, Goddard, & Riives, 1983), by permission).

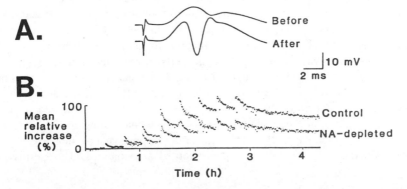

train of stimuli can produce an enhancement of these responses which persists without decrement for hours.

LTP has been studied intensively in the hippocampus because of its possible role in learning and memory. Nevertheless, the mechanism underlying this phenomenon has remained elusive. Although enhanced release of transmitter during LTP has been observed, it is unlikely that this alone can account for all aspects of the phenomenon. The interaction of the transmitter with postsynaptic (or presynaptic) receptors also appears to be necessary for induction of LTP; blocking chemical synaptic transmission with low-calcium solutions or blocking transmitter receptors with a specific antagonist abolishes the ability to induce LTP (Dunwiddie et al., 1978). Trains of stimuli have been shown to result in morphological alteration in postsynaptic sites (Fifkova & van Harreveld, 1977), and intracellular injection of a calcium-chelating agent into a postsynaptic cell prevents LTP in that cell (Lynch et al., 1983). Thus, there is evidence for both presynaptic and postsynaptic changes during LTP.

As a test for generalized postsynaptic changes during hippocampal LTP, several investigators have examined the effect of tetanization of one pathway (the conditioning pathway) on subsequent postsynaptic responses elicited by a putative transmitter or a nontetanized pathway (the test pathway). A finding of enhanced test responses (i.e., heterosynaptic facilitation) would argue that LTP involves an overall increase in excitability of the postsynaptic neuron. To test this idea, glutamate, a powerful pyramidal cell excitant and a proposed hippocampal neurotransmitter, was iontophoresed at several sites before and after the induction of LTP (Lynch et al., 1976). Instead of an increase in the response to glutamate, a lasting decrease in the response was noted. Electrical stimulation of two pathways (Fig. 13.2A) during LTP revealed that only responses to the tetanized (conditioned) pathway are enhanced (Andersen et al., 1977), and that responses to stimulation of other pathways are concurrently depressed (heterosynaptic depression; Dunwiddie & Lynch, 1978; Lynch et al., 1977) Subsequent reports have suggested that heterosynaptic depression decays more rapidly than LTP. However, Abraham and Goddard (1983) have found that this effect can last for several hours. Such results suggest that while LTP is confined to the tetanized or conditioned pathway, generalized effects of repetitive stimulation can be detected throughout the neuron for long periods. Heterosynaptic depression could be a mechanism whereby the efficacy of transmission through the tetanized pathway is further augmented relative to that in untetanized pathways, increasing the signal-to-noise ratio beyond that attained solely by LTP.

In support of the involvement of hippocampal neuronal plasticity in learning phenomena are recent reports that stimulation of pairs of inputs to hippocampal cells can produce LTP under conditions in which stimulation of one pathway alone cannot elicit the response. This is formally analogous to associative learning paradigms. Utilizating two pathways to dentate granule cells in the anesthetized rat, a massive ipsilateral input and a weak contralateral input, Levy and Steward (1979) found that LTP can be induced in the weak input only if trains of stimuli are delivered simultaneously to both pathways. No heterosynaptic potentiation is observed in response to the weak input if the train is delivered solely to the strong ipsilateral pathway; therefore, the associative LTP is not a generalized postsynaptic increase in responsiveness. On the contrary, following induction of associative LTP, repetitive simu-

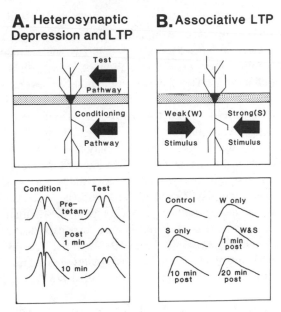

Fig. 13.2. Schematic diagrams showing characteristics and forms of LTP. The experimental arrangement (upper boxes) and representative data (lower boxes) are illustrated for experiments on heterosynaptic depression, homosynaptic LTP (A) and associative LTP (B). Upper boxes in both A and B depict a pyramidal neuron and the stimulated pathways. (A) Examples of heterosynaptic depression and LTP. Repetitive stimulation of one input (conditioning pathway) produced subsequent enhancement of extracellularly recorded population spikes to stimulation of the conditioned pathway (homosynaptic LTP) and reduction of responses to a second (test) pathway (heterosynaptic depression). Although responses are only shown here for 10 minutes after the conditioning stimuli, heterosynaptic depression could last for several hours (adapted from Lynch, Dunwiddie, & Gribkoff, 1977, by permission). (B) Example of associative LTP. Stimulus trains applied to a weak input (W), a strong input (S), or both were used to demonstrate associative LTP. Intracellularly recorded EPSPs are shown to a single stimulus of the weak input. Trains delivered to either the weak or strong inputs alone did not produce LTP. Pairing both inputs caused a form of LTP that depended on this association and did not result from a general increase in excitability or changes in electrical properties of the cell membrane (adapted from Barrionuevo & Brown, 1983, by permission).

lation of the strong ipsilateral pathway reverses the associatively conditioned LTP of the weak input. Furthering the analogy to behavioral conditioning, a weak form of heterosynaptic depression produced by stimulation of the strong input could act as an "extinction" mechanism to reverse the LTP. Barrioneuvo and Brown (1983) have found that associative LTP can be induced in hippocampal CA1 neurons *in vitro* (Fig.13.2B) and have shown that intracellularly recorded passive membrane properties are not altered during associative LTP. Future studies and refinements should reveal more information concerning the mechanisms of this form of LTP, and the degree to which this neuromodulatory phenomenon actually participates in behavioral associative conditioning.

LTP in Other Systems

The unique nature of the response of hippocampal neurons to repetitive stimulation was emphasized in early studies. It is now thought, however, that LTP is not confined to the hippocampal formation. Stimulation of many pathways has produced post-tetanic potentiation and LTP of evoked potentials in several target neurons of the rat limbic forebrain (Racine & Milgram, 1983; Racine et al., 1983). These neurons reside not only in the hippocampal subfields, but also in the amygdala, pyriform cortex, subiculum, and septal nuclei. This indicates the widespread nature of this phenomenon, although hippocampal neurons display the greatest degree and duration of LTP. Lee (1982) showed that LTP can also be induced in cerebral cortical neurons in *in vitro* slices. In this preparation, LTP remains stable during a 4-hour recording period, indicating that a long-lasting change in transmission can occur in these cells. Similarly, in the cat medial geniculate nucleus, repetitive stimulation of appropriate pathways can produce an increase in postsynaptic responsiveness that is maintained in excess of 1 hour (Gerren & Weinberger, 1983). Thus, one important, emerging concept is that long-lasting enhancement of postsynaptic responses, induced by afferent stimulation, is more widespread in the mammalian brain than previously appreciated.

While hippocampal LTP has received the greatest attention, a form of LTP in rat superior cervical ganglion was reported by Dunant and Dolivo (1968) many years prior to the discovery of the analogous hippocampal phenomenon. A single train of

Fig. 13.3. Long-term potentiation in the mammalian superior cervical ganglion. Upper traces show postsynaptic responses to preganglionic electrical stimuli before and after a train (tetanus) of conditioning stimuli. The postsynaptic responses were recorded extracellularly in an *in vitro* experiment. Lower graph depicts results of experiment in which a single train of stimuli produced long-lasting enhancement of subsequent responses (from Briggs, Brown, & McAfee, 1985, by permission).

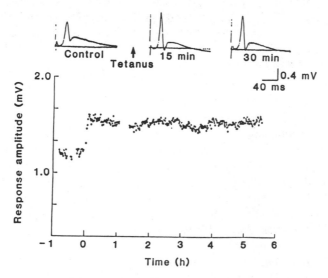

stimuli to the preganglionic nerve results in prolonged (>30 min) enhancement of the postganglionic EPSP. They found that the presynaptic spike is not altered during most of this period, that the degree of potentiation is dependent on the concentration of extracellular calcium available, and that the phenomenon is not a result of increased postsynaptic response to the transmitter. Recent studies of LTP in this system have revealed that enhancement of the nicotinic cholinergic fast EPSP is long-lasting (> 1 hr), calcium-dependent, specific to the tetanized fibers, and does not require synaptic transmission for its initiation (Fig. 13.3) (Brown & McAfee, 1982; Briggs et al., 1985a). Application of muscarinic cholinergic antagonists does not block LTP, suggesting that it is not a result of an underlying muscarinic slow EPSP. Direct measurements have shown increased acetylcholine release during the period of enhanced EPSPs (Briggs et al., 1985). A similar form of LTP has been reported in frog sympathetic ganglion, where the nicotinic fast EPSP is potentiated for several hours after a high-frequency train of preganglionic stimuli (Koyano et al., 1985). In this ganglion an increase in quantal size and/or quantal content accompanies LTP. LTP at synapses in sympathetic ganglia, therefore, appears similar to LTP at central synapses. Although this evidence again demonstrates that LTP is not unique to the cells of the mammalian hippocampus, it still remains to be shown that the duration of LTP in other systems approaches that seen in the hippocampus *in vivo*. It may be that this type of long-lasting sensitization is a common mechanism for enhancing the relative importance of frequently used afferents. Associative LTP, on the other hand, may be more rare.

Catecholamines and LTP

Several recent studies have suggested an involvement of catecholamines in some forms of hippocampal synaptic plasticity. Hippocampal catecholamines may directly modulate short-term synaptic plasticity, and also play a supportive role in the development and maintenance of longer-lasting forms. For example, depletion of endogenous norepinephrine decreases the magnitude of LTP observed *in vivo* (Bliss et al., 1983) (Fig. 13.1B). Haas and Rose (1984) found that the inhibitory effect of spike afterhyperpolarization is reduced during LTP, and catecholamines can also produce this effect. In addition, direct application of norepinephrine *in vitro* increases the probability of induction of hippocampal LTP, and enhances its magnitude and duration.

Specific adrenergic antagonists, on the other hand, can block LTP (Hopkins & Johnston, 1984). This evidence strongly suggests that LTP, or at least the degree to which it is expressed, is a consequence of the release of endogenous catecholamine by electrical stimulation. Pharmacological blockage of catecholamine receptors in superior cervical ganglion, however, did not affect LTP in this system, suggesting that different mechanisms may produce or maintain LTP in other systems.

Catecholamines have profound modulatory effects on hippocampal neurons. Norepinephrine produces a selective enhancement of the response to depolarizing current pulses (Langmoen et al., 1981), suggesting an action on one or more voltage-dependent conductances. Furthermore, as described in Chapter 9, low concentrations of norepinephrine specifically reduce or abolish the calcium-dependent potassium conductance that mediates spike afterhyperpolarization and accommodation (Madison

& Nicoll, 1982). Extracellular application of a membrane soluble cyclic AMP analogue also reduces the afterhyperpolarization and spike accommodation (Newberry &
Nicoll, 1984). While an initial report suggested that dopamine and cyclic AMP *aug-
ment* the afterhypolarization (Benardo & Prince, 1982), other work argues that dopamine acts similarly to norepinephrine (Gribkoff & Ashe, 1984a,b), and that some
of its actions are probably mediated by adrenergic receptors. In addition, intracellular
injection of cyclic AMP and the catalytic subunit of cyclic AMP-dependent protein
kinase has been shown to mimic some effects of catecholamines, including a reduction
of the afterhyperpolarization and spike accommodation (Gribkoff et al., 1984). Different catecholamines therefore produce similar effects on synaptic transmission and
membrane properties in hippocampal neurons, and cyclic AMP appears to mediate
some of these neuromodulatory effects. At present it is unknown which, if any, of
these effects of catecholamines may contribute to LTP.

Future Studies of LTP

Although LTP has been well characterized, there is little direct evidence that LTP
contributes to behavioral phenomena such as learning. Most studies of LTP have
relied on electrical stimulation that produces synchronous, repetitive discharge of
many presynaptic fibers. Such simultaneous repetitive firing of many cells probably
does not occur during the normal operation of the central nervous system, but does
resemble discharges observed prior to and during seizures. While the work on associative LTP is suggestive of a role in learning, behavioral paradigms demonstrate
associative learning when many seconds separate single pairs of stimuli, unlike the
close pairing of stimulus trains required in LTP studies. Future research would ben-
efit by determining the results of activiation of fewer afferents, such as those that
may occur during particular behavioral conditioning paradigms. In addition, it will
be most useful to analyze intracellularly recorded synaptic potentials or voltage clamp
currents during LTP, rather than the complex extracellular responses. For example,
a recent study of LTP using the single-electrode voltage-clamp technique has shown
that LTP results in an enhanced synaptic conductance, which produces larger EPSPs
(Barrionuevo et al., 1986). It seems clear that a finer analysis of LTP under more
physiological conditions is required, an approach currently employed by several lab-
oratories.

Another aspect of LTP that must be studied in greater detail is its biochemical
mechanism. Among the mechanisms that have been hypothesized are changes in the
number of functional postsynaptic receptors (Lynch & Baudry, 1984) and the possible involvement of cyclic nucleotides and cyclic AMP-dependent protein kinase (e.g.,
via catecholamines, as discussed above). LTP may also be associated with changes
in the phosphorylation state of proteins that are substrates for protein kinase C. Phorbol esters, which activate this enzyme, reportedly enhance LTP (Routtenberg et al.,
1985; Lovinger et al., 1985); they also block a calcium-dependent potassium conductance and reduce a late hyperpolarizing synaptic response (Baraban et al., 1985).
These avenues of research, when coupled with detailed knowledge of the aspects of
synaptic transmission affected during LTP, should eventually lead to a better understanding of long-lasting synaptic plasticity at the molecular level.

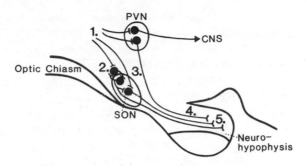

Fig. 13.4. Schematic view of the magnocellular neuroendocrine system showing possible sites of modulation. (1) Extrinsic sources of modulatory influence can include other hypothalamic nuclei as well as areas outside the hypothalamus (e.g., catecholamine neurons from brain stem). (2) Modulation of local circuits in and near the supraoptic and paraventricular nuclei (SON and PVN) can occur by both extrinsic and intranuclear sources. (3) Intranuclear modulation in both the SON and PVN can result from the local release of peptide by magnocellular neurons. (4) Neuromodulators (e.g., opioid peptides) can also act on the neurohypophysis. (5) The net effect of all neuromodulatory actions is to alter secretion of the neurohypophysial peptides, oxytocin and vasopressin. Some of the magnocellular neurons of the paraventricular nucleus project to sites in the central nervous system (CNS), where they presumably have a neuromodulatory influence on central target neurons.

TRANSITION OF CELL DISCHARGE PATTERN IN BURSTING NEURONS

Magnocellular Neuroendocrine System

Neuroendocrine cells in the vertebrate nervous system produce and release peptides that act as hormones and also as neurotransmitters/neuromodulators. The release of vasopressin and oxytocin from the mammalian hypothalamus is a phenomenon whose anatomical basis and physiological significance is relatively well understood; therefore, this is rapidly becoming recognized as an excellent model system for investigating modulation. Figure 13.4 illustrates the loci of possible neuromodulatory control in the magnocellular nuclei of the hypothalamus and in the neurohypophysis.

The magnocellular neurons located in the supraoptic and paraventricular nuclei of mammals synthesize and release peptide neurohormones into the general circulation. Magnocellular neurons in both nuclei send their axons into the neurohypophysis. With appropriate physiological activation, they release oxytocin and vasopressin into the perivascular spaces surrounding fenestrated capillaries (Fig. 13.4). After entering the general circulation, these peptides act on known target tissues and regulate basic reproductive, renal, and cardiovascular functions. Oxytocinergic and vasopressinergic magnocellular neurons in the paraventricular nucleus also project widely in the central nervous system, where they probably play a modulatory role.

The magnocellular neurons discharge in characteristic bursting patterns *in vivo* in response to physiological stimuli that promote neurohypophysial peptide release.

In the absence of stimulation, magnocellular neuron discharge is slow and unpatterned. With osmotic stimulation, one type of magnocellular neuron fires in a fast-continuous pattern that is punctuated by short, high-frequency bursts in lactating rats; the second type of magnocellular neuron responds by firing in prolonged bursts that are separated by silent periods (Brimble & Dyball, 1977). The fast-continuous type of magnocellular neuron has been shown to fire a synchronous, high-frequency burst immediately preceding the rise in intramammary pressure that accompanies the milk ejection reflex in lactating rats, strongly suggesting that this cell type releases oxytocin (Wakerley & Lincoln, 1973). The phasically discharging magnocellular neuron is thought to be vasopressinergic, and recent studies have demonstrated that the characteristic phasic pattern is optimal for hormone release from the neurohypophysis (Bicknell & Leng, 1981; Shaw et al., 1984).

Immunocytochemical techniques coupled with intracellular recording and staining have demonstrated that vasopressinergic magnocellular neurons retain their ability to fire in the characteristic phasic pattern *in vitro* (Yamashita et al., 1983; Cobbett et al., 1986). Phasic bursting can be observed after blockade of chemical synaptic transmission (Hatton, 1982), and intracellular studies have provided additional evidence that phasic bursting is an intrinsic property of these neurons (Andrew & Dudek, 1984a). Bursting appears to involve slow oscillations in membrane potential; a depolarizing afterpotential follows each spike, and summation of these depolarizations results in a maintained depolarization that promotes further spiking (Andrew & Dudek, 1984a). Spike frequency adaptation during the burst, and the eventual termination of the burst, may result from a calcium-activated potassium conductance (Andrew & Dudek, 1984b). While the ability of these cells to fire in a phasic bursting pattern is intrinsic, synaptic and other extrinsic stimuli appear to modulate the characteristic discharge pattern, as in the case of *Aplysia* bag cell neurons and neuron R15 (see Chapters 6 and 7).

Application of neurotransmitters, such as acetylcholine and norepinephrine, markedly affects vasopressin release and regulates phasic discharge. Figure 13.5 shows preliminary results concerning the action of norepinephrine on magnocellular neurons, including the intiation of phasic discharge. Acetylcholine application and stimulation of cholinergic afferents can also enhance phasic discharge in the supraoptic nucleus (Bioulac et al., 1978; Hatton et al., 1983). These substances may simply depolarize these neurons, thus activating intrinsic conductance mechanisms; they may also directly affect the conductances responsible for depolarizing afterpotentials and afterhyperpolarizations, and thereby modulate the characteristics of phasic bursts. Future pharmacological studies with intracellular recording techniques will need to consider slow modulatory actions on the intrinsic conductance mechanisms that mediate bursting (see Chapter 6).

Interestingly, the peptides released by these cells may also influence their own firing pattern. Interconnections between magnocellular neurons may occur within the supraoptic and paraventricular nuclei (e.g., see Theodosis, 1985). Iontophoresis of oxytocin excites magnocellular neurons in paraventricular nucleus (Moss et al., 1972), while application of an oxytocin antagonist depresses the burst discharge of oxytocinergic paraventricular neurons that occurs in response to suckling (Freund-Mercier & Richard, 1984). *In vitro* studies in supraoptic nucleus showed that vasopressin pro-

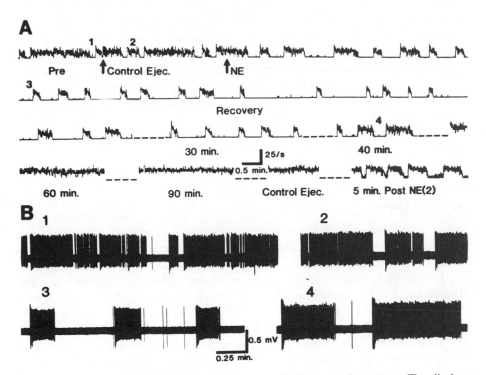

Fig. 13.5. Action of norepinephrine on firing pattern of supraoptic neurons. The discharge pattern of a neuron in the supraoptic nucleus was recorded extracellularly from a slice of rat hypothalamus. (A) Ratemeter record before and after focal application of control solution and norepinephrine (NE) near the recorded cell. Norepinephrine initiated phasic bursting; recovery was not complete until >40 minutes after drug application. (B) Action potentials recorded from neuron contributing to ratemeter records of A. Numbers refer to points in the previous ratemeter record (Gribkoff & Dudek, unpublished observations).

duces a direct, sodium-dependent depolarization that decreases spontaneous discharge. Vasopressin increases cyclic AMP levels, and a membrane-soluble cyclic AMP analogue produces a depolarization similar to the one caused by vasopressin (Abe et al., 1983). The significance of this autoregulation of peptide release is not understood, but continued study should reveal the mechanism by which neurohypophysial peptides influence their own secretion.

It is possible that the release of peptides may be modulated directly, independent of changes in electrical properties. The mammalian neurohypophysis, containing the axons and terminals of the magnocellular cells, is an ideal model system for studying the modulation of release. The absence of neuronal cell bodies, and the finding that fibers containing possible neuromodulators (such as opioid peptides and dopamine) are present in this structure, have allowed the investigation of the modulation of hormone release. Opiates have recently been shown to regulate the release of oxytocin from the isolated neurohypophysis, an effect that involves a direct action on the axon terminals. In an initial study, Clarke and others (1979) found that morphine decreased and naloxone increased the rise in intramammary pressure resulting from oxytocin release, indicating that opiates depress some component of the milk ejection reflex. To determine the locus of action, they recorded from oxytocinergic cells in the hypothalamus, and found that morphine had no effect on their electrical response to physiological stimuli that normally cause oxytocin release, although release from the neurohypophysis was reduced. Subsequent investigation with the isolated neuro-hypophysis showed that opiates inhibit secretion of oxytocin (but not vasopressin), presumably by altering some aspect of excitation-secretion coupling (Bicknell & Leng, 1982).

Rhythmic Bursting in Neurons of the Nucleus Tractus Solitarius

Recent studies on neuromodulation of burst discharges have dealt with peptidergic regulation of a central neuronal network within the nucleus tractus solitarius, which is involved with rhythmic breathing movements. Extracellular recording had previously localized respiratory neurons in this region, and immunocytochemical staining had identified thyrotropin-releasing hormone (TRH) in the same region. Application of TRH to the brain stem increases respiratory rate and minute ventilation. Dekin, Richerson, and Getting (1985) have used intracellular recording in a brain stem slice preparation to study the effects of TRH on putative respiratory neurons. Before TRH application, the neurons displayed nonrhythmic activity. TRH induced 70% of the neurons to develop depolarizing afterpotentials and eventually to fire in a rhythmic bursting pattern (Fig. 13.6). Steady injected currents and current-evoked spike trains modified the bursting pattern, and the voltage-dependent oscillations were tetrodotoxin-resistant; therefore, TRH appears to transform these neurons into endogenous bursters. Further studies are required to specify the actual mechanism by which TRH converts the firing pattern of the putative respiratory neurons into a rhythmic burst discharge.

Epileptiform Bursting

Epilepsy is a neurological disorder that could well involve imbalances in neuromodulatory inputs to populations of cortical neurons. For example, slow pharmacological actions on voltage-dependent conductances via second messenger systems could be a critical aspect of epileptogenesis. The ability to study these phenomena in numerous animal phyla and at many neurobiological levels—from the single channel to the neuronal network—may provide insights into how dysfunctions of neuromodulatory mechanisms underlie neurological disorders.

Epileptiform activity may be induced experimentally in hippocampal pyramidal cells. While individual cells fire brief bursts under "normal" conditions, perfusion of the *in vitro* hippocampal slice with agents that block GABA-ergic inhibition (e.g., picrotoxin, bicuculline, and penicillin) results in spontaneous and synchronous bursts of population spikes. Thus pharmacological removal of inhibitory mechanisms leaves a network of hippocampal neurons that show epileptiform activity. Acetylcholine perfusion of penicillin-treated hippocampal slices (Fig. 13.7) enhanced the duration

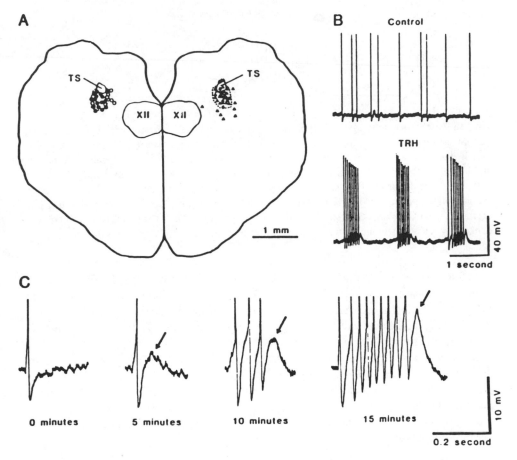

Fig. 13.6. Modulation by thyrotropin-releasing hormone of discharge pattern of neuron in nucleus tractus solitarius. (A) Schematic diagram of cross section of brain stem. The right side depicts a map of the dorsal respiratory group near the tractus solitarius (TS); triangles show the distribution of identified respiratory neurons, and the dashed line bounds region of highest density of respiratory neurons. The left side indicates locations of neurons studied in a slice preparation of the nucleus tractus solitarius; closed circles indicate cells that responded to thyrotropin-releasing hormone (TRH), open circles show loci of unresponsive cells. (B) Effect of TRH on neuron firing. Unpatterned activity occurred prior to TRH (control), while phasic bursting was observed during exposure to TRH. (C) A depolarizing afterpotential and bursting in this same neuron was observed during exposure to TRH (from Dekin, Richerson, & Getting, 1985, by permission).

of epileptiform bursts (Kriegstein, Suppes, & Prince, 1983) and dopamine dampened the discharges (Suppes et al., 1985). These agents probably alter epileptiform bursting by acting on slow intrinsic conductance mechanisms that may in turn be dependent on second messengers (such as cyclic nucleotides) or membrane voltage. Thus, agents such as acetylcholine and dopamine may have complex neuromodulatory effects on hippocampal epileptogenesis, as they do on other bursting neurons.

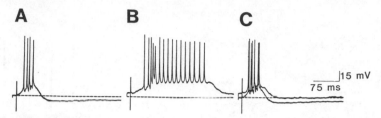

Fig. 13.7. Enhancement by acetylcholine of penicillin-induced bursting of hippocampal pyramidal neuron. The traces show an intracellularly recorded response to orthodromic stimulation in the presence of 3.5 mM sodium penicillin. (A) Response prior to focal acetycholine
application. (B) Response during pressure application of acetylcholine from microelectrode
with large tip diameter. (C) Response 60 seconds (depolarized trace) and 5 minutes after
acetylcholine application (baseline trace). Acetylcholine produced an increase in the duration
of the evoked depolarization shift, thus greatly increasing the number of action potentials
evoked by a single stimulus (adapted from Kriegstein, Suppes, & Prince, 1983).

Synchronous epileptiform field bursts also occur in hippocampal slices with ionic
rather than pharmacological manipulation; lowering extracellular calcium in the medium, which blocks evoked chemical synaptic transmission, can produce synchronous bursting in virtually every region of the hippocampus (see Dudek et al., in press,
for review). This system may prove useful in examining the mechanisms of action
of neuromodulatory agents on a spontaneously bursting population of mammalian
neurons (Haas et al., 1984). Acetylcholine, norepinephrine, and dopamine increase
the frequency of these field bursts at nanomolar to micromolar concentrations; these
neuromodulatory effects are consistent with the blocking actions of these agents on
afterhyperpolarizations, which are thought to be mediated by calcium-dependent potassium conductance.

CONCLUSIONS

Previous chapters have provided detailed discussions of neuromodulatory phenomena
at the single-channel and molecular level in "simple" systems. This chapter has used
selected examples in an attempt to impart a feeling for the ubiquitous nature and the
complexity of neuromodulatory events in the mammalian brain. Because of technical
limitations, most of the research has concentrated more on the phenomena and less
on the underlying mechanisms, but recent advances in neurophysiological techniques
should make it possible to approach some of the important questions that arise from
such studies. The task for the future is to apply the lessons, learned from studies of
invertebrates and other model systems, toward an understanding of analogous events
in the mammalian brain.

REFERENCES

Abe, H., Inoue, M., Matsuo. T., and Ogata. N. (1983) The effects of vasopressin on electrical
activity in the guinea-pig supraoptic nucleus *in vitro. J. Physiol London 331*, 665–685.

Abraham, W.C., and Goddard, G.V. (1983) Asymmetric relationships between homosynaptic long-term potentiation and heterosynaptic long-term depression. *Nature 305*, 717–719.

Andersen, P., Sundberg, S.H., Sveen, O., and Wigstrom, H. (1977) Specific longlasting potentiation of synaptic transmission in hippocampal slices. *Nature 266*, 736–737.

Andrew, R.D. and Dudek, F.E. (1983) Burst discharge in mammalian neuroendocrine cells involves an intrinsic regenerative mechanism. *Science 221*, 1050–1052.

Andrew, R.D. and Dudek, F.E. (1984a) Analysis of intracellularly recorded phasic bursting by mammalian neuroendoctrine cells. *J. Neurophysiol. 51*, 552–565.

Andrew, R.D. and Dudek, F.E. (1984b) Intrinsic inhibition in magnocellular neuroendocrine cells of rat hypothalamus. *J. Physiol. London 353*, 171–185.

Baraban, J.M., Snyder, S.H., and Alger, B.E. (1985) Protein kinase C regulates ionic conductance in hippocampal pyramidal neurons: Electrophysiological effects of phorbol esters. *Proc. Natl. Acad. Sci. USA 82*, 2538–2542.

Barrionuevo, G. and Brown, T.H. (1983) Associative long-term potentiation in hippocampal slices. *Proc. Natl. Acad. Sci. U.S.A. 80*, 7347–7351.

Barrionuevo, G., Kelso, S.R., Johnston, D., and Brown, T.H. (1986) Conductance mechanisms responsible for long-term potentiation in monosynaptic and isolated excitatory synaptic inputs to hippocampus. *J. Neurophysiol. 55*, 540–550.

Benardo, L.S. and Prince D.A. (1982) Dopamine action on hippocampal pyramidal cells. *J. Neurosci. 2*, 415–423.

Bicknell, R.J. and Leng, G. (1981) Relative efficiency of neuronal firing patterns for vasopressin release *in vitro*. *Neuroendocrinology 33*, 295–299.

Bicknell, R.J. and Leng, G. (1982) Endogenous opiates regulate oxytocin but not vasopressin secretion from neurohypophysis. *Nature 298*, 161–162.

Bioulac, B., Gaffori, O., Harris, M., and Vincent, J.-D. (1978) Effects of acetylcholine, sodium glutamate and GABA on the discharge of supraoptic neurons in the rat. *Brain Res. 154*, 159–162.

Bliss, T.V.P. and Gardner-Medwin, A. (1973) Long-lasting potentiation of synaptic transmission in the dentate area of unanesthetized rabbit following stimulation of the perforant path. *J. Physiol. London 232*, 357–374.

Bliss, T.V.P., Goddard, G.V., and Riives, M. (1983) Reduction of long-term potentiation in the dentate gyrus of the rat following selective depletion of monoamines. *J. Physiol. London 334*, 475–491.

Briggs, C.A., Brown, T.H., and McAfee, D.A. (1985a) Neurophysiology and pharmacology of long-term potentiation in the rat sympathetic ganglion. *J. Physiol. London 359*, 503–521.

Briggs, C.A., McAfee, D.A., and McCaman, R.E. (1985b) Long-term potentiation of synaptic acetylcholine release in the superior cervical ganglion of the rat. *J. Physiol. London 363*, 181–190.

Brimble, M.J. and Dyball, R.E.J. (1977) Characterization of the response of oxytocin and vasopressin secreting neurones in the supraoptic nucleus to osmotic stimulation. *J. Physiol. London 271*, 253–271.

Brown, T.H. and McAfee,D.A. (1982) Long-term synaptic potentiation in the superior cervical ganglion. *Science 215*, 1411–1413.

Clarke, G., Wood. P., Merrick, L., and Lincoln, P.W. (1979) Opiate inhibition of peptide release from the neurohumoral terminals of hypothalamic neurones. *Nature 282*, 746–748.

Cobbett, P., Smithson, K.G., and Hatton, G.I. (1986) Immunoreactivity to vasopressin- but not oxytocin-associated neurophysin antiserum in phasic neurons of rat hypothalamic paraventricular nucleus. *Brain Res. 362*, 7–16.

Day, T.A., Randle, J.C.R., and Renaud, L.P. (1985) Opposing α- and β-adrenergic mecha-

nisms mediate dose-dependent actions of noradrenaline on supraoptic vasopressin neurones *in vitro*. *Brain Res. 358*, 171–179.

Dekin, M.S., Richerson, G.B., and Getting, P.A. (1985) Thyrotropin—releasing hormone
induces rhythmic bursting in neurons of the nucleus tractus solitarius. *Science 229*, 67–
69.

Douglas, R.M. and Goddard, G.V. (1975) Long-term potentiation of the perforant path-granule
cell synapse in the rat hippocampus. *Brain Res. 86*, 205–215.

Dudek, F.E., Snow, R.W., and Taylor, C.P. (In press) Role of electrical interactions in syn-
chronization of epileptiform bursts. In *Basic Mechanisms of the Epilepsies: Molecular
and Cellular Approaches* (Advances in Neurology, V. 44) (eds. A.V. Delgado-Escueta,
A.A. Ward, Jr., D.M. Woodbury and R.J. Porter), Raven press, New York.

Dunwiddie, T. and Lynch, G. (1978) Long-term potentiation and depression of synaptic responses in the rat hippocampus: localization and frequency dependency. *J. Physiol.
London 276*, 353–367.

Dunwiddie, T., Madison, D., and Lynch, G. (1978) Synaptic transmission is required for
initiation of long-term potentiation. *Brain Res. 150*, 413–417.

Dunant, Y. and Dolivo, M. (1968) Plasticity of synaptic functions in the excised sympathetic
ganglion of the rat. *Brain Res. 10*, 271–273.

Fifkova, E. and Van Harreveld, A. (1977) Long-lasting morphological changes in dendritic
spines of dentate granule cells following stimulation of the entorhinal area. *J. Neuro-
cytol. 6*, 211–230.

Freund-Mercier, M. and Richard, P. (1984) Electrophysiological evidence for facilitatory control of oxytocin neurones by oxytocin during suckling in the rat. *J. Physiol. London
352*, 447–466.

Gerren, R.A. and Weinberger, N.M. (1983) Long-term potentiation in the magnocellular medial geniculate nucleus of the anesthetized cat. *Brain Res. 265*, 138–142.

Gribkoff, V.K. and Ashe, J.H. (1984a) Modulation by dopamine of population responses and
cell membrane properties of hippocampal CA1 neurons in vitro. *Brain Res. 292*, 327–
338.

Gribkoff, V.K. and Ashe, J.H. (1984b) Modulation by dopamine of population spikes in area
CA_1 hippocampal neurons elicited by paired stimulus pulses. *Cell. Molec. Neurobiol.
4*, 177–183.

Gribkoff, V.K., Ashe, J.H., Fletcher, W.H., and Lekawa, M.E. (1984) Dopamine, cyclic
AMP, and protein kinase produce a similar long-lasting increase in input resistance in
hippocampal CA1 neurons. *Soc. Neurosci. Absts. 10*, 898.

Haas, H.L., Jefferys, J.G.R., Slater, N.T., and Carpenter, D.O. (1984) Modulation of low
calcium induced field bursts in the hippocampus by monoamines and cholinomimetics.
Pflugers Arch. 400, 28–33.

Haas, H.L. and Rose, G. (1984) The role of inhibitory mechanisms in hippocampal long-term
potentiation. *Neurosci. Lett. 47*, 301–306.

Hatton, G.I. (1982) Phasic bursting activity of rat paraventricular neurones in the absence of
synaptic transmission. *J. Physiol. London 327*, 273–284.

Hatton, G.I., Ho, Y.W., and Mason, W.T. (1983) Synaptic activation of phasic bursting in
rat supraoptic nucleus neurones recorded in hypothalamic slices. *J. Physiol. London
345*, 297–317.

Hopkins, W.F. and Johnston, D. (1984) Frequency-dependent noradrenergic modulation of
long-term potentiation in the hippocampus. *Science 226*, 350–352.

Koyano, K., Kuba, K., and Minota, S. (1985) Long-term potentiation of transmitter release
induced by repetitive presynaptic activities in bull-frog sympathetic ganglia. *J. Physiol.
London 359*, 219–233.

Kriegstein, A.R., Suppes, T., and Prince, D.A. (1983) Cholinergic enhancement of penicillin-induced epileptiform discharges in pyramidal neurons of the guinea pig hippocampus. *Brain Res. 266*, 137–142.

Langmoen, I.A., Segal, M., and Andersen, P. (1981) Mechanisms of norepinephrine actions on hippocampal pyramidal cells *in vitro. Brain Res. 208*, 349–362.

Lee, K.S. (1982) Sustained enhancement of evoked potentials following brief, high-frequency stimulation of the cerebral cortex *in vitro. Brain Res. 239*, 617–623.

Levy, W.B. and Steward, O. (1979) Synapses as associative memory elements in the hippocampal formation. *Brain Res. 175*, 233–245.

Lovinger, D., Colley, P., Linden, D.J., Murakami, K. and Routtenberg, A. (1985) Phorbol ester, which induces protein kinase C (PKC) translocation to the membrane, prevents decay of long-term potentiation. *Soc. Neurosci. Abstr. 11*, 927.

Lynch, G., and Baudry, M. (1984) The biochemistry of memory: A new and specific hypothesis. *Science 224*, 1057–1063.

Lynch, G., Larson, J., Kelso, S., Barrionuevo, G., and Schottler, F. (1983) Intracellular injections of EGTA block induction of hippocampal long-term potentiation. *Nature 305*, 719–721.

Lynch, G.S., Dunwiddie, T., and Gribkoff, V. (1977) Heterosynaptic depression: a postsynaptic correlate of long-term potentiation. *Nature 266*, 737–739.

Lynch, G.S., Gribkoff, V.K. and Deadwyler, S.A. (1976) Long-term potentiation is accompanied by a reduction in dendritic responsiveness to glutamic acid. *Nature 263*, 151–153.

Madison, D.V., and Nicoll, R.A. (1982) Noradrenaline blocks accomodation of pyramidal cell discharge in the hippocampus. *Nature 299*, 636–638.

Moos, F., Freund-Mercier, M.J., Guerné, Y., Guerné, J.M., Stoeckel, M.E., and Richard, P. (1984) Release of oxytocin and vasopressin by magnocellular nuclei *in vitro:* specific facilitatory effect of oxytocin on its own release. *J. Endocrinol. 102*, 63–72.

Moss, R.L., Dyball, R.E.J., and Cross, B.A. (1972) Excitation of antidromically identified paraventricular neurons by iontophoretically applied ocytocin. *Exptl. Neurol. 34*, 95–102.

Newberry, N.R. and Nicoll, R.A. (1984) A bicuculline-resistant inhibitory postsynaptic potential in rat hippocampal pyramidal cells *in vitro. J. Physiol. London 348*, 239–254.

Racine, R.J. and Milgram, N.W. (1983) Short-term potentiation phenomena in the rat limbic forebrain. *Brain Res. 260*, 201–216.

Racine, R.J., Milgram, N.W., and Hafner, S. (1983) Long-term potentiation phenomena in the rat limbic forebrain. *Brain Res. 260*, 217–231.

Renaud, L.P., Day, T.A., Randle, J.C.R., and Bourque, C.W. (1985) *In vivo* and *in vitro* electrophysiological evidence that central noradrenergic pathways enhance the activity of vasopressinergic neurosecretory cells. In *Vasopressin*, (ed., R.W. Schrier) Raven Press, New York, pp. 385–394.

Routtenberg, A., Lovinger, D. and Steward, O. (1985) Selective increase in the phosphorylation of a 47-kDa protein (F1) directly related to long-term potentiation. *Behav. Neural Biol. 43*, 3–11.

Shaw, F.D., Bicknell, R.J., and Dyball, R.E.J. (1984) Facilitation of vasopressin release from the neurohypophysis by application of electrical stimuli in bursts. *Neuroendocrinology 39*, 371–376.

Sklar, A.H. and Schrier, R.W. (1983) Central nervous system mediators of vasopressin release. *Physiol. Rev. 63*, 1243–1280.

Sladek, C.D. (1983) Regulation of vasopressin release by neurotransmitters, neuropeptides and osmotic stimuli. In *The Neurohypophysis: Structure, Function and Control, Progress in Brain Res., Vol. 60* (eds. B.A. Cross, G. Leng), Elsevier, Amsterdam, pp. 71–90.

Snyder, S.H. (1985) Adenosine as a neuromodulator. *Ann. Rev. Neurosci. 8*, 103–124.

Suppes, T., Kriegstein, A.R., and Prince, D.A. (1985) The influence of dopamine on epilep-
    tiform burst activity in hippocampal pyramidal neurons. *Brain Res. 326,* 273–280.
Theodosis, D.T (1985) Oxytocin-immunoreactive terminals synapse on oxytocin neurones in
    the supraoptic nucleus. *Nature 313,* 682–684.
Wakerley, J.B. and Lincoln, D.W. (1973) The milk ejection reflex of the rat: a 20-to-40 fold
    acceleration in the firing of paraventricular neurones during oxytocin release. *J. Endo-
    crinol. 57,* 477–493.
Yamashita, H., Inenaga, K., Kawata, M., and Sano, Y. (1983) Phasically firing neurons in
    the supraoptic nucleus of the rat hypothalamus: immunocytochemical and electrophys-
    iological studies. *Neurosci. Lett. 37,* 87–92.

Index